REFERENCE EDITION

ENDOCRINE BOARD REVIEW 2024

Frances J. Hayes, MB BCh, BAO
Program Chair
Associate Clinical Chief of the Division of Reproductive Endocrinology
Massachusetts General Hospital
Associate Professor of Medicine
Harvard Medical School

John D. Carmichael, MD
Clinical Chief
Division of Endocrinology, Diabetes, and Metabolism
Co-Director, USC Pituitary Center
Associate Professor of Clinical Medicine
Keck School of Medicine of the University of Southern California

Natalie E. Cusano, MD, MS
Professor of Medicine
Zucker School of Medicine at Hofstra/Northwell
Director of the Bone Metabolism Program
Division of Endocrinology at Lenox Hill Hospital

Kanishka Desai, MD
Clinical Associate Professor of Medicine
Endocrinology, Gerontology, and Metabolism
Stanford University

Tobias Else, MD
Associate Professor of Internal Medicine
Division of Metabolism, Endocrinology, and Diabetes
University of Michigan

Jacqueline Jonklaas, MD, PhD, MPH
Professor
Division of Endocrinology
Georgetown University Medical Center

Sangeeta R. Kashyap, MD
Assistant Chief of Clinical Affairs
Division of Endocrinology, Diabetes, and Metabolism
Weill Cornell Medicine
New York Presbyterian

Margaret Flynn Lippincott, MD
Assistant Professor of Medicine
Harvard Medical School
Physician Investigator
Reproductive Endocrine Unit
Massachusetts General Hospital

Marie E. McDonnell, MD
Chief, Diabetes Section
Division of Endocrinology Diabetes and Hypertension
Brigham and Women's Hospital
Associate Professor of Medicine
Harvard Medical School

Stephanie Page, MD, PhD
Professor/Head, Division of Metabolism, Endocrinology, and Nutrition
Co-Director, UW Medicine Diabetes Institute
Robert B. McMillen Professor of Lipid Research
University of Washington School of Medicine

Anne L. Peters, MD
Professor of Clinical Medicine
Keck School of Medicine of the University of Southern California

Abbie L. Young, MS, CGC, ELS(D)
Medical Editor

Endocrine Society
2055 L Street NW, Suite 600, Washington, DC 20036
1-888-ENDOCRINE • www.endocrine.org

ENDOCRINE SOCIETY

The Endocrine Society is the world's largest, oldest, and most active organization working to advance the clinical practice of endocrinology and hormone research. Founded in 1916, the Society now has more than 18,000 global members across a range of disciplines. The Society has earned an international reputation for excellence in the quality of its peer-reviewed journals, educational resources, meetings, and programs that improve public health through the practice and science of endocrinology.

For between-edition updates, visit us at:
https://www.endocrine.org/education-and-training/book-updates

Other publications:
endocrine.org/publications

The statements and opinions expressed in this publication are those of the individual authors and do not necessarily reflect the views of the Endocrine Society. The Endocrine Society is not responsible or liable in any way for the currency of the information, for any errors, omissions, or inaccuracies, or for any consequences arising therefrom. With respect to any drugs mentioned, the reader is advised to refer to the appropriate medical literature and the product information currently provided by the manufacturer to verify appropriate dosage, method and duration of administration, and other relevant information. In all instances, it is the responsibility of the treating physician or other health care professional, relying on independent experience and expertise, as well as knowledge of the patient, to determine the best treatment for the patient.

ISBN: 978-1-936704-43-9
Library of Congress Control Number: 2024942276

On the Cover: © Shutterstock. Close-up a stethoscope on laptop. Computed tomography on digitally on a laptop. Selective focus.

OVERVIEW

The Endocrine Board Review (EBR) 16th Edition (2024) is a board examination preparation book designed both for endocrine fellows who have completed or are nearing completion of their fellowship and are preparing to sit for the board certification exam, and for practicing endocrinologists in search of a comprehensive self-assessment of endocrinology, either to prepare for recertification or to update their practice. EBR consists of approximately 220 case-based, American Board of Internal Medicine (ABIM) style, multiple-choice questions. Each section follows the ABIM Endocrinology, Diabetes, and Metabolism Certification Examination blueprint, covering the breadth and depth of the certification and recertification examinations. Each case is discussed comprehensively with detailed answer explanations and references.

The EBR 16th Edition (2024) reference book is intended primarily for consultation and self-assessment of knowledge relating to endocrinology. As a reference book, educational credits are not available upon completion of the multiple-choice questions included. For information on educational products that include educational credit, please visit endocrine.org/store.

LEARNING OBJECTIVES

Upon completion of this educational activity, learners will be able to demonstrate enhanced medical knowledge and clinical skills across all major areas of endocrinology; apply knowledge and skills in diagnosing, managing, and treating a wide spectrum of endocrine disorders; and successfully complete the board examination for certification or recertification in the subspecialty of endocrinology, diabetes, and metabolism.

TARGET AUDIENCE

This activity should be of substantial interest to endocrinologists, internists, and endocrine fellows preparing for the board examination or recertification; or endocrinologists and other health care practitioners seeking a review in endocrinology.

STATEMENT OF INDEPENDENCE

The Endocrine Society has a policy of ensuring that the content and quality of this educational activity are balanced, independent, objective, and scientifically rigorous. The scientific content of this activity was developed under the supervision of the Endocrine Society's EBR faculty. There are no commercial supporters of this activity and no commercial entities have had an influence over the planning of this activity.

DISCLOSURE POLICY

The faculty, committee members, and staff who are in position to control the content of this activity are required to disclose to the Endocrine Society and to learners any relevant financial relationship(s) of the individual or spouse/partner that have occurred within the last 12 months with any commercial interest(s) whose products or services are related to the content. Financial relationships are defined by remuneration in any amount from the commercial interest(s) in the form of grants; research support; consulting fees; salary; ownership interest (eg, stocks, stock options, or ownership interest excluding diversified mutual funds); honoraria or other payments for participation in speakers' bureaus, advisory boards, or boards of directors; or other financial benefits. The intent of this disclosure is not to prevent planners with relevant financial relationships from planning or delivery of content, but rather to provide learners with information that allows them to make their own judgments of whether these financial relationships may have influenced the educational activity with regard to exposition or conclusion.

The Endocrine Society has reviewed all disclosures and resolved or managed all identified conflicts of interest, as applicable.

The faculty reported the following relevant financial relationship(s) during the content development process for this activity:

John D. Carmichael, MD, has served as an advisory board member for Camurus, Novo Nordisk, Recordati, and Xeris. He is also a member of the American Association of Clinical Endocrinologists (Pituitary, Adrenal, and Neuroendocrine Disease State Network) and the Pituitary Society.

Natalie E. Cusano, MD, MS, has served as a research investigator for Shire/Takeda, a speaker for Alexion Pharmaceuticals, and a consultant for Ascendis Pharma. She has also spoken for Alexion and serves on the Editorial Board for Endocrine Practice.

Tobias Else, MD, has served as a co-investigator for Corcept Pharmaceuticals and Merck, an advisory board member for Merck and Lantheus, and a committee member for VHL Alliance.

Sangeeta R. Kashyap, MD, has served as a consultant and coinvestigator to GI Dynamics; she has received research support from Fractyl, Inc; and she is chief medical officer of Gila Therapeutics.

Marie E. McDonnell, MD, has served as a trial event adjudicator for a trial conducted by Eisai and receives research funding from Lilly, Inc, that is paid to her institution.

Stephanie Page, MD, PhD, is an editor at UpToDate and has served as a consultant to Pharmajor International.

Anne L. Peters, MD, has served as an advisory board member for Abbott Diabetes Care, Medscape, Novo Nordisk, Vertex, and Zealand and as a consultant for Blue Circle Health. She has received research support from Dexcom, Insulet, and Abbott Diabetes Care. She has stock options in Omada Health and Teladoc.

The following faculty reported no relevant financial relationships: Kaniksha Desai, MD; Frances J. Hayes, MB BCh, BAO; Jacqueline Jonklaas, MD, PhD, MPH; and Margaret Flynn Lippincott, MD

The medical editor for this activity reported no relevant financial relationships: Abbie L. Young, MS, CGC, ELS(D)

Endocrine Society staff associated with the development of content for this activity reported no relevant financial relationships.

DISCLAIMERS

The information presented in this activity represents the opinion of the faculty and is not necessarily the official position of the Endocrine Society.

Use of professional judgment:

The educational content in this activity relates to basic principles of diagnosis and therapy and does not substitute for individual patient assessment based on the health care provider's examination of the patient and consideration of laboratory data and other factors unique to the patient. Standards in medicine change as new data become available.

Drugs and dosages:

When prescribing medications, the physician is advised to check the product information sheet accompanying each drug to verify conditions of use and to identify any changes in drug dosage schedule or contraindications.

POLICY ON UNLABELED/OFF-LABEL USE

The Endocrine Society has determined that disclosure of unlabeled/off-label or investigational use of commercial product(s) is informative for audiences and therefore requires this information to be disclosed to the learners at the beginning of the presentation. Uses of specific therapeutic agents, devices, and other products discussed in this educational activity may not be the same as those indicated in product labeling approved by the Food and Drug Administration (FDA). The Endocrine Society requires that any discussions of such "off-label" use be based on scientific research that conforms to generally accepted standards of experimental design, data collection, and data analysis. Before recommending or prescribing any therapeutic agent or device, learners should review the complete prescribing information, including indications, contraindications, warnings, precautions, and adverse events.

ACKNOWLEDGMENT OF COMMERCIAL SUPPORT

The activity is not supported by educational grant(s) or other funds from any commercial supporters.

Publication Date: August 2024

Contents

For between-edition updates, visit us at: https://www.endocrine.org/education-and-training/book-updates.

LABORATORY REFERENCE RANGES

Reference ranges vary among laboratories. Conventional units are listed first with SI units in parentheses.

Lipid Values

High-density lipoprotein (HDL) cholesterol

- Optimal --- >60 mg/dL (SI: >1.55 mmol/L)
- Normal --- 40-60 mg/dL (SI: 1.04-1.55 mmol/L)
- Low --- <40 mg/dL (SI: <1.04 mmol/L)

Low-density lipoprotein (LDL) cholesterol

- Optimal --- <100 mg/dL (SI: <2.59 mmol/L) (for primary prevention); <70 mg/dL (SI: <1.81 mmol/L) (for secondary prevention)
- Low --- 100-129 mg/dL (SI: 2.59-3.34 mmol/L)
- Borderline-high --- 130-159 mg/dL (SI: 3.37-4.12 mmol/L)
- High --- 160-189 mg/dL (SI: 4.14-4.90 mmol/L)
- Very high --- ≥190 mg/dL (SI: ≥4.92 mmol/L)

Non-HDL cholesterol

- Optimal --- <130 mg/dL (SI: <3.37 mmol/L)
- Borderline-high --- 130-159 mg/dL (SI: 3.37-4.12 mmol/L)
- High --- ≥240 mg/dL (SI: ≥6.22 mmol/L)

Total cholesterol

- Optimal --- <200 mg/dL (SI: <5.18 mmol/L)
- Borderline-high --- 200-239 mg/dL (SI: 5.18-6.19 mmol/L)
- High --- ≥240 mg/dL (SI: ≥6.22 mmol/L)

Triglycerides

- Optimal --- <150 mg/dL (SI: <1.70 mmol/L)
- Borderline-high --- 150-199 mg/dL (SI: 1.70-2.25 mmol/L)
- High --- 200-499 mg/dL (SI: 2.26-5.64 mmol/L)
- Very high --- ≥500 mg/dL (SI: ≥5.65 mmol/L)

Lipoprotein (a) --- ≤30 mg/dL (SI: ≤1.07 µmol/L)

Apolipoprotein B --- 50-110 mg/dL (SI: 0.5-1.1 g/L)

Hematologic Values

Erythrocyte sedimentation rate --- 0-20 mm/h

Haptoglobin --- 30-200 mg/dL (SI: 300-2000 mg/L)

Hematocrit --- 41%-51% (SI: 0.41-0.51) (male); 35%-45% (SI: 0.35-0.45) (female)

Hemoglobin A_{1c} --- 4.0%-5.6% (20-38 mmol/mol)

Hemoglobin --- 13.8-17.2 g/dL (SI: 138-172 g/L) (male); 12.1-15.1 g/dL (SI: 121-151 g/L) (female)

International normalized ratio --- 0.8-1.2

Mean corpuscular volume (MCV) --- 80-100 μm^3 (SI: 80-100 fL)

Platelet count --- 150-450 x 10^3/µL (SI: 150-450 x 10^9/L)

Protein (total) --- 6.3-7.9 g/dL (SI: 63-79 g/L)

Reticulocyte count --- 0.5%-1.5% of red blood cells (SI: 0.005-0.015)

White blood cell count --- 4500-11,000/µL (SI: 4.5-11.0 x 10^9/L)

Thyroid Values

Thyroglobulin --- 3-42 ng/mL (SI: 3-42 µg/L) (after surgery and radioactive iodine treatment: <0.1 ng/mL [SI: <0.1 µg/L])

Thyroglobulin antibodies --- ≤4.0 IU/mL (SI: ≤4.0 kIU/L)

Thyrotropin (TSH) --- 0.5-5.0 mIU/L

Thyrotropin-receptor antibodies (TRAb) --- ≤1.75 IU/L

Thyroid-stimulating immunoglobulin --- ≤120% of basal activity

Thyroperoxidase (TPO) antibodies --- <2.0 IU/mL (SI: <2.0 kIU/L)

Thyroxine (T_4) (free) --- 0.8-1.8 ng/dL (SI: 10.30-23.17 pmol/L)

Thyroxine (T_4) (total) --- 5.5-12.5 µg/dL (SI: 70.79-160.88 nmol/L)

Free thyroxine (T_4) index --- 4-12

Triiodothyronine (T_3) (free) --- 2.3-4.2 pg/mL (SI: 3.53-6.45 pmol/L)

Triiodothyronine (T_3) (total) --- 70-200 ng/dL (SI: 1.08-3.08 nmol/L)

Triiodothyronine (T_3), reverse --- 10-24 ng/dL (SI: 0.15-0.37 nmol/L)

Triiodothyronine uptake, resin --- 25%-38%

Radioactive iodine uptake --- 3%-16% (6 hours); 15%-30% (24 hours)

Endocrine Values

Serum

Aldosterone --- 4-21 ng/dL (SI: 111.0-582.5 pmol/L)

Alkaline phosphatase --- 50-120 U/L (SI: 0.84-2.00 µkat/L)

Alkaline phosphatase (bone-specific) --- ≤20 µg/L (adult male); ≤14 µg/L (premenopausal female); ≤22 µg/L (postmenopausal female)

Androstenedione --- 65-210 ng/dL (SI: 2.27-7.33 nmol/L) (adult male); 30-200 ng/dL (SI:1.05-6.98 nmol/L) (adult female)

Antimullerian hormone --- 0.7-19.0 ng/mL (SI: 5.0-135.7 pmol/L) (male, >12 years); 0.9-9.5 ng/mL (SI: 6.4-67.9 pmol/L) (female, 13-45 years); <1.0 ng/mL (SI: <7.1 pmol/L) (female, >45 years)

Calcitonin --- <16 pg/mL (SI: <4.67 pmol/L) (basal, male); <8 pg/mL (SI: <2.34 pmol/L) (basal, female); ≤130 pg/mL (SI: ≤37.96 pmol/L) (peak calcium infusion, male); ≤90 pg/mL (SI: ≤26.28 pmol/L) (peak calcium infusion, female)

Carcinoembryonic antigen --- <2.5 ng/mL (SI: <2.5 µg/L)

Chromogranin A --- <93 ng/mL (SI: <93 µg/L)

Corticosterone--- 53-1560 ng/dL (SI: 1.53-45.08 nmol/L) (>18 years)

Corticotropin (ACTH) ---------- 10-60 pg/mL (SI: 2.2-13.2 pmol/L)

Cortisol (8 AM) -------------- 5-25 µg/dL (SI: 137.9-689.7 nmol/L)

Cortisol (4 PM)----------------2-14 µg/dL (SI: 55.2-386.2 nmol/L)

C-peptide-------------------- 0.5-2.0 ng/mL (SI: 0.17-0.66 nmol/L)

C-reactive protein -----------0.8-3.1 mg/L (SI: 7.62-29.52 nmol/L)

Cross-linked N-telopeptide of type 1 collagen --------------------

5.4-24.2 nmol BCE/mmol creat (male);

6.2-19.0 nmol BCE/mmol creat (female)

Dehydroepiandrosterone sulfate (DHEA-S)

Patient Age	Female	Male
18-29 years	44-332 µg/dL (SI: 1.19-9.00 µmol/L)	89-457 µg/dL (SI: 2.41-12.38 µmol/L)
30-39 years	31-228 µg/dL (SI: 0.84-6.78 µmol/L)	65-334 µg/dL (SI: 1.76-9.05 µmol/L)
40-49 years	18-244 µg/dL (SI: 0.49-6.61 µmol/L)	48-244 µg/dL (SI: 1.30-6.61 µmol/L)
50-59 years	15-200 µg/dL (SI: 0.41-5.42 µmol/L)	35-179 µg/dL (SI: 0.95-4.85 µmol/L)
≥60 years	15-157 µg/dL (SI: 0.41-4.25 µmol/L)	25-131 µg/dL (SI: 0.68-3.55 µmol/L)

Deoxycorticosterone ----<10 ng/dL (SI: <0.30 nmol/L) (>18 years)

1,25-Dihydroxyvitamin D_3---- 16-65 pg/mL (SI: 41.6-169.0 pmol/L)

Estradiol -------------10-40 pg/mL (SI: 36.7-146.8 pmol/L) (male);

10-180 pg/mL (SI: 36.7-660.8 pmol/L) (follicular, female);

100-300 pg/mL (SI: 367.1-1101.3 pmol/L) (midcycle, female);

40-200 pg/mL (SI: 146.8-734.2 pmol/L) (luteal, female);

<20 pg/mL (SI: <73.4 pmol/L) (postmenopausal, female)

Estrone --------------10-60 pg/mL (SI: 37.0-221.9 pmol/L) (male);

17-200 pg/mL (SI: 62.9-739.6 pmol/L) (premenopausal female);

7-40 pg/mL (SI: 25.9-147.9 pmol/L) (postmenopausal female)

α-Fetoprotein ------------------------------ <6 ng/mL (SI: <6 µg/L)

Follicle-stimulating hormone (FSH) ------------------------------

1.0-13.0 mIU/mL (SI: 1.0-13.0 IU/L) (male);

<3.0 mIU/mL (SI: <3.0 IU/L) (prepuberty, female);

2.0-12.0 mIU/mL (SI: 2.0-12.0 IU/L) (follicular, female);

4.0-36.0 mIU/mL (SI: 4.0-36.0 IU/L) (midcycle, female);

1.0-9.0 mIU/mL (SI: 1.0-9.0 IU/L) (luteal, female);

>30.0 mIU/mL (SI: >30.0 IU/L) (postmenopausal, female)

Free fatty acids -------------- 10.6-18.0 mg/dL (SI: 0.4-0.7 nmol/L)

Gastrin------------------------------- <100 pg/mL (SI: <100 ng/L)

Growth hormone (GH)--- 0.01-0.97 ng/mL (SI: 0.01-0.97 µg/L) (male);

0.01-3.61 ng/mL (SI: 0.01-3.61 µg/L) (female)

Homocysteine ----------------------- ≤1.76 mg/L (SI: ≤13 µmol/L)

β-Human chorionic gonadotropin (β-hCG) -----------------------

<3.0 mIU/mL (SI: <3.0 IU/L) (nonpregnant female);

>25 mIU/mL SI: >25 IU/L) indicates a positive pregnancy test

β-Hydroxybutyrate ----------------<3.0 mg/dL (SI: <288.2 µmol/L)

17-Hydroxypregnenolone --- 29-189 ng/dL (SI: 0.87-5.69 nmol/L)

17α-Hydroxyprogesterone ---------------------------------------

<220 ng/dL (SI: <6.67 nmol/L) (adult male);

<80 ng/dL (SI: <2.42 nmol/L) (follicular, female);

<285 ng/dL (SI: <8.64 nmol/L) (luteal, female);

<51 ng/dL (SI: <1.55 nmol/L) (postmenopausal, female)

25-Hydroxyvitamin D ---

<20 ng/mL (SI: <49.9 nmol/L) (deficiency);

21-29 ng/mL (SI: 52.4-72.4 nmol/L) (insufficiency);

30-80 ng/mL (SI: 74.9-199.7 nmol/L) (optimal levels);

>80 ng/mL (SI: >199.7 nmol/L) (toxicity possible)

Inhibin B -------------------------15-300 pg/mL (SI: 15-300 ng/L)

Insulinlike growth factor 1 (IGF-1)

Patient Age	Female	Male
18 years	162-541 ng/mL (SI: 21.2-70.9 nmol/L)	170-640 ng/mL (SI: 22.3-83.8 nmol/L)
19 years	138-442 ng/mL (SI: 18.1-57.9 nmol/L)	147-527 ng/mL (SI: 19.3-69.0 nmol/L)
20 years	122-384 ng/mL (SI: 16.0-50.3 nmol/L)	132-457 ng/mL (SI: 17.3-59.9 nmol/L)
21-25 years	116-341 ng/mL (SI: 15.2-44.7 nmol/L)	116-341 ng/mL (SI: 15.2-44.7 nmol/L)
26-30 years	117-321 ng/mL (SI: 15.3-42.1 nmol/L)	117-321 ng/mL (SI: 15.3-42.1 nmol/L)
31-35 years	113-297 ng/mL (SI: 14.8-38.9 nmol/L)	113-297 ng/mL (SI: 14.8-38.9 nmol/L)
36-40 years	106-277 ng/mL (SI: 13.9-36.3 nmol/L)	106-277 ng/mL (SI: 13.9-36.3 nmol/L)
41-45 years	98-261 ng/mL (SI: 12.8-34.2 nmol/L)	98-261 ng/mL (SI: 12.8-34.2 nmol/L)
46-50 years	91-246 ng/mL (SI: 11.9-32.2 nmol/L)	91-246 ng/mL (SI: 11.9-32.2 nmol/L)
51-55 years	84-233 ng/mL (SI: 11.0-30.5 nmol/L)	84-233 ng/mL (SI: 11.0-30.5 nmol/L)
56-60 years	78-220 ng/mL (SI: 10.2-28.8 nmol/L)	78-220 ng/mL (SI: 10.2-28.8 nmol/L)
61-65 years	72-207 ng/mL (SI: 9.4-27.1 nmol/L)	72-207 ng/mL (SI: 9.4-27.1 nmol/L)
66-70 years	67-195 ng/mL (SI: 8.8-25.5 nmol/L)	67-195 ng/mL (SI: 8.8-25.5 nmol/L)
71-75 years	62-184 ng/mL (SI: 8.1-24.1 nmol/L)	62-184 ng/mL (SI: 8.1-24.1 nmol/L)
76-80 years	57-172 ng/mL (SI: 7.5-22.5 nmol/L)	57-172 ng/mL (SI: 7.5-22.5 nmol/L)
>80 years	53-162 ng/mL (SI: 6.9-21.2 nmol/L)	53-162 ng/mL (SI: 6.9-21.2 nmol/L)

Insulinlike growth factor binding protein 3 ---------- 2.5-4.8 mg/L

Insulin ---------- 1.4-14.0 μIU/mL (SI: 9.7-97.2 pmol/L)

Islet-cell antibody assay ----------

0 Juvenile Diabetes Foundation units

Luteinizing hormone (LH) ----------

1.0-9.0 mIU/mL (SI: 1.0-9.0 IU/L) (male);

<1.0 mIU/mL (SI: <1.0 IU/L) (prepuberty, female);

1.0-18.0 mIU/mL (SI: 1.0-18.0 IU/L) (follicular, female);

20.0-80.0 mIU/mL (SI: 20.0-80.0 IU/L) (midcycle, female);

0.5-18.0 mIU/mL (SI: 0.5-18.0 IU/L) (luteal, female);

>30.0 mIU/mL (SI: >30.0 IU/L) (postmenopausal, female)

Metanephrines (plasma fractionated)

Metanephrine ---------- <99 pg/mL (SI: <0.50 nmol/L)

Normetanephrine ---------- <165 pg/mL (SI: <0.90 nmol/L)

75-g oral glucose tolerance test blood glucose values ----------

60-100 mg/dL (SI: 3.3-5.6 mmol/L) (fasting);

<200 mg/dL (SI: <11.1 mmol/L) (1 hour);

<140 mg/dL (SI: <7.8 mmol/L) (2 hour);

between 140-200 mg/dL (SI: 7.8-11.1 mmol/L) is considered impaired glucose tolerance or prediabetes; greater than 200 mg/dL (SI: >11.1 mmol/L) is a sign of diabetes mellitus

50-g oral glucose tolerance test for gestational diabetes ----------

<140 mg/dL (SI: <7.8 mmol/L) (1 hour)

100-g oral glucose tolerance test for gestational diabetes ----------

<95 mg/dL (SI: <5.3 mmol/L) (fasting);

<180 mg/dL (SI: <10.0 mmol/L) (1 hour);

<155 mg/dL (SI: <8.6 mmol/L) (2 hour);

<140 mg/dL (SI: <7.8 mmol/L) (3 hour)

Osteocalcin ---------- 9.0-42.0 ng/mL (SI: 9.0-42.0 μg/L)

Parathyroid hormone, intact (PTH) - 10-65 pg/mL (SI: 10-65 ng/L)

Parathyroid hormone–related protein (PTHrP) ---------- <2.0 pmol/L

Progesterone ---------- ≤1.2 ng/mL (SI: ≤3.8 nmol/L) (male);

≤1.0 ng/mL (SI: ≤3.2 nmol/L) (follicular, female);

2.0-20.0 ng/mL (SI: 6.4-63.6 nmol/L) (luteal, female);

≤1.1 ng/mL (SI: ≤3.5 nmol/L) (postmenopausal, female);

>10.0 ng/mL (SI: >31.8 nmol/L) (evidence of ovulatory adequacy)

Proinsulin ---------- 26.5-176.4 pg/mL (SI: 3.0-20.0 pmol/L)

Prolactin ---------- 4-23 ng/mL (SI: 0.17-1.00 nmol/L) (male);

4-30 ng/mL (SI: 0.17-1.30 nmol/L) (nonlactating female);

10-200 ng/mL (SI: 0.43-8.70 nmol/L) (lactating female)

Prostate-specific antigen (PSA) ----------

<2.0 ng/mL (SI: <2.0 μg/L) (≤40 years);

<2.8 ng/mL (SI: <2.8 μg/L) (≤50 years);

<3.8 ng/mL (SI: <3.8 μg/L) (≤60 years);

<5.3 ng/mL (SI: <5.3 μg/L) (≤70 years);

<7.0 ng/mL (SI: <7.0 μg/L) (≤79 years);

<7.2 ng/mL (SI: <7.2 μg/L) (≥80 years)

Renin activity, plasma, sodium replete, ambulatory ----------

0.6-4.3 ng/mL per h

Renin, direct concentration ---------- 4-44 pg/mL (SI: 0.1-1.0 pmol/L)

Sex hormone–binding globulin (SHBG) ----------

1.1-6.7 μg/mL (SI: 10-60 nmol/L) (male);

2.2-14.6 μg/mL (SI: 20-130 nmol/L) (female)

α-Subunit of pituitary glycoprotein hormones ----------

<1.2 ng/mL (SI: <1.2 μg/L)

Testosterone (bioavailable) ----------

0.8-4.0 ng/dL (SI: 0.03-0.14 nmol/L)

(20-50 years, female on oral estrogen);

0.8-10.0 ng/dL (SI: 0.03-0.35 nmol/L)

(20-50 years, female not on oral estrogen);

83.0-257.0 ng/dL (SI: 2.88-8.92 nmol/L) (male 20-29 years);

72.0-235.0 ng/dL (SI: 2.50-8.15 nmol/L) (male 30-39 years);

61.0-213.0 ng/dL (SI: 2.12-7.39 nmol/L) (male 40-49 years);

50.0-190.0 ng/dL (SI: 1.74-6.59 nmol/L) (male 50-59 years);

40.0-168.0 ng/dL (SI: 1.39-5.83 nmol/L) (male 60-69 years)

Testosterone (free) -- 9.0-30.0 ng/dL (SI: 0.31-1.04 nmol/L) (male);

0.3-1.9 ng/dL (SI: 0.01-0.07 nmol/L) (female)

Testosterone (total) - 300-900 ng/dL (SI: 10.4-31.2 nmol/L) (male);

8-60 ng/dL (SI: 0.3-2.1 nmol/L) (female)

Vitamin B_{12} ---------- 180-914 pg/mL (SI: 133-674 pmol/L)

Chemistry Values

Alanine aminotransferase ---------- 10-40 U/L (SI: 0.17-0.67 μkat/L)

Albumin ---------- 3.5-5.0 g/dL (SI: 35-50 g/L)

Amylase ---------- 26-102 U/L (SI: 0.43-1.70 μkat/L)

Anion gap ---------- 3-11 mEq/L (SI: 3-11 mmol/L)

Aspartate aminotransferase ---------- 20-48 U/L (SI: 0.33-0.80 μkat/L)

Bicarbonate ---------- 21-28 mEq/L (SI: 21-28 mmol/L)

Bilirubin (total) ---------- 0.3-1.2 mg/dL (SI: 5.1-20.5 μmol/L)

Blood gases

Po_2, arterial blood ---------- 80-100 mm Hg (SI: 10.6-13.3 kPa)

Pco_2, arterial blood ---------- 35-45 mm Hg (SI: 4.7-6.0 kPa)

Blood pH ---------- 7.35-7.45

Calcium ---------- 8.2-10.2 mg/dL (SI: 2.1-2.6 mmol/L)

Calcium (ionized) ---------- 4.60-5.08 mg/dL (SI: 1.2-1.3 mmol/L)

Carbon dioxide ---------- 22-28 mEq/L (SI: 22-28 mmol/L)

CD_4 cell count ---------- 500-1400/μL (SI: 0.5-1.4 x 10^9/L)

Chloride ---------- 96-106 mEq/L (SI: 96-106 mmol/L)

Creatine kinase ---------- 50-200 U/L (SI: 0.84-3.34 μkat/L)

Creatinine ---------- 0.7-1.3 mg/dL (SI: 61.9-114.9 μmol/L) (male);

0.6-1.1 mg/dL (SI: 53.0-97.2 μmol/L) (female)

Ferritin ---------- 15-200 ng/mL (SI: 33.7-449.4 pmol/L)

Folate ---------- ≥4.0 ng/mL (SI: ≥4.0 μg/L)

Glucose ---------- 70-99 mg/dL (SI: 3.9-5.5 mmol/L)

γ-Glutamyltransferase ----------- 2-30 U/L (SI: 0.03-0.50 µkat/L)

Iron --

50-150 µg/dL (SI: 9.0-26.8 µmol/L) (male);

35-145 µg/dL (SI: 6.3-26.0 µmol/L) (female)

Lactate dehydrogenase --------- 100-200 U/L (SI: 1.7-3.3 µkat/L)

Lactic acid -------------------5.4-20.7 mg/dL (SI: 0.6-2.3 mmol/L)

Lipase -------------------------- 10-73 U/L (SI: 0.17-1.22 µkat/L)

Magnesium ------------------- 1.5-2.3 mg/dL (SI: 0.6-0.9 mmol/L)

Osmolality ------------275-295 mOsm/kg (SI: 275-295 mmol/kg)

Phosphate -------------------- 2.3-4.7 mg/dL (SI: 0.7-1.5 mmol/L)

Potassium -------------------- 3.5-5.0 mEq/L (SI: 3.5-5.0 mmol/L)

Prothrombin time --------------------------------------8.3-10.8 s

Serum urea nitrogen-------------8-23 mg/dL (SI: 2.9-8.2 mmol/L)

Sodium ------------------- 136-142 mEq/L (SI: 136-142 mmol/L)

Transferrin saturation ---------------------------------- 14%-50%

Troponin I ------------------------------ <0.6 ng/mL (SI: <0.6 µg/L)

Tryptase --------------------------- <11.5 ng/mL (SI: <11.5 µg/L)

Uric acid ----------------- 3.5-7.0 mg/dL (SI: 208.2-416.4 µmol/L)

Urine

Albumin----------30-300 µg/mg creat (SI: 3.4-33.9 µg/mol creat)

Albumin-to-creatinine ratio ---------------------- <30 mg/g creat

Aldosterone------------------- 3-20 µg/24 h (SI: 8.3-55.4 nmol/d)

(should be <12 µg/24 h [SI: <33.2 nmol/d] with oral sodium loading—confirmed with 24-hour urinary sodium >200 mEq)

Calcium ------------------- 100-300 mg/24 h (SI: 2.5-7.5 mmol/d)

Catecholamine fractionation

Normotensive normal ranges:

Dopamine ------------------ <400 µg/24 h (SI: <2610 nmol/d)

Epinephrine --------------------<21 µg/24 h (SI: <115 nmol/d)

Norepinephrine ----------------<80 µg/24 h (SI: <473 nmol/d)

Citrate ---------------- 320-1240 mg/24 h (SI: 16.7-64.5 mmol/d)

Cortisol ------------------------ 4-50 µg/24 h (SI: 11-138 nmol/d)

Cortisol following dexamethasone-suppression test

(low-dose: 2 day, 2 mg daily)---- <10 µg/24 h (SI: <27.6 nmol/d)

Creatinine------------------- 1.0-2.0 g/24 h (SI: 8.8-17.7 mmol/d)

Glomerular filtration rate (estimated) ---- >60 mL/min per 1.73 m^2

5-Hydroxyindole acetic acid---2-9 mg/24 h (SI: 10.5-47.1 µmol/d)

Iodine (random)-->100 µg/L

17-Ketosteroids----6.0-21.0 mg/24 h (SI: 20.8-72.9 µmol/d) (male);

4.0-17.0 mg/24 h (SI: 13.9-59.0 µmol/d) (female)

Metanephrine fractionation

Normotensive normal ranges:

Metanephrine-------- <261 µg/24 h (SI: <1323 nmol/d) (male);

<180 µg/24 h (SI: <913 nmol/d) (female)

Normetanephrine-------------------- age and sex dependent

Total metanephrine------------------ age and sex dependent

Osmolality --------- 150-1150 mOsm/kg (SI: 150-1150 mmol/kg)

Oxalate -------------------------- <40 mg/24 h (SI: <456 mmol/d)

Phosphate ----------------- 0.9-1.3 g/24 h (SI: 29.1-42.0 mmol/d)

Potassium -------------------17-77 mEq/24 h (SI: 17-77 mmol/d)

Sodium -------------------40-217 mEq/24 h (SI: 40-217 mmol/d)

Uric acid -------------------------<800 mg/24 h (SI: <4.7 mmol/d)

Saliva

Cortisol (salivary), midnight --------- <0.13 µg/dL (SI: <3.6 nmol/L)

Semen

Semen analysis------------->20 million sperm/mL; >50% motility

COMMON ABBREVIATIONS USED IN ENDOCRINE BOARD REVIEW

ACTH = corticotropin
ACE inhibitor = angiotensin-converting enzyme inhibitor
ALT = alanine aminotransferase
AST = aspartate aminotransferase
BMI = body mass index
CNS = central nervous system
CT = computed tomography
DHEA = dehydroepiandrosterone
DHEA-S = dehydroepiandrosterone sulfate
DNA = deoxyribonucleic acid
DPP-4 inhibitor = dipeptidyl-peptidase 4 inhibitor
DXA = dual-energy x-ray absorptiometry
FDA = Food and Drug Administration
FGF-23 = fibroblast growth factor 23
FNA = fine-needle aspiration
FSH = follicle-stimulating hormone
GH = growth hormone
GHRH = growth hormone–releasing hormone
GLP-1 receptor agonist = glucagonlike peptide 1 receptor agonist
GnRH = gonadotropin-releasing hormone
hCG = human chorionic gonadotropin
HDL = high-density lipoprotein
HIV = human immunodeficiency virus
HMG-CoA reductase inhibitor = 3-hydroxy-3-methylglutaryl coenzyme A reductase inhibitor
IGF-1 = insulinlike growth factor 1
LDL = low-density lipoprotein
LH = luteinizing hormone
MCV = mean corpuscular volume
MIBG = *meta*-iodobenzylguanidine
MRI = magnetic resonance imaging
NPH insulin = neutral protamine Hagedorn insulin
PCSK9 inhibitor = proprotein convertase subtilisin/kexin 9 inhibitor
PET = positron emission tomography
PSA = prostate-specific antigen
PTH = parathyroid hormone
PTHrP = parathyroid hormone–related protein
SGLT-2 inhibitor = sodium-glucose cotransporter 2 inhibitor
SHBG = sex hormone–binding globulin
T_3 = triiodothyronine
T_4 = thyroxine
TPO antibodies = thyroperoxidase antibodies
TRH = thyrotropin-releasing hormone
TRAb = TSH-receptor antibodies
TSH = thyrotropin
VLDL = very low-density lipoprotein

ENDOCRINE BOARD REVIEW

QUESTIONS

Adrenal Board Review

Tobias Else, MD

1 A 59-year-old woman is referred for further evaluation of an incidentally discovered adrenal mass. She presented with lower abdominal/pelvic pain, and CT did not show any unusual findings other than the adrenal lesion, measuring 3.8 × 2.8 cm.

She has a history of breast cancer diagnosed 10 years ago, which was treated with lumpectomy, radiation therapy, and tamoxifen. Postoperatively, she had a deep venous thrombosis with a small pulmonary embolism, and she took anticoagulation therapy for 2 years. She does not have hypertension, hypokalemia, or diabetes. Her BMI is 23.3 kg/m^2.

Her primary care physician ordered washout CT, which showed a homogeneous adrenal mass with peripheral areas of minor calcification (*see image*). The mass had attenuation values of 24 Hounsfield units (unenhanced), 27 Hounsfield units (early phase), and 26 Hounsfield units (delayed phase).

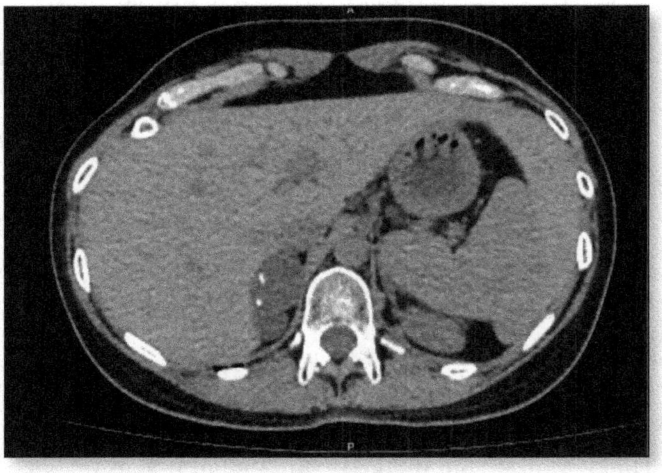

Laboratory test results:

Potassium = 4.8 mEq/L (3.5-5.0 mEq/L) (SI: 4.8 mmol/L [3.5-5.0 mmol/L])
Sodium = 141 mEq/L (136-142 mEq/L) (SI: 141 mmol/L [136-142 mmol/L])
Plasma normetanephrine = 132 pg/mL (<165 pg/mL) (SI: <0.72 nmol/L [<0.90 nmol/L])
Plasma metanephrine = <40 pg/mL (<99 pg/mL) (SI: <0.20 nmol/L [<0.50 nmol/L])
Cortisol (following 1 mg dexamethasone) = 0.8 µg/dL (SI: 22.1 nmol/L)

Which of the following is the best next step in this patient's care?

A. Perform ^{18}FDG-PET
B. Measure cortisol following cosyntropin stimulation
C. Reassure her of the benign character of the adrenal mass
D. Refer for biopsy for the adrenal mass
E. Refer for right adrenalectomy

2 A 56-year-old woman with type 2 diabetes seeks advice regarding prednisone taper. She recently had an episode of a severe urticarial rash of unknown etiology. Following recommendations by her dermatologist, she started 60 mg of prednisone daily, and over the course of 4 weeks, she has tapered this to 5 mg daily (which has been her dose for the last 7 days). She reports that her blood glucose values were initially slightly increased after starting prednisone, but they have now normalized. Her dermatologist recommended stopping prednisone without further taper, but she is concerned about possible adrenal insufficiency.

Which of the following is the best recommendation now?

A. Educate about symptoms and signs of adrenal insufficiency; ask her to call if she has any symptoms after stopping prednisone
B. Measure 8 AM cortisol
C. Measure 8 AM cortisol and ACTH
D. Perform a cosyntropin-stimulation test
E. Switch hydrocortisone, 15 mg in the morning and 5 mg in the early afternoon, and taper hydrocortisone by 5 mg every 2 weeks

3 A 24-year-old woman had genetic testing because of a family history of breast cancer in her mother and maternal grandmother. A large next-generation sequencing panel revealed a pathogenic variant in *SDHA*, c.91C>T, p.R31X. She has been referred by a genetic counselor for further evaluation and management.

The patient does not have a personal or family history of pheochromocytoma, paraganglioma, kidney cancer, or gastrointestinal stroma tumor. Review of systems is negative.

On physical examination, she is a thin, healthy appearing woman. Her blood pressure is 110/77 mm Hg, and pulse rate is 69 beats/min. Her cranial nerves are intact, and there are no palpable neck or abdominal tumors.

Which of the following is the best recommendation regarding initial workup and future surveillance?

A. Additional genetic testing to confirm the presence of the *SDHA*, c.91C>T, p.R31X variant
B. Annual Ga-DOTATATE PET and plasma metanephrine measurement
C. Annual plasma metanephrine measurement
D. Annual whole-body MRI and plasma metanephrine measurement
E. Reassure the patient she has a very low tumor risk and that surveillance recommendations are not mandatory

4 A 21-year-old woman is referred because of low potassium levels and hypertension. Her primary care physician ordered biochemical screening for primary aldosteronism:

Aldosterone (immunoassay) = 14 ng/dL (4-21 ng/dL) (SI: 388.4 pmol/L [111.0-582.5 pmol/L])
Plasma renin activity = <0.6 ng/mL per h (0.6-4.3 ng/mL per h)
Potassium = 2.8 mEq/L (3.5-5.0 mEq/L) (SI: 2.8 mmol/L [3.5-5.0 mmol/L])
Sodium = 136 mEq/L (136-142 mEq/L) (SI: 136 mmol/L [136-142 mmol/L])

She reports that she has always had elevated blood pressure. Her blood pressure today is 159/98 mm Hg. On review of systems, she says that she has never had a period and that she has only minimal pubic hair growth and no breast development, which is confirmed on physical examination. She is not aware of anyone in her family with absent periods or infertility.

Which of the following is the best next step to determine this patient's definitive diagnosis?

A. Measure 8 AM ACTH, cortisol, deoxycorticosterone, and 11-deoxycortisol
B. Measure aldosterone in a 24-hour urine collection
C. Perform abdominal CT
D. Perform a progesterone challenge
E. Perform cosyntropin-stimulation testing with measurement of 17-hydroxyprogesterone

5 A 48-year-old man is referred after an adrenal mass was incidentally identified during evaluation of sigmoid diverticulitis. Review of imaging shows a 3.2-cm homogeneous adrenal mass with a density of 8 Hounsfield units.

The patient recently changed his job to a more sedentary position and has gained about 10 lb (4.5 kg) over the course of the last 12 months. He feels well. He does not have hypertension, and he takes no medication.

On physical examination, his blood pressure is 132/81 mm Hg and pulse rate is 77 beats/min. His height is 74.8 in (190 cm), and weight is 231 lb (105 kg) (BMI = 29.0 kg/m^2). He has an overall athletic appearance with mild central fat distribution, normal muscle tone and strength, and no plethora or striae.

Laboratory test results at the time of discharge from the recent hospitalization:

Potassium = 4.4 mEq/L (3.5-5.0 mEq/L)
(SI: 4.4 mmol/L [3.5-5.0 mmol/L])
Sodium = 138 mEq/L (136-142 mEq/L)
(SI: 138 mmol/L [136-142 mmol/L])

Which of the following is the best next step in this patient's diagnostic workup?

A. Measure 8 AM aldosterone and metanephrine and perform a 1-mg dexamethasone-suppression test with measurement of cortisol and dexamethasone
B. Measure 8 AM cortisol and ACTH and obtain 3 midnight salivary cortisol measurements
C. Perform a 1-mg dexamethasone-suppression test with measurement of cortisol and dexamethasone
D. Perform a 1-mg dexamethasone-suppression test with measurement of cortisol only
E. Perform ^{18}FDG-PET

6 A 32-year-old woman presents for follow-up of prolactinoma, for which she takes cabergoline. She states she has been healthy most of her life but had an adrenalectomy for a 5.4-cm adrenal mass at age 2 years, which was discovered during evaluation of virilization. She does not have children. She has 2 healthy brothers. Her father died at age 40 years in an accident, and she does not have any information about the paternal side of her family. Her mother was an only child and had a diagnosis of bilateral breast cancer at age 32 years. Her maternal grandparents are alive and well in their 90s. Her maternal grandmother had a diagnosis of hyperparathyroidism at age 74 years and osteosarcoma at age 29 years.

Which of the following hereditary conditions is most likely present in this family?

A. Hereditary breast and ovarian cancer due to pathogenic variants in *BRCA1* or *BRCA2*
B. Li-Fraumeni syndrome
C. Lynch syndrome
D. McCune-Albright syndrome
E. Multiple endocrine neoplasia type 1

7 A 72-year-old man is referred for evaluation of possible Cushing syndrome. He had recent onset of subjective muscle weakness and experienced a weight gain of 15 lb (6.8 kg) over the last year. He has also developed a new diagnosis of diabetes (hemoglobin A_{1c} = 7.9% [63 mmol/mol]) and hypertension, which is currently treated with amlodipine, 10 mg daily.

On physical examination, he has slight redness of his face, facial rounding, small violaceous striae, and mildly atrophic skin. His height is 73.2 in (186 cm), and weight is 218 lb (99 kg) (BMI = 28.6 kg/m^2).

Laboratory evaluation at the initial visit shows hypokalemia, neutrophilia, and lymphocytopenia.

He calls 10 days after a 1-mg dexamethasone-suppression test was ordered to discuss the results. He apologizes that he did not immediately do the test. He had been diagnosed with COVID-19 3 days after his clinic visit, and his primary care provider then treated successfully him with nirmatrelvir and ritonavir (Paxlovid). He immediately did the dexamethasone-suppression test when he felt better (when a COVID-19 home test was negative and he felt well enough to go to the blood draw station).

His cortisol value was 1.8 mg/dL (49.7 nmol/L) (8 AM blood draw).

Which of the following is the best next step in this patient's diagnostic workup?

A. Measure 8 AM ACTH and cortisol
B. Obtain panel measurements for synthetic steroids
C. Perform pituitary MRI
D. Recommend no further diagnostic testing
E. Repeat the 1-mg dexamethasone-suppression test

8 A 55-year-old woman is referred after undergoing surgery (R0 resection) for a 6.8-cm adrenal mass 2 weeks ago. The pathological diagnosis was a 6.8-cm adrenocortical carcinoma, stage 2, with a Ki67 index of 18%. She feels well, other than some soreness around the incision site. She had no symptoms of hormone excess before surgery, but formal testing has not yet been pursued.

Physical examination findings are unremarkable, with no hirsutism, plethora, central fat distribution, muscle weakness, striae, or skin atrophy.

Her cortisol concentration (8 AM) is 17.4 ug/dL (480.0 nmol/L).

She is advised to travel to an academic center, but she prefers to stay local and obtain her care at this clinic.

Which of the following plans is the best next step in this patient's care?

A. Recommend no further follow-up; instruct her to return to clinic with any new symptoms
B. Refer for radiation therapy to the tumor bed
C. Refer for adjuvant cytotoxic chemotherapy, followed by mitotane for at least 2 years
D. Refer for adjuvant immunotherapy with pembrolizumab, followed by mitotane for at least 2 years
E. Start therapy with mitotane and continue for at least 2 years

9 A 23-year-old woman is referred for evaluation of unwanted facial hair, acne, and irregular menses. She developed pubic hair and body odor at age 5 years and was the tallest girl in her class until she stopped growing at age 11 years. She developed acne and facial hair at age 10 years, and menarche was at age 12 years. Her menses have always been irregular, and she has not menstruated for 8 months.

On physical examination, she has coarse terminal hairs and shaved stubble on her chin, upper lip, and sides of her face and acne on her forehead. Findings on pelvic examination, including external genitalia, are normal. She has no moon facies, dermal atrophy, myopathy, striae, or acanthosis nigricans. Her blood pressure is 120/80 mm Hg, and BMI is 23 kg/m^2.

Screening laboratory test results (sample drawn at 1 PM):

Serum cortisol = 6.0 µg/dL (2-14 µg/dL) (SI: 166 nmol/L [55-386 nmol/L])
Serum DHEA-S = 380 µg/dL (44-332 µg/dL) (SI: 10.3 µmol/L [1.2-9.0 µmol/L])
Serum 17-hydroxyprogesterone = 300 ng/dL (<80 ng/dL [follicular]) (SI: 9.1 nmol/L [<2.4 nmol/L])
Serum total testosterone = 75 ng/dL (8-60 ng/dL) (SI: 2.6 nmol/L [0.3-2.1 nmol/L])
SHBG = 1.0 µg/mL (2.2-14.6 µg/mL) (SI: 8.9 nmol/L [20-130 nmol/L])
Serum prolactin = 10 ng/mL (4-30 ng/mL) (SI: 0.4 nmol/L [0.2-1.3 nmol/L])
Serum glucose = 70 mg/dL (70-99 mg/dL) (SI: 3.9 mmol/L [3.9-5.5 mmol/L])

Which of the following is the most appropriate next step in this patient's evaluation?

A. Adrenal-directed CT
B. Cosyntropin-stimulation test measuring 17-hydroxyprogesterone and cortisol
C. No further testing
D. Plasma ACTH measurement
E. Serum 11-deoxycortisol measurement

10 A 25-year-old woman with a well-documented diagnosis of nonclassic 21-hydroxylase deficiency (21-OHD) would like to start a family. Her cosyntropin-stimulated 17-hydroxyprogesterone concentration is 3400 ng/dL (103.0 nmol/L), and her cortisol concentration is 21 µg/dL (579.3 nmol/L). She has not had DNA testing for genotyping. No members of her family or her husband's family have classic 21-OHD, there is no suspicious family history, and neither the patient nor her husband is of an ethnicity with an unusually high prevalence of classic or nonclassic 21-OHD. She asks about the risk of having an affected child.

How would you counsel the patient regarding the risk of having a child with classic 21-OHD?

A. Her risk of having a child with *classic* 21-OHD is <0.01%
B. Her risk of having a child with *classic* 21-OHD is >0.5%
C. She cannot have a child with *classic* 21-OHD because she has the *nonclassic* form
D. She can have a child with *classic* 21-OHD only if her partner also has a clinical diagnosis of *nonclassic* 21-OHD
E. There is a 50% risk the patient's child will have 21-OHD

11 A 24-year-old man is referred by a urologist for evaluation before surgery for testicular masses. The patient gives a history of taking hydrocortisone and fludrocortisone throughout childhood, but he stopped all medications at age 21 years.

On physical examination, he is a normal-appearing young man with a blood pressure of 106/72 mm Hg and pulse rate of 84 beats/min. Both testes have firm, irregular masses that are 2 to 3 cm in maximal dimension. His 8 AM cortisol concentration is 4 μg/dL (110.4 nmol/L) by immunoassay. Semen analysis documents azoospermia.

Which of the following is the most likely pattern of laboratory test results in this patient?

Answer	Testosterone	Androstenedione	LH
A.	↑	↑	↑
B.	↓	↓	↓
C.	Normal	↑	↓
D.	↓	↓	↑
E.	Normal	Normal	Normal

12 A 49-year-old woman with a history of estrogen receptor–positive breast cancer diagnosed 3 years earlier is referred for evaluation of an adrenal mass. Her only medication is tamoxifen. She has no evidence of breast cancer recurrence, but recent abdominal CT shows a 2.8-cm right adrenal nodule with an attenuation value of 46 Hounsfield units. FDG-PET demonstrates accumulation of FDG in the right adrenal nodule, but no significant accumulation in other sites. The patient is asymptomatic and has never had hypertension.

On physical examination, her height is 64 in (162.6 cm) and weight is 110 lb (50 kg) (BMI = 18.9 kg/m^2). Her blood pressure is 122/76 mm Hg, and pulse rate is 68 beats/min.

The cortisol concentration after an overnight 1-mg dexamethasone-suppression test is 2.2 μg/dL (SI: 60.7 nmol/L).

Which of the following is the best next step in this patient's management?

A. High-dose dexamethasone-suppression test
B. Measurement of plasma free fractionated metanephrines
C. Measurement of serum aldosterone and plasma renin activity
D. Percutaneous CT-guided aspiration biopsy of the right adrenal nodule
E. Surgical removal of the right adrenal nodule

13 An endocrine consult is requested for a 69-year-old woman who is in the medical intensive care unit for hypovolemic shock from urosepsis. Before hospital admission her only medications were metformin, 1000 mg daily; lisinopril, 20 mg daily; and atorvastatin, 5 mg daily. She remains intubated and has been treated with pressors and saline boluses for 3 days. Her systolic blood pressure is 85 mm Hg, and pulse rate is 118 beats/min. The team has performed a cosyntropin-stimulation test and asks for assistance with result interpretation.

Results of cosyntropin-stimulation testing:
Basal serum cortisol = 9.4 μg/dL (5-25 μg/dL) (SI: 259 nmol/L [138-690 nmol/L])
Stimulated serum cortisol = 13.4 μg/dL (SI: 370 nmol/L)
Serum glucose = 134 mg/dL (70-99 mg/dL) (SI: 7.4 mmol/L [3.9-5.5 mmol/L])
Serum albumin = 2.3 g/dL (3.5-5.0 g/dL) (SI: 23 g/L [35-50 g/L])

Which of the following is the best next step in this patient's evaluation and management?

A. Low-dose cosyntropin-stimulation test
B. No further testing
C. Plasma ACTH measurement
D. Serum DHEA-S measurement
E. Synthetic steroid measurement

14 A 43-year-old woman is seen for follow-up of Cushing disease. She initially presented with hypertension, hypokalemia, muscle weakness, hirsutism, oligomenorrhea, and weight gain over the last 2 years. She underwent transsphenoidal surgery 6 weeks ago.

Preoperative laboratory test results:

Late-night salivary cortisol = 0.82 μg/dL (<0.13 μg/dL) (SI: 22.6 nmol/L [<3.6 nmol/L])
Urinary free cortisol = 850 μg/24 h (4-50 μg/24 h) (SI: 2346 nmol/d [11-138 nmol/d])
Basal plasma ACTH = 102 pg/mL (10-60 pg/mL) (SI: 22.4 pmol/L [2.2-13.2 pmol/L])

Postoperatively, serial morning cortisol values were less than 0.5 μg/dL (<13.8 nmol/L). She takes hydrocortisone, 25 mg on arising and 10 mg in the early afternoon.

Her blood pressure has normalized, and she has lost 8 lb (3.6 kg). She describes diffuse muscle aches, fatigue, and anorexia. She states, "I am sleeping all day and feel worse than when I had Cushing's."

On physical examination, her blood pressure is 120/80 mm Hg and pulse rate is 70 beats/min without orthostatic changes. Her cushingoid features are beginning to resolve.

Laboratory test results:

Serum sodium = 136 mEq/L (136-142 mEq/L) (SI: 136 mmol/L [136-142 mmol/L])
Serum potassium = 4.4 mEq/L (3.5-5.0 mEq/L) (SI: 4.4 mmol/L [3.5-5.0 mmol/L])
Fasting glucose = 80 mg/dL (70-99 mg/dL) (SI: 4.4 mmol/L [3.9-5.5 mmol/L])
Serum cortisol (8 AM) before first dose of hydrocortisone = <0.5 μg/dL (5-25 μg/dL) (SI: <13.8 nmol/L [137.9-689.7 nmol/L])
DHEA-S = <15 μg/dL (18-244 μg/dL) (SI: <0.41 μmol/L [0.49-6.61 μmol/L])
Basal plasma ACTH = <4 pg/mL (10-60 pg/mL) (SI: <0.9 pmol/L [2.2-13.2 pmol/L])

Which of the following should be done next to address her symptoms?

A. Add DHEA, 25 mg daily
B. Add fludrocortisone, 0.1 mg daily
C. Increase the hydrocortisone dosage to 40 mg on arising and 20 mg in the early afternoon
D. Measure late-night salivary cortisol
E. Perform another pituitary MRI

15 A general surgeon requests a consult to evaluate a 68-year-old woman for adrenal insufficiency. The patient had a left hemicolectomy for colon cancer with construction of a transient colostomy the night before. Overnight she had episodes of hypotension with blood pressure as low as 90/50 mm Hg (baseline blood pressure is 130/80 mm Hg), mild fever, tachycardia of 110 beats/min, and increased output through her colostomy. She was treated with intravenous fluids and 50 mg of tramadol. She developed mild hyponatremia, and a morning cortisol concentration was documented to be 0.9 μg/dL (24.8 nmol/L).

She does not smoke cigarettes and was healthy before her surgery. She has a diagnosis of mild hypertension and diet-controlled diabetes (most recent hemoglobin A_{1c} = 6.8% [51 mmol/mol]).

She is resting comfortably and does not have any nausea. She would like to eat.

On physical examination, she does not appear ill. She has obesity (BMI = 32 kg/m^2). Her blood pressure is 124/85 mm Hg, and pulse rate is 90 beats/min.

Her most recent basic metabolic profile:

Sodium = 133 mEq/L (136-142 mEq/L) (SI: 133 mmol/L [136-142 mmol/L])
Potassium = 3.8 mEq/L (3.5-5.0 mEq/L) (SI: 3.8 mmol/L [3.5-5.0 mmol/L])
Glucose = 168 mg/dL (70-99 mg/dL) (SI: 9.3 mmol/L [3.9-5.5 mmol/L])
Serum creatinine = 0.7 mg/dL (0.6-1.1 mg/dL) (SI: 61.9 μmol/L [53.0-97.2 μmol/L])

Which of the following is the most likely cause of this patient's low cortisol level?

A. Delayed effect of inhaled anesthetics
B. Medication given as a prophylaxis for postoperative nausea
C. Metastasis from the colon cancer
D. Overnight use of tramadol
E. Primary autoimmune adrenal insufficiency

16 A 57-year-old man is seen for an annual visit for management of hypothyroidism.

On physical examination, he is a healthy appearing, overweight (BMI = 26.0 kg/m^2), middle-aged man. His blood pressure today, however, is 162/102 mm Hg, and pulse rate is 74 beats/min. His thyroid gland is small and firm, and other examination findings are normal.

Routine laboratory test results:

Sodium = 141 mEq/L (136-142 mEq/L) (SI: 141 mmol/L [136-142 mmol/L])
Potassium = 2.8 mEq/L (3.5-5.0 mEq/L) (SI: 2.8 mmol/L [3.5-5.0 mmol/L])
TSH = 1.2 mIU/L (0.5-5.0 mIU/L)
Serum cortisol after 1 mg dexamethasone = <0.2 μg/dL (SI: <5.5 nmol/L)

During a thorough dietary history, the patient states that he is now taking a daily weight-loss supplement containing extract of authentic licorice.

Which of the following biochemical profiles is expected?

Answer	Plasma renin activity	Serum aldosterone
A.	↑	↑
B.	↓	↑
C.	↑	↓
D.	↓	↓
E.	Normal	Normal

17 A nephrology colleague asks for an opinion regarding a 32-year-old woman who underwent successful left laparoscopic adrenalectomy for a 2.1-cm aldosterone-secreting adenoma 4 months earlier. The patient had presented with hypokalemia (potassium = 2.9 mEq/L [2.9 mmol/L]) and severe hypertension (initial blood pressure = 162/102 mm Hg). She was not seen by an endocrinologist before surgery. After surgery, her hypokalemia resolved, and her blood pressure normalized without any medications. Since her operation, she has been easily fatigued and has had a decreased appetite; she has lost 6.5 lb (3 kg). Her only medication is an oral contraceptive.

On physical examination, she is a healthy appearing woman with obesity (BMI = 31.3 kg/m^2). Her blood pressure is 124/82 mm Hg, and pulse rate is 82 beats/min. She has upper-body obesity, with increased supraclavicular and dorsocervical fat. The rest of her examination findings are normal.

Laboratory test results (sample drawn in the morning):

Sodium = 134 mEq/L (136-142 mEq/L) (SI: 134 mmol/L [136-142 mmol/L])
Potassium = 4.7 mEq/L (3.5-5.0 mEq/L) (SI: 4.7 mmol/L [3.5-5.0 mmol/L])
Glucose = 91 mg/dL (70-99 mg/dL) (SI: 5.1 mmol/L [3.9-5.5 mmol/L])
Creatinine = 0.8 mg/dL (0.6-1.1 mg/dL) (SI: 70.7 μmol/L [53.0-97.2 μmol/L])
Cortisol = 3.8 μg/dL (5-25 μg/dL) (SI: 105 nmol/L [137.9-689.7 nmol/L])
Plasma ACTH = 98 pg/mL (10-60 pg/mL) (SI: 21.6 pmol/L [2.2-13.2 pmol/L])
Aldosterone = 5 ng/dL (4-21 ng/dL) (SI: 138.7 pmol/L [111.0-582.5 pmol/L])
Plasma renin activity = 4.2 ng/mL per h (0.6-4.3 ng/mL per h)

In addition to initiating hydrocortisone replacement therapy, which of the following is the best recommendation?

A. Adrenal protocol CT
B. DHEA-S measurement
C. Measurement of 21-hydroxylase antibodies
D. MRI of the pituitary gland
E. No further diagnostic studies

18 A 46-year-old woman with primary adrenal insufficiency and Hashimoto thyroiditis presents for follow-up. She takes hydrocortisone, 15 mg, upon awakening, and 5 mg in the early afternoon. She takes fludrocortisone, 0.1 mg every other day, and levothyroxine, 100 mcg daily. She reports some forgetfulness, minor lower-extremity weakness, and slipping of her footwear when walking. She has not had any diarrhea.

On physical examination, her blood pressure is 123/78 mm Hg and pulse rate is 72 beats/min. She appears tanned (slightly more than on previous examinations), but no skin lesions are noted. Her ankle reflexes are diminished, and vibration sense is absent in the toes.

Laboratory test results:

Hemoglobin = 12.4 g/dL (12.1-15.1 g/dL) (SI: 124 g/L [121-151 g/L])
Mean corpuscular volume = 98 μm^3 (80-100 μm^3) (SI: 98 fL [80-100 fL])
White blood cell count = 4200/µL (4500-11,000/µL) (SI: 4.2 × 10^9/L [4.5-11.0 × 10^9/L]) (normal differential)
TSH = 5.2 mIU/L (0.5-5.0 mIU/L)
ACTH = 210 pg/mL (10-60 pg/mL) (SI: 46.2 pmol/L [2.2-13.2 pmol/L])
Renin (mass) = 20 pg/mL (4-44 pg/mL)
Vitamin B_{12} = 190 pg/mL (180-914 pg/mL) (SI: 140 pmol/L [133-674 pmol/L])
Folate = 4.5 ng/mL (≥4.0 ng/mL) (SI: 4.5 µg/L [≥4.0 µg/L])
Tissue transglutaminase-IgA, negative
Tissue transglutaminase-IgG, negative

Which of the following is the best next test in this patient's diagnostic workup?

A. Esophagogastroduodenoscopy with deep duodenal biopsy
B. Free T_4 measurement
C. Genetic testing for adrenoleukodystrophy
D. Homocysteine and methylmalonic acid measurement
E. Total IgA measurement

19 A 59-year-old woman is referred for a second opinion regarding primary aldosteronism. She developed resistant hypertension in her early 50s and was found to be hypokalemic 6 months ago on routine blood testing.

Screening laboratory test results:

Sodium = 142 mEq/L (136-142 mEq/L) (SI: 142 mmol/L [136-142 mmol/L])
Potassium = 3.2 mEq/L (3.5-5.0 mEq/L) (SI: 3.2 mmol/L [3.5-5.0 mmol/L])
Serum aldosterone = 22 ng/dL (4-21 ng/dL) (SI: 610.3 pmol/L [111.0-582.5 pmol/L])
Plasma renin activity = <0.6 ng/mL per h (0.6-4.3 ng/mL per h)

Confirmatory laboratory testing:

Urinary sodium = 240 mEq/24 h (SI: 240 mmol/d)
Urinary aldosterone = 24 µg/24 h (SI: 66.6 nmol/d)

CT shows normal glands.

She undergoes adrenal venous sampling with continuous infusion of cosyntropin at a rate of 50 mcg per h. The results are shown (*see table*).

Measurement	Right adrenal vein	Left adrenal vein	Inferior vena cava
Aldosterone	36 ng/dL (SI: 998.6 pmol/L)	6400 ng/dL (SI: 177,536 pmol/L)	34 ng/dL (SI: 943.2 pmol/L)
Cortisol	21 µg/dL SI: 579.4 nmol/L)	2000 µg/dL (SI: 55,176 nmol/L)	19 µg/dL (SI: 524.2 nmol/L)
Aldosterone-to-cortisol ratio	1.7	3.2	1.8

She is told that the source is the left adrenal gland based on the high left adrenal vein aldosterone concentration and the aldosterone-to-cortisol ratio.

How should the results of the adrenal venous sampling study be interpreted?

A. Both adrenal glands are sources (bilateral, idiopathic hyperaldosteronism)
B. Insufficient information to interpret whether the study was successful
C. Left adrenal gland is the source (left adenoma)
D. Right adrenal gland is the source (right adenoma)
E. Unable to localize

20 A 25-year-old woman is referred for evaluation of possible Cushing syndrome. She has gained 20 lb (9.1 kg) in the past 5 months with associated facial fullness and plethora. She has new-onset hypertension and oligomenorrhea. She is not taking any medications.

On physical examination, she is a cushingoid-appearing young woman. Her blood pressure is 142/94 mm Hg, pulse rate is 76 beats/min, and BMI is 28.1 kg/m². She has substantial supraclavicular and dorsocervical fat accumulation.

She brings the following test results:

Sodium = 141 mEq/L (136-142 mEq/L) (SI: 141 mmol/L [136-142 mmol/L])
Potassium = 3.7 mEq/L (3.5-5.0 mEq/L) (SI: 3.7 mmol/L [3.5-5.0 mmol/L])
Fasting glucose = 99 mg/dL (70-99 mg/dL) (SI: 5.5 mmol/L [3.9-5.5 mmol/L])
Late-night salivary cortisol = 0.41 µg/dL (<0.13 µg/dL) (SI: 11.3 nmol/L [<3.6 nmol/L])
Urinary free cortisol = 129 µg/24 h (4-50 µg/24 h) (SI: 356 nmol/d [11-138 nmol/d])
Serum cortisol (8 AM) = 17.6 µg/dL (5-25 µg/dL) (SI: 485.5 nmol/L [137.9-389.7 nmol/L])
Serum cortisol (8 AM) after overnight 1-mg dexamethasone-suppression test = 17.4 µg/dL (SI: 480.0 nmol/L)
DHEA-S = 5.0 µg/dL (44-332 µg/dL) (SI: 0.14 µmol/L [1.19-9.00 µmol/L])
Basal plasma ACTH = 14.0 pg/mL (10-60 pg/mL) (SI: 3.1 pmol/L [2.2-13.2 pmol/L])

Pituitary MRI shows a 2-mm hypodense lesion in the left side of the pituitary gland. She has been referred to a neurosurgeon who has scheduled transsphenoidal pituitary surgery.

Which of the following is the best recommendation?

A. Bilateral inferior petrosal ACTH sampling
B. CT of the adrenal glands
C. CT of the chest
D. Ga-DOTATATE PET-CT
E. Pituitary surgery as scheduled

21 A 59-year-old man is referred for evaluation of an adrenal nodule and possible adrenal insufficiency. He had a recent abdominal CT for pain as part of an emergency department evaluation. The homogeneous nodule measures 1.2 cm and has a density of −2 Hounsfield units. No previous imaging is available.

The patient has chronic back pain and has received multiple facet joint injections over the last 3 years. He has been on long-term opioid therapy with oxycodone extended release, 20 mg daily, for the last 5 years. He also takes carbamazepine and gabapentin as adjunct pain medications. He had steady weight gain of 62 lb (28.2 kg) over the last 3 years. He has hypertension that is currently treated with amlodipine, 5 mg daily, and hydrochlorothiazide, 25 mg daily. Type 2 diabetes was diagnosed 2 years ago. He was initially treated with lifestyle changes but was subsequently prescribed glipizide and metformin. His last hemoglobin A_{1c} measurement 6 months ago was 7.1% (54 mmol/mol). He has no nausea, vomiting, or diarrhea. Aside from chronic back pain, he has no other symptoms.

On physical examination, he appears healthy. His blood pressure is 138/77 mm Hg, pulse rate is 68 beats/min, and temperature is 98.1°F (36.7°C). His height is 71.5 in (182 cm), and weight is 262 lb (119 kg) (BMI = 36.0 kg/m²). He has central fat distribution and normal muscle strength. There is no bruising and no increased pigmentation.

Laboratory test results (sample drawn while fasting at 8 AM):

Sodium = 140 mEq/L (136-142 mEq/L) (SI: 140 mmol/L [136-142 mmol/L])
Potassium = 4.2 mEq/L (3.5-5.0 mEq/L) (SI: 4.2 mmol/L [3.5-5.0 mmol/L])
Plasma ACTH = 22 pg/mL (10-60 pg/mL) (SI: 4.8 pmol/L [2.2-13.2 pmol/L])
Cortisol = 1.4 μg/dL (5-25 μg/dL) (SI: 38.6 nmol/L [137.9-689.7 nmol/L])
Plasma renin activity = 3.1 ng/mL per h (0.6-4.3 ng/mL per h)
Aldosterone = 14.8 ng/dL (4-21 ng/dL) (SI: 410.6 pmol/L [111.0-582.5 pmol/L])
Hemoglobin A_{1c} = 8.1% (4.0%-5.6%) (SI: 65 mmol/mol [20-38 mmol/mol])

Which of the following is the best next step in this patient's care?

A. Counsel to seek alternatives to facet injections
B. Discuss alternatives to opioid medication
C. Measure 24-hour urinary aldosterone after 3 days of salt loading
D. Perform a cosyntropin-stimulation test
E. Start hydrocortisone replacement with 10 mg in the morning and 5 mg in the early afternoon

22 A primary care physician refers a 45-year-old man with bilateral adrenal enlargement. The physician is concerned about the possibility of bilateral pheochromocytoma because laboratory testing documented slightly elevated plasma metanephrines. The patient's CT is shown, demonstrating adrenal enlargement *(see image, arrows).*

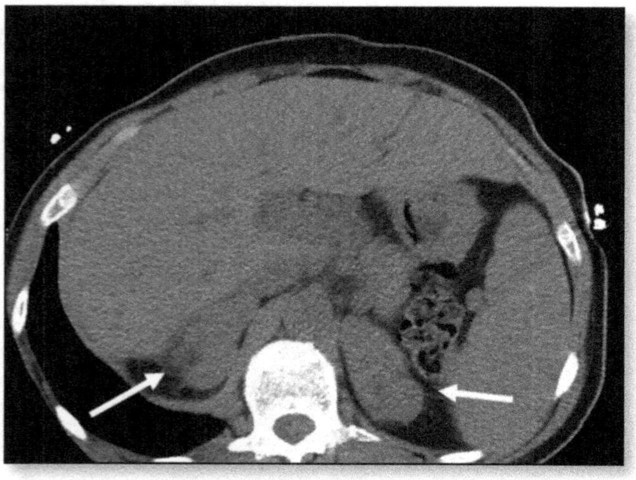

The patient's appetite has been poor, and he has lost 11 lb (5 kg) in the past 3 months. He has no family history of endocrinopathy. He is not taking any medications.

On physical examination, his blood pressure is 100/68 mm Hg with a pulse rate of 96 beats/min while seated, and blood pressure is 88/50 mm Hg with a pulse rate of 120 beats/min while standing. The rest of the examination findings are unremarkable.

Initial laboratory test results:

Plasma normetanephrine = 225 pg/mL (<165 pg/mL) (SI: <1.23 nmol/L [<0.90 nmol/L])
Plasma metanephrine = <40 pg/mL (<99 pg/mL) (SI: <0.21 nmol/L [<0.50 nmol/L])

After examining the patient, the following additional laboratory tests are ordered (sample drawn at 8 AM):

Sodium = 131 mEq/L (136-142 mEq/L) (SI: 131 mmol/L [136-142 mmol/L])
Potassium = 4.4 mEq/L (3.5-5.0 mEq/L) (SI: 4.4 mmol/L [3.5-5.0 mmol/L])
Aldosterone = 4 ng/dL (4-21 ng/dL) (SI: 111 pmol/L [111.0-582.5 pmol/L])
Plasma renin activity = 17 ng/mL per h (0.6-4.3 ng/mL per h)
Plasma ACTH = 212 pg/mL (10-60 pg/mL) (SI: 46.6 pmol/L [2.2-13.2 pmol/L])
Cortisol = 3.2 μg/dL (5-25 μg/dL) (SI: 88.3 nmol/L [137.9-389.7 nmol/L])

Which of the following diagnostic tests is most likely to be helpful in the further diagnosis and management of this patient?

A. Bilateral adrenal venous sampling for cortisol, aldosterone, and catecholamines
B. CT-guided percutaneous adrenal biopsy
C. Pituitary-directed MRI
D. Measurement of 21-hydroxylase antibodies
E. Measurement of 24-hour urinary free cortisol

Bone Board Review

Natalie E. Cusano, MD, MS

1 A 75-year-old woman is admitted to the hospital with a 3-day history of nausea, vomiting, epigastric pain, lethargy, and delirium. She is unable to provide her medical history, but her medical record includes stage 1 breast cancer diagnosed at age 65 years (status post lumpectomy and radiation therapy), osteoporosis, hypothyroidism, and stage 3 chronic kidney disease (baseline estimated glomerular filtration rate = 57 mL/min per 1.73 m^2). Her home medication list includes alendronate, 70 mg weekly; levothyroxine, 75 mcg daily; calcium carbonate, 600 mg twice daily; cholecalciferol, 2000 international units (50 mcg) daily; and famotidine, 20 mg twice daily.

On physical examination, she is lethargic, oriented only to person, and has very dry mucous membranes.

Findings on chest x-ray and abdominal CT are normal.

Initial laboratory test results:

Calcium = 17.1 mg/dL (8.2-10.2 mg/dL) (SI: 4.3 mmol/L [2.1-2.6 mmol/L])
Phosphate = 3.5 mg/dL (2.3-4.7 mg/dL) (SI: 1.1 mmol/L [0.7-1.5 mmol/L])
Potassium = 3.0 mEq/L (3.5-5.0 mEq/L) (SI: 3.0 mmol/L [3.5-5.0 mmol/L])
Bicarbonate = 33 mEq/L (21-28 mEq/L) (SI: 33 mmol/L [21-28 mmol/L])
Serum urea nitrogen = 50 mg/dL (8-23 mg/dL) (SI: 17.9 mmol/L [2.9-8.2 mmol/L])
Creatinine = 3.5 mg/dL (0.6-1.1 mg/dL) (SI: 309.4 μmol/L [53.0-97.2 μmol/L])
PTH = <10 pg/mL (10-65 pg/mL) (SI: <1.1 pmol/L [1.1-6.9 pmol/L])
PTHrP = <2.0 pmol/L (<2.0 pmol/L)
25-Hydroxyvitamin D = 90 ng/mL (30-80 ng/mL) (SI: 224.6 nmol/L [74.9-199.7 nmol/L])
TSH = 0.1 mIU/L (0.5-5.0 mIU/L)
Venous blood gas pH = 7.45
Other laboratory test results, pending

Which of the following diagnoses best explains her clinical presentation?

A. Dehydration
B. Humeral hypercalcemia of malignancy
C. Milk-alkali syndrome
D. Thyrotoxicosis
E. Vitamin D intoxication

2 A 55-year-old woman with a history of hypothyroidism and lumbar spinal fusion surgery presents for routine follow-up. Her mother had a history of a hip fracture, prompting recent bone density screening that is notable for T-scores of −1.3 at the lumbar spine (L1-L4), −2.3 at the femoral neck, and −1.6 at the total hip. She has no personal history of fracture. Menopause occurred at age 51 years, and she currently has mild hot flashes but no other menopausal symptoms. She consumes 3 servings of dairy per day supplemented with vitamin D. Her 25-hydroxyvitamin D concentration is 31 ng/mL (30-80 ng/mL [optimal]) (SI: 77.4 nmol/L [74.9-199.7 nmol/L]).

Which of the following is the best next step?

A. Repeat DXA in 2 years
B. Review her bone density images
C. Start ibandronate, 150 mg monthly
D. Start supplementation with calcium and vitamin D
E. Start transdermal estradiol and oral progesterone

3 *Which of the following sets of laboratory results would be typical for a patient with hypercalcemia due to granulomatous disease, such as sarcoidosis or foreign body granuloma?*

	PTH	Phosphate	1,25-Dihydroxy-vitamin D
A.	<10 pg/mL (SI: <1.06 pmol/L)	2.0 mg/dL (SI: 0.65 mmol/L)	45 pg/mL (SI: 117 pmol/L)
B	10 pg/mL (SI: 1.06 pmol/L)	4.7 mg/dL (SI: 1.52 mmol/L)	45 pg/mL (SI: 117 pmol/L)
C.	15 pg/mL (SI: 1.59 pmol/L)	4.7 mg/dL (SI: 1.52 mmol/L)	80 pg/mL (SI: 208 mmol/L)
D.	30 pg/mL (SI: 3.18 pmol/L)	5.0 mg/dL (SI: 1.62 mmol/L)	90 pg/mL (SI: 234 mmol/L)
E.	70 pg/mL (SI: 7.43 pmol/L)	2.0 mg/dL (SI: 0.65 mmol/L)	90 pg/mL (SI: 234 mmol/L)

Reference ranges: intact PTH, 0-65 pg/mL (SI: 1.06-6.90 pmol/L); phosphate, 2.3-4.7 mg/dL (SI: 0.74-1.52 mmol/L); 1,25-dihydroxyvitamin D, 16-65 pg/mL (SI: 41.6-169.0 pmol/L).

4 A 66-year-old woman is sent to the emergency department by her primary care provider for hypocalcemia. She had seen her physician due to numbness and tingling around her lips, fingers, and toes. She has a history of osteoporosis treated with alendronate, 70 mg weekly, and gastroesophageal reflux disease in good control with omeprazole, 40 mg daily. She has had no changes to her medications in the past 3 years.

On physical examination, she has a positive Chvostek sign. She has no neck scars, mucocutaneous candidiasis, or vitiligo.

Her family history is unremarkable.

Laboratory test results:

Potassium = 2.7 mEq/L (3.5-5.0 mEq/L) (SI: 2.7 mmol/L [3.5-5.0 mmol/L])
Serum calcium = 6.7 mg/dL (8.2-10.2 mg/dL) (SI: 1.7 mmol/L [2.1-2.6 mmol/L])
Magnesium = 0.6 mg/dL (1.5-2.3 mg/dL) (SI: 0.25 mmol/L [0.6-0.9 mmol/L])
Albumin = 3.8 g/dL (3.5-5.0 g/dL) (SI: 38 g/L [35-50 g/L])
PTH = <3 pg/mL (10-65 pg/mL) (SI: <0.32 pmol/L [1.06-6.90 pmol/L])
25-Hydroxyvitamin D = 10 ng/mL (30-80 ng/mL [optimal]) (SI: 25.0 nmol/L [74.9-199.7 nmol/L])

Which of the following is the most likely primary cause of this patient's hypocalcemia?

A. Alendronate
B. Hypokalemia
C. Idiopathic hypoparathyroidism
D. Omeprazole
E. Vitamin D deficiency

5 A 75-year-old woman with osteoporosis presents to establish care. Until now, her care has been managed by her primary care provider. She started alendronate, 70 mg weekly, 5 years ago after experiencing a right hip fracture from a fall from standing height. Bone density testing at that time was notable for T-scores of −1.8 at the lumbar spine, −2.7 at the femoral neck, and −2.4 at the total hip (left hip values). Her most recent bone density was overall unchanged. She has been taking alendronate as prescribed and is tolerating it well. She had a cerebrovascular accident 8 months ago with residual right-sided weakness.

Physical examination findings are unremarkable.

Metabolic evaluation for secondary causes of bone loss is unremarkable.

Which of the following is the best course of action?

A. Continue alendronate
B. Continue alendronate and add teriparatide
C. Discontinue alendronate and start intravenous ibandronate
D. Discontinue alendronate and start romosozumab
E. Discontinue alendronate due to duration of use

6 A 28-year-old woman is admitted to the hospital with pyelonephritis. The intern says the patient has a history of a bone disease and has recently started some form of treatment with which she is unfamiliar. There is concern because her alkaline phosphatase concentration is 15,562 U/L (50-120 U/L) (SI: 259.89 μkat/L [0.84-2.00 μkat/L]).

Which of the following is this patient's most likely underlying diagnosis?

A. Fibrous dysplasia
B. Hypophosphatasia
C. Paget disease
D. Primary hyperparathyroidism
E. X-linked hypophosphatemic rickets

7 *Which of the following represents the typical laboratory profile for a patient with X-linked hypophosphatemic rickets?*

	Calcium	Phosphate	PTH	25-Hydroxy-vitamin D	1,25-Dihydroxy-vitamin D
A.	N/↓	↓/N	↑	↓	N/↓/↑
B.	↓	↓/N	↑	N/↑	↓
C.	↓	↓/N	↑	N/↑	N/↑
D.	↓	↑	↓	N	↓
E.	N	↓	N/↑	N	N/↓

8 A 62-year-old woman presents for evaluation of primary hyperparathyroidism. She has a history of hypertension well controlled on amlodipine and is otherwise healthy. She has had hypercalcemia with inappropriately normal PTH concentrations over the past year, with previously normal serum calcium concentrations. She has no history of fracture, abdominal pain, constipation, or other symptoms of hypercalcemia. She has 2 servings of dairy per day and is taking vitamin D, 2000 international units (50 mcg) daily. Her family history is negative for calcium disorders or endocrine tumors.

On physical examination, her height is 64 in (162.6 cm) and weight is 135 lb (61.2 kg) (BMI = 23.2 kg/m^2). She has lost 2 in (5.1 cm) in height. There are no dysmorphic features.

Kidney ultrasonography demonstrates no nephrolithiasis. Bone mineral density is notable for T-scores of −1.8 at the lumbar spine, −1.9 at the femoral neck, −2.0 at the total hip, and −2.1 at the distal radius, with FRAX scores below the treatment threshold. She is not interested in parathyroid surgery unless clinically indicated.

Laboratory test results:

Serum calcium = 11.1 mg/dL (8.2-10.2 mg/dL) (SI: 2.78 mmol/L [2.1-2.6 mmol/L])
Serum PTH = 120 pg/mL (10-65 pg/mL) (SI: <12.73 pmol/L [1.06-6.90 pmol/L])
Albumin = 3.8 g/dL (3.5-5.0 g/dL) (SI: 38 g/L [35-50 g/L])
Phosphate = 3.0 mg/dL (2.3-4.7 mg/dL) (SI: 1.0 mmol/L [0.7-1.5 mmol/L])
Creatinine = 0.6 mg/dL (0.6-1.1 mg/dL) (SI: 53.0 μmol/L [53.0-97.2 μmol/L])
25-Hydroxyvitamin D = 34 ng/mL (30-80 ng/mL [optimal]) (SI: 84.9 nmol/L [74.9-199.7 nmol/L])
Urinary calcium = 200 mg/24 h (100-250 mg/24 h) (SI: 5.0 mmol/d [2.5-7.5 mmol/d])

Which of the following is the best next step?

A. Order parathyroid sestamibi
B. Order thoracic and lumbar spine radiographs
C. Restrict calcium intake
D. Start alendronate
E. Start cinacalcet

9 A 65-year-old woman with a history of controlled type 1 diabetes presents for routine monitoring. She inquires about bone density testing. She has a history of a childhood right wrist fracture after falling out of a tree and an ankle fracture after being struck by a bicycle at age 62 years. Her mother had a history of osteoporosis and vertebral fracture; there is no parental history of hip fracture. She quit smoking cigarettes at age 60 years and does not drink alcohol. She has osteopenia on bone density testing, and a FRAX score is subsequently calculated.

Which of the following has the greatest impact on this patient's fracture risk as calculated by FRAX after bone density testing?

A. Age
B. Family history
C. Previous fracture
D. Secondary osteoporosis (type 1 diabetes)
E. Tobacco use

10 A 65-year-old woman with a history of osteoporosis and a lumbar vertebral fracture is starting denosumab therapy.

Which of the following represents the approximate expected changes to her lumbar spine bone density and vertebral fracture risk at 36 months based on the pivotal clinical trial leading to drug approval?

Answer	Lumbar spine bone density	Vertebral fracture risk reduction
A.	+4%	50%
B.	+4%	70%
C.	+9%	50%
D.	+9%	70%
E.	+15%	90%

11 A 57-year-old woman sustains a rib fracture after tripping on a rug and falling. She has no personal history of fracture. Her mother has a history of hip fracture. She is healthy other than asthma treated with albuterol as needed. Menopause occurred at age 51 years, and she currently has no hot flashes or other menopausal symptoms. She consumes 3 servings of dairy per day supplemented with vitamin D. Assessment of bone mineral density is notable for T-scores of −2.0 at the lumbar spine, −1.8 at the femoral neck, and −1.6 at the total hip. Metabolic evaluation for secondary causes of bone loss is unremarkable.

Her 25-hydroxyvitamin D concentration is 31 ng/mL (30-80 ng/mL [optimal]) (SI: 77.4 nmol/L [74.9-199.7 nmol/L]).

Which of the following is the best next step in this patient's management?

A. Calculate her FRAX score
B. Repeat bone density assessment in 2 years
C. Start alendronate
D. Start calcium supplementation with vitamin D
E. Start hormone therapy

12 A 28-year-old G1P0 woman at 11 weeks' gestation presents with nausea and vomiting. She recalls being told she had mild hypercalcemia a few years ago, but she did not follow-up at that time. She is tired but arousable.

Laboratory test results:

Serum calcium = 13.9 mg/dL (8.2-10.2 mg/dL) (SI: 3.5 mmol/L [2.1-2.6 mmol/L])
PTH = 75 pg/mL (10-65 pg/mL) (SI: 75 ng/L [10-65 ng/L])
25-Hydroxyvitamin D = 26 ng/mL (30-80 ng/mL [optimal]) (SI: 64.9 nmol/L [74.9-199.7 nmol/L])
1,25-Dihydroxyvitamin D = 82 pg/mL (16-65 pg/mL) (SI: 213.2 pmol/L [41.6-169.0 pmol/L])
Creatinine = 0.8 mg/dL (0.6-1.1 mg/dL) (SI: 70.7 µmol/L [53.0-97.2 µmol/L])
Albumin = 3.4 g/dL (3.5-5.0 g/dL) (SI: 34 g/L [35-50 g/L])
Phosphate = 3.0 mg/dL (2.3-4.7 mg/dL) (SI: 1.0 mmol/L [0.7-1.5 mmol/L])
Urinary calcium = 321 mg/24 h (100-250 mg/24 h) (SI: 8.0 mmol/d [2.5-7.5 mmol/d])

Her serum-corrected calcium level remains elevated at 12.9 mg/dL (3.2 mmol/L) after intravenous fluids. Her nausea has improved.

Which of the following is the best next step for management of this patient's disorder?

A. Cinacalcet
B. Denosumab
C. Parathyroidectomy in the second trimester
D. Parathyroidectomy now
E. Prednisone

13 A 65-year-old woman with a history of multiple low-trauma vertebral fractures is initiating treatment with romosozumab. She inquires about monitoring for treatment effect.

What are the expected changes in bone turnover markers with this therapy?

Answer	Bone formation	Bone resorption
A.	↑	⟷
B.	↑	↑
C.	↑	↓
D.	⟷	↓
E.	↓	↓

14 A 28-year-old woman is referred by her primary care physician for endocrine evaluation after abnormal findings are noted on an x-ray performed because of right shoulder pain (*see image*). She has a history of precocious puberty and recurrent ovarian cysts. Previous evaluation by a pediatric endocrinologist when she was a child did not result in a clear diagnosis.

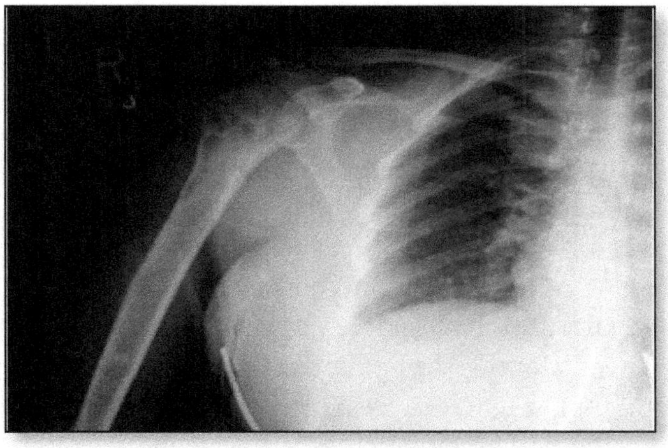

Used with permission of Mayo Foundation for Medical Education and Research, all rights reserved.

On physical examination, her height is 61 in (154.9 cm) and weight is 130 lb (59 kg) (BMI = 24.6 kg/m^2). She has normal facies and an enlarged and nodular thyroid gland.

Laboratory test results:

TSH = 0.2 mIU/L (0.5-5.0 mIU/L)
Calcium, normal
PTH, normal
Alkaline phosphatase, normal
Phosphate, normal
25-Hydroxyvitamin D, normal
1,25-Dihydroxyvitamin D, normal

Kidney function is normal.

Which of the following best explains this patient's clinical presentation?

A. Albright hereditary osteodystrophy
B. Fibrodysplasia ossificans progressiva
C. McCune-Albright syndrome
D. Monostotic fibrous dysplasia
E. Oncogenic osteomalacia (tumor-induced osteomalacia)

15 A 51-year-old man with newly diagnosed HIV infection is admitted to the hospital with nausea, vomiting, and altered mental status. According to friends, he has been ill for 3 months with fever, weight loss, night sweats, malaise, and cough. He is an undocumented immigrant who has avoided seeking traditional medical care because of concerns about deportation. He is found to have active pulmonary *Mycobacterium bovis* with multiple opacities on chest x-ray. He has been taking an over-the-counter vitamin supplement found in the Dominican Republic and upper Manhattan that contains massive doses of vitamin D (864,000 international units) and vitamin A (123,000 international units) in a 5-mL bottle (much higher than the listed dosage).

On physical examination, he is a lethargic, cachectic man with tachycardia and diffuse lymphadenopathy.

Laboratory test results:

Calcium = 17.1 mg/dL (8.2-10.2 mg/dL) (SI: 4.3 mmol/L [2.1-2.6 mmol/L])
Albumin = 3.3 g/dL (3.5-5.0 g/dL) (SI: 33 g/L [35-50 g/dL])
Intact PTH = <10 pg/mL (10-65 pg/mL) (SI: <1.06 ng/L [1.06-6.90 pmol/L])
PTHrP, undetectable
25-Hydroxyvitamin D = 525 ng/mL (30-80 ng/mL [optimal]) (SI: 1310.4 nmol/L [74.9-199.7 nmol/L])

1,25-Dihydroxyvitamin D = >180 pg/mL (16-65 pg/mL) (SI: >468 pmol/L [41.6-169.0 pmol/L])

Over what timeframe is this patient's 25-hydroxyvitamin D concentration expected to decrease to around 30 ng/mL (74.9 nmol/L)?

A. 2 to 3 days
B. 2 to 3 weeks
C. 2 to 3 months
D. 8 to 12 months
E. 24 to 36 months

16 An 82-year-old woman has a history of multiple medical problems, including primary hyperparathyroidism. Despite a history of nephrolithiasis and meeting criteria for parathyroidectomy, she has declined surgery. Her bone mineral density is notable for T-scores of −1.8 at the lumbar spine, −2.1 at the femoral neck, −1.8 at the total hip, and −2.4 at the distal radius. Her serum calcium concentration has been in the range of 11.3 to 11.6 mg/dL (2.8-2.9 mmol/L) with symptoms of nausea and constipation. Therapy with cinacalcet is considered.

What are the expected effects of cinacalcet on this patient's biochemical and bone density parameters?

Answer	Serum calcium	PTH	Bone density
A.	↓↓	⟷	↑
B	↓	⟷	⟷
C.	↓↓	↓	⟷
D.	↓↓	↓	↑
E.	↓	↓	↑

17 A 55-year-old woman with postoperative hypoparathyroidism presents for follow-up. She has a history of Graves disease. At age 39 years, she underwent total thyroidectomy, which was complicated by hypoparathyroidism. She currently takes levothyroxine, 125 mcg daily; calcium, 500 mg 3 times daily; and calcitriol, 0.25 mcg twice daily. She has no symptoms of hypocalcemia and otherwise feels well.

Laboratory test results:

Serum calcium = 8.0 mg/dL (8.2-10.2 mg/dL) (SI: 2.0 mmol/L [2.1-2.6 mmol/L])
25-Hydroxyvitamin D = 31 ng/mL (30-80 ng/mL [optimal]) (SI: 77.4 nmol/L [74.9-199.7 nmol/L])
Creatinine = 1.3 mg/dL (0.6-1.1 mg/dL) (SI: 114.9 μmol/L [53.0-97.2 μmol/L])
Albumin = 3.8 g/dL (3.5-5.0 g/dL) (SI: 38 g/L [35-50 g/L])
Phosphate = 4.7 mg/dL (2.3-4.7 mg/dL) (SI: 1.5 mmol/L [0.7-1.5 mmol/L])

Which of the following is the best next step for monitoring this patient?

A. Bone density assessment
B. Dental examination
C. Imaging of the basal ganglia
D. Kidney ultrasonography
E. Measurement of intraocular pressure

18 A 19-year-old woman presents for follow-up of hypoparathyroidism. She was initially diagnosed at age 9 years after a seizure from severe hypocalcemia and has been maintained on calcium and calcitriol ever since. Over the past several months, she has noted anorexia, 10-lb (4.5-kg) weight loss, weakness, and dizziness.

Physical examination reveals a supine blood pressure of 80/60 mm Hg, pulse rate of 120 beats/min, and dystrophic fingernails and toenails.

Which of the following laboratory measurements is key to this patient's diagnosis?

A. Serum ceruloplasmin
B. Serum iron studies
C. Serum morning cortisol
D. Serum TSH
E. Transglutaminase antibodies

19 A 72-year-old man presents for evaluation after diagnosis of an L1 fracture that occurred when lifting a heavy package. He has osteoarthritis of the spine. He underwent pelvic irradiation for bladder cancer 5 years ago. He is otherwise in good health. He regularly attends follow-up appointments with his oncologist.

On physical examination, he has tenderness over his lower spine. Four years ago, DXA revealed T-scores of −2.0 at the lumbar spine and −1.5 at the femoral neck with FRAX scores that did not meet treatment thresholds.

Current laboratory test results, including complete blood cell count, routine chemistries, alkaline phosphatase, PSA, 25-hydroxyvitamin D, serum/urine protein electrophoresis, and PTH, are normal. Serum testosterone on a morning specimen is 270 ng/dL (300-900 ng/dL) (SI: 9.4 nmol/L [10.4-31.2 nmol/L]). SHBG is within the reference range.

Which of the following is the best next step in this patient's care?

A. Begin alendronate
B. Begin teriparatide
C. Begin testosterone
D. Obtain another DXA before considering therapy
E. Refer for bone biopsy and possible kyphoplasty at L1

20 Paget disease of bone was recently diagnosed in a 72-year-old woman with chronic left hip pain. Her alkaline phosphatase concentration is 250 U/L (40-120 U/L) (SI: 4.2 μkat/L [0.7-2.0 μkat/L]), and her γ-glutamyltranspeptidase level is normal. Bone scan shows intense increased uptake in the left ilium, acetabulum, and femoral head. Radiographs show Paget disease in her left hemipelvis and femoral head, as well as moderate degenerative arthritis in the left hip. Treatment with zoledronic acid is recommended. She wonders what to expect in the next few years.

Which of the following is most likely to occur?

A. Hearing loss due to Paget disease
B. Osteonecrosis of the femoral neck
C. Spread of Paget disease to the right hip
D. Total resolution of all hip pain
E. Worsening arthritis in the hip

21 A 45-year-old woman presents with bilateral hip pain and the radiographic findings shown (*see image*). She underwent Roux-en-Y gastric bypass surgery for obesity 3 years ago and has lost more than 100 lb (>45.5 kg).

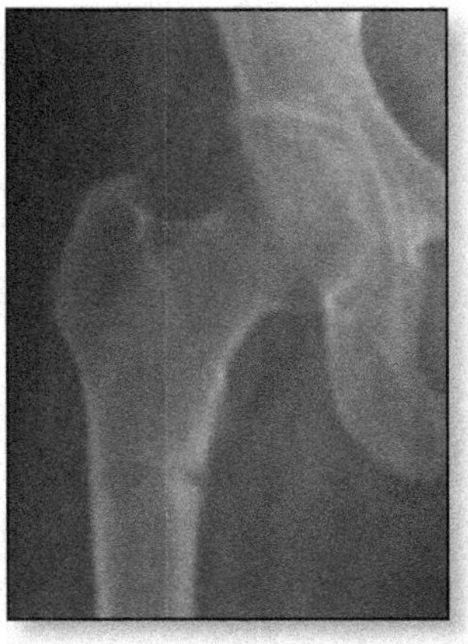

Laboratory test results:

Serum calcium = 8.2 mg/dL (8.2-10.2 mg/dL) (SI: 2.1 mmol/L [2.1-2.6 mmol/L])
Phosphate = 2.2 mg/dL (2.3-4.7 mg/dL) (SI: 0.7 mmol/L [0.7-1.5 mmol/L])
Creatinine = 0.9 mg/dL (0.7-1.3 mg/dL) (SI: 79.6 μmol/L [61.9-114.9 μmol/L])
Serum alkaline phosphatase = 346 U/L (50-120 U/L) (SI: 5.78 μkat/L [0.84-2.00 μkat/L])

Measurement of which of the following is most likely to provide this patient's diagnosis?

A. 1,25-Dihydroxyvitamin D
B. 25-Hydroxyvitamin D
C. C-telopeptide
D. FGF-23
E. Intact PTH

22 A 55-year-old man with rheumatoid arthritis has been on a stable dosage of methotrexate and prednisone, 5 mg daily, for the past 3 years. DXA performed last month shows his lowest T-score to be −2.0 at the femoral neck. According to the FRAX calculator adjusted for glucocorticoid use, his risk for major osteoporosis-related fracture is 12% and his risk for hip fracture is 1.1%. His only other health issue is Barrett esophagus for which he takes long-term proton-pump inhibitor therapy.

In addition to optimizing calcium and vitamin D, which of the following is the first-line therapeutic intervention?

A. Denosumab
B. Ibandronate
C. Teriparatide
D. Zoledronic acid
E. No intervention needed now

23 A 53-year-old man has had a single episode of a calcium-containing kidney stone. His workup reveals normal serum calcium and PTH levels, with a 24-hour urinary calcium excretion of 335 mg/24 h (100-300 mg/24 h) (SI: 8.4 mmol/d [2.5-7.5 mmol/d]). Levels of 24-hour urinary oxalate, uric acid, sodium, and citrate are normal. His urine volume is 1650 mL/24 h. Kidney stone analysis documents calcium oxalate.

Which of the following recommendations would provide the greatest reduction in his risk of future calcium oxalate stone disease?

A. Hydrochlorothiazide
B. Increased fluid intake
C. Potassium citrate
D. Reduced dietary oxalate
E. Reduced dietary sodium

24 An emergency department physician calls for advice regarding a 28-year-old woman with a 5-year history of postsurgical hypoparathyroidism. She presented with perioral numbness and tingling and muscle spasms. She has been nonadherent to her regimen of oral calcium and calcitriol. Her weight is 154 lb (70 kg).

Laboratory test results:

Calcium = 6.5 mg/dL (8.2-10.2 mg/dL) (SI: 1.6 mmol/L [2.1-2.6 mmol/L])
Albumin = 3.8 mg/dL (3.5-5.0 g/dL) (SI: 38 g/L [35-50 g/L])
Phosphate = 5.3 mg/dL (2.3-4.7 mg/dL) (SI: 1.7 mmol/L [0.7-1.5 mmol/L])
Magnesium = 1.9 mg/dL (1.5-2.3 mg/dL) (SI: 0.78 mmol/L [0.6-0.9 mmol/L])
Creatinine = 0.9 mg/dL (0.6-1.1 mg/dL) (SI: 79.6 μmol/L [53.0-97.2 μmol/L])

In addition to restarting treatment with oral calcium and calcitriol, which additional treatment would be best?

Answer	Initial therapy	Subsequent therapy
A.	Intravenous bolus of 100 mg calcium chloride	Continuous calcium chloride infusion of 0.5 mg/kg per h
B.	Intravenous bolus of 1 g calcium chloride	Continuous calcium chloride infusion of 2 mg/kg per h
C.	Intravenous bolus of 150 mg calcium gluconate	Continuous calcium gluconate infusion of 1 mg/kg per h
D.	Intravenous bolus of 150 mg calcium gluconate	Continuous calcium gluconate infusion of 1 mg/kg per h + teriparatide 20 mcg subcutaneously daily
E.	Intravenous bolus of 500 mg calcium gluconate	Continuous calcium gluconate infusion to achieve a total dose of 2000 mg calcium over 24 hours

25 A 62-year-old man is referred for evaluation of muscle and bone pain, fatigue, weakness, spontaneous fractures, and difficulty walking. Symptoms began 4 years ago. Physical examination reveals diffuse bony tenderness, proximal muscle weakness, and ataxic gait. DXA documents T-scores of −3 to −4 at all sites.

Laboratory test results:

- Chemistry panel, normal
- Serum 25-hydroxyvitamin D = 28 ng/mL (30-80 ng/mL [optimal]) (SI: 69.9 nmol/L [62.4-199.7 nmol/L])
- Serum 1,25-dihydroxyvitamin D = 12 pg/mL (16-65 pg/mL) (SI: 31.2 pmol/L [41.6-169.0 pmol/L])
- PTH = 98 pg/mL (10-65 pg/mL) (SI: 10.4 pmol/L [1.1-6.9 pmol/L])
- Serum phosphate = measurements ranging from 1.1 to 1.3 mg/dL (2.3-4.7 mg/dL) (SI: 0.36 to 0.42 mmol/L [0.74-1.52 mmol/L])
- Maximum tubular phosphate reabsorption (phosphorus tubule maximum/glomerular filtration rate), low

Which of the following is the key diagnostic test to order next?

A. 24-Hour urine collection for calcium, electrolytes, amino acids, glucose, and creatinine
B. 24,25-Dihydroxyvitamin D measurement
C. FGF-23 measurement
D. *PHEX* gene testing
E. Sestamibi scan

26 A 20-year-old woman is referred from orthopedics after a recent tibial stress fracture. Her fracture has successfully healed, and she has resumed regular activities. She runs 25 miles per week, with no increase in physical activity before her fracture. She follows a healthy diet rich in protein and fiber, although she avoids fats. She has amenorrhea.

Physical examination is notable for a BMI of 19.1 kg/m^2 and is otherwise normal, including findings on pelvic examination.

Bone density is significant for Z-scores of −2.6 at the lumbar spine, −1.6 at the femoral neck, and −1.5 at the total hip.

Laboratory evaluation is notable for low levels of estradiol and FSH but is otherwise negative for secondary causes of amenorrhea and bone loss.

Which of the following is the best treatment for this patient's bone health?

A. Alendronate, 70 mg weekly
B. Combined oral contraceptive pill
C. Denosumab, 60 mg subcutaneously every 6 months
D. Teriparatide, 20 mcg daily
E. Working with a dietician to resolve energy deficiency

27 A 64-year-old man with end-stage kidney disease due to hypertension has been receiving hemodialysis for 10 years. He is referred for evaluation because of multiple vertebral fractures and a femoral neck T-score of −3.8 on DXA. Long-term medications include calcitriol, 0.5 mcg twice daily, and cinacalcet, 90 mg twice daily.

Laboratory test results:

- Serum calcium = 8.1 mg/dL (8.2-10.2 mg/dL) (SI: 2.0 mmol/L [2.1-2.6 mmol/L])
- Phosphate = 5.2 mg/dL (2.3-4.7 mg/dL) (SI: 1.7 mmol/L [0.7-1.5 mmol/L])
- 25-Hydroxyvitamin D = 24 ng/mL (25-80 ng/mL [optimal]) (SI: 59.9 nmol/L [62.4-199.7 nmol/L])
- PTH = 78 pg/mL (10-65 pg/mL) (SI: 8.3 pmol/L [1.1-6.9 pmol/L])
- Total alkaline phosphatase = 48 U/L (50-120 U/L) (SI: 0.80 μkat/L [0.84-2.00 μkat/L])

An iliac crest biopsy is done after double-tetracycline labeling.

While awaiting bone biopsy results, which of the following changes in management should be made immediately?

A. Begin denosumab
B. Begin teriparatide
C. Decrease the calcitriol dosage
D. Decrease the cinacalcet dosage
E. Increase the calcitriol dosage

28 A 28-year-old man is referred after an acute episode of renal colic. Imaging studies show bilateral kidney stones. Metabolic evaluation is consistent with primary hyperparathyroidism as illustrated by the following laboratory test results:

Serum calcium = 11.9 mg/dL (8.2-10.2 mg/dL) (SI: 2.98 mmol/L [2.1-2.6 mmol/L])
Serum PTH = 112 pg/mL (10-65 pg/mL) (SI: 112 ng/L [10-65 ng/L])
Urinary calcium excretion = 400 mg/24 h (100-300 mg/24 h) (SI: 10 mmol/d [2.5-7.5 mmol/d])

Following a sestamibi scan demonstrating a "probable" adenoma in the right lower pole, the patient undergoes minimally invasive parathyroidectomy with resection of 1 enlarged parathyroid gland. Pathologic examination confirms a hyperplastic adenoma. Two weeks later, he returns for blood work while taking elemental calcium, 600 mg twice daily.

Laboratory test results 2 weeks after surgery:

Calcium = 11.8 mg/dL (8.2-10.2 mg/dL) (SI: 2.95 mmol/L [2.1-2.6 mmol/L])
Phosphate = 2.2 mg/dL (2.3-4.7 mg/dL) (SI: 0.7 mmol/L [0.7-1.5 mmol/L])
Albumin = 4.2 g/dL (3.5-5.0 g/dL) (SI: 42 g/L [35-50 g/L])
PTH = 120 pg/mL (10-65 pg/mL) (SI: 12.7 pmol/L [1.1-6.9 pmol/L])
Serum creatinine = 1.0 mg/dL (0.7-1.3 mg/dL) (SI: 88.4 μmol/L [61.9-114.9 μmol/L])

Which of the following is the best next step?

A. 4D CT of the neck
B. Cessation of calcium supplementation and recheck of laboratory tests in 1 month
C. Genetic testing for pathogenic variants in the calcium-sensing receptor gene (*CASR*)
D. Genetic testing for pathogenic variants in the multiple endocrine neoplasia type 1 gene (*MEN1*)
E. Repeated sestamibi scan

29 A 45-year-old woman with a history of postoperative hypoparathyroidism following total thyroidectomy for benign goiter presents to the emergency department with perioral numbness and tingling. Her treatment regimen for hypoparathyroidism has remained stable over many years and includes calcium carbonate, 600 mg 3 times daily; calcitriol, 0.5 mcg twice daily; and vitamin D, 1000 international units daily. She states that she has had good treatment adherence. Her medical history is otherwise remarkable only for gastroesophageal reflux disease, and 3 days ago her treatment was changed from ranitidine to omeprazole, 20 mg twice daily.

Laboratory test results:

Serum calcium = 6.8 mg/dL (8.2-10.2 mg/dL) (SI: 1.7 mmol/L [2.1-2.6 mmol/L])
Albumin = 3.8 mg/dL (3.5-5.0 g/dL) (SI: 38 g/L [35-50 g/L])
Intact PTH = <3 pg/mL (10-65 pg/mL) (SI: 0.3 pmol/L [1.1-6.9 pmol/L])
25-Hydroxyvitamin D = 32 ng/mL (30-80 ng/mL [optimal]) (SI: 79.9 nmol/L [62.4-199.7 nmol/L])
Phosphate = 5.3 mg/dL (2.3-4.7 mg/dL) (SI: 1.7 mmol/L [0.7-1.5 mmol/L])
Magnesium = 1.5 mg/dL (1.5-2.3 mg/dL) (SI: 0.6 mmol/L [0.6-0.9 mmol/L])

In addition to intravenous calcium gluconate infusion and calcitriol, 0.5 mg twice daily, which of the following therapies should she receive?

A. Calcium carbonate, 600 mg 4 times daily
B. Calcium carbonate, 600 mg 4 times daily, and hydrochlorothiazide, 25 mg daily
C. Calcium citrate, 600 mg 4 times daily
D. PTH (1-34), 20 mcg subcutaneously twice daily, and calcium carbonate, 600 mg 4 times daily
E. rhPTH (1-84), 100 mcg subcutaneously daily, and calcium carbonate, 600 mg 4 times daily

30 A 57-year-old woman seeks advice regarding osteoporosis and fractures. She entered menopause 5 years ago and has not taken hormone therapy. During childhood, she sustained several long-bone fractures that were attributed to her active lifestyle and participation in sports. Her last childhood fracture was at age 15 years. Since menopause, however, she has sustained fractures at the wrist, humerus, and femur in low-trauma falls. Recent DXA reveals T-scores of −3.0 at the spine, −2.8 at the femoral neck, and −2.7 at the total hip. Her mother was diagnosed with osteoporosis at age 65 years.

On physical examination, she is a well-appearing woman with no dysmorphic features. Her height is 65 in (165.1 cm). Sclerae appear slightly greyish. She has no joint deformities or laxity. Her dentition appears normal. She wears bilateral hearing aids.

Laboratory test results:

Complete blood cell count, normal
Electrolytes, normal
Calcium, normal
Creatinine, normal
Liver function tests, normal
Alkaline phosphatase, normal
Phosphate, normal
TSH, normal
25-Hydroxyvitamin D, normal
1,25-Dihydroxyvitamin D, normal
Intact PTH, normal

Sequencing which of the following genes will establish the diagnosis?

A. LDL receptor-related protein 5 gene (*LRP5*)
B. Osteoprotegerin gene (*TNFRSF11B*)
C. Phosphate-regulating endopeptidase gene (*PHEX*)
D. Sclerostin gene (*SOST*)
E. Type 1 collagen α 1 and 2 genes (*COL1A1*/*COL1A2*)

31 A 61-year-old man is referred for evaluation of possible Paget disease. He was found to have an elevated alkaline phosphatase level on recent laboratory studies done before cataract surgery. He had bariatric surgery 15 years ago and takes cholecalciferol, 2000 international units daily. He has no chronic medical problems and has not seen a physician in the past 5 years. He feels generally well.

Laboratory test results:

Alkaline phosphatase = 220 U/L (50-120 U/L) (SI: 3.7 μkat/L [0.8-2.0 μkat/L])
Serum calcium = 8.6 mg/dL (8.2-10.2 mg/dL) (SI: 2.2 mmol/L [2.1-2.6 mmol/L])
Serum creatinine = 1.3 mg/dL (0.7-1.3 mg/dL) (SI: 114.9 μmol/L [61.9-114.9 mmol/L])
γ-Glutamyltranspeptidase, normal

Which of the following is the best next step in this patient's evaluation?

A. 1,25-Dihydroxyvitamin D measurement
B. 25-Hydroxyvitamin D measurement
C. Serum C-telopeptide measurement
D. Skeletal survey
E. Whole-body bone scan

32 A 21-year-old woman is referred for a second opinion regarding hypercalcemia. She was noted to have a serum calcium concentration of 12.5 mg/dL (3.1 mmol/L) in the emergency department after presenting with nausea and vomiting due to gastrointestinal illness. Hypercalcemia has persisted in the subsequent months after recovery with calcium concentrations ranging from 11.9 to 12.3 mg/dL (3.0-3.1 mmol/L). She is otherwise healthy and has no history of kidney stones or fractures. She brings the following laboratory test results to her appointment:

Serum calcium = 12.3 mg/dL (8.2-10.2 mg/dL) (SI: 3.1 mmol/L [2.1-2.6 mmol/L])
PTH = 60 pg/mL (10-65 pg/mL) (SI: 6.4 pmol/L [1.1-6.9 pmol/L])
25-Hydroxyvitamin D = 31 ng/mL (30-80 ng/mL [optimal]) (SI: 77.4 nmol/L [74.9-199.7 nmol/L])
Magnesium = 2.3 mg/dL (1.5-2.3 mg/dL) (SI: 0.95 mmol/L [0.6-0.9 mmol/L])
Phosphate = 2.3 mg/dL (2.3-4.7 mg/dL) (SI: 0.7 mmol/L [0.7-1.5 mmol/L])
24-hour urinary calcium clearance-to-creatinine clearance ratio = 0.006
Calcium-sensing receptor (*CASR*) gene testing, negative for pathogenic variants

Her mother is normocalcemic. Her father is deceased, and she has no siblings or children. Neck ultrasonography and parathyroid sestamibi scan are negative for parathyroid abnormalities.

Which of the following is the best next step?

A. 4D CT of the neck and mediastinum
B. Genetic testing for *GNA11* and *AP2S1* pathogenic variants
C. Genetic testing for *PHEX* pathogenic variants
D. MRI of the neck and mediastinum
E. Referral to a surgeon for 4-gland parathyroid exploration

33 A 72-year-old man is referred for evaluation of hypercalcemia incidentally noted on routine laboratory testing. He feels well and has no concerns. He was treated for tuberculosis 40 years ago, and a basal cell skin cancer was excised 20 years ago. There is no personal or family history of hypercalcemia. Physical examination findings are unremarkable.

Laboratory test results:

Serum calcium = 11.1 mg/dL (8.2-10.2 mg/dL) (SI: 2.8 mmol/L [2.1-2.6 mmol/L])
PTH = 40 pg/mL (10-65 pg/mL) (SI: 4.2 pmol/L [1.1-6.9 pmol/L])
25-Hydroxyvitamin D = 18 ng/mL (30-80 ng/mL [optimal]) (SI: 44.9 nmol/L [74.9-199.7 nmol/L])
1,25-Dihydroxyvitamin D = 75 pg/mL (16-65 pg/mL) (SI: 195 pmol/L [41.6-169.0 pmol/L])
Creatinine = 1.2 mg/dL (0.7-1.3 mg/dL) (SI: 106.1 µmol/L [61.9-114.9 µmol/L])
Urinary calcium = 90 mg/24 h (100-300 mg/24 h) (SI: 2.3 mmol/d [2.5-7.5 mmol/d])
24-Hour urine calcium clearance-to-creatinine clearance ratio = 0.011

Which of the following is the most likely cause of this patient's hypercalcemia?

A. Calcitriol toxicity
B. Familial hypocalciuric hypercalcemia
C. Granulomatous disease
D. Hypercalcemia of malignancy
E. Primary hyperparathyroidism

Diabetes Mellitus, Section 1 Board Review

Anne Peters, MD

1 A 32-year-old woman with a 15-year history of type 1 diabetes would like to start using a tubeless automated insulin delivery (AID) system. Her glucose values have always been high, and her hemoglobin A_{1c} values range from 10.0% to 12.0% (86-108 mmol/mol). Her continuous glucose monitoring data are shown (*see image*). She has moderately severe diabetic nonproliferative retinopathy and a urinary albumin-to-creatinine ratio of 65 mg/g.

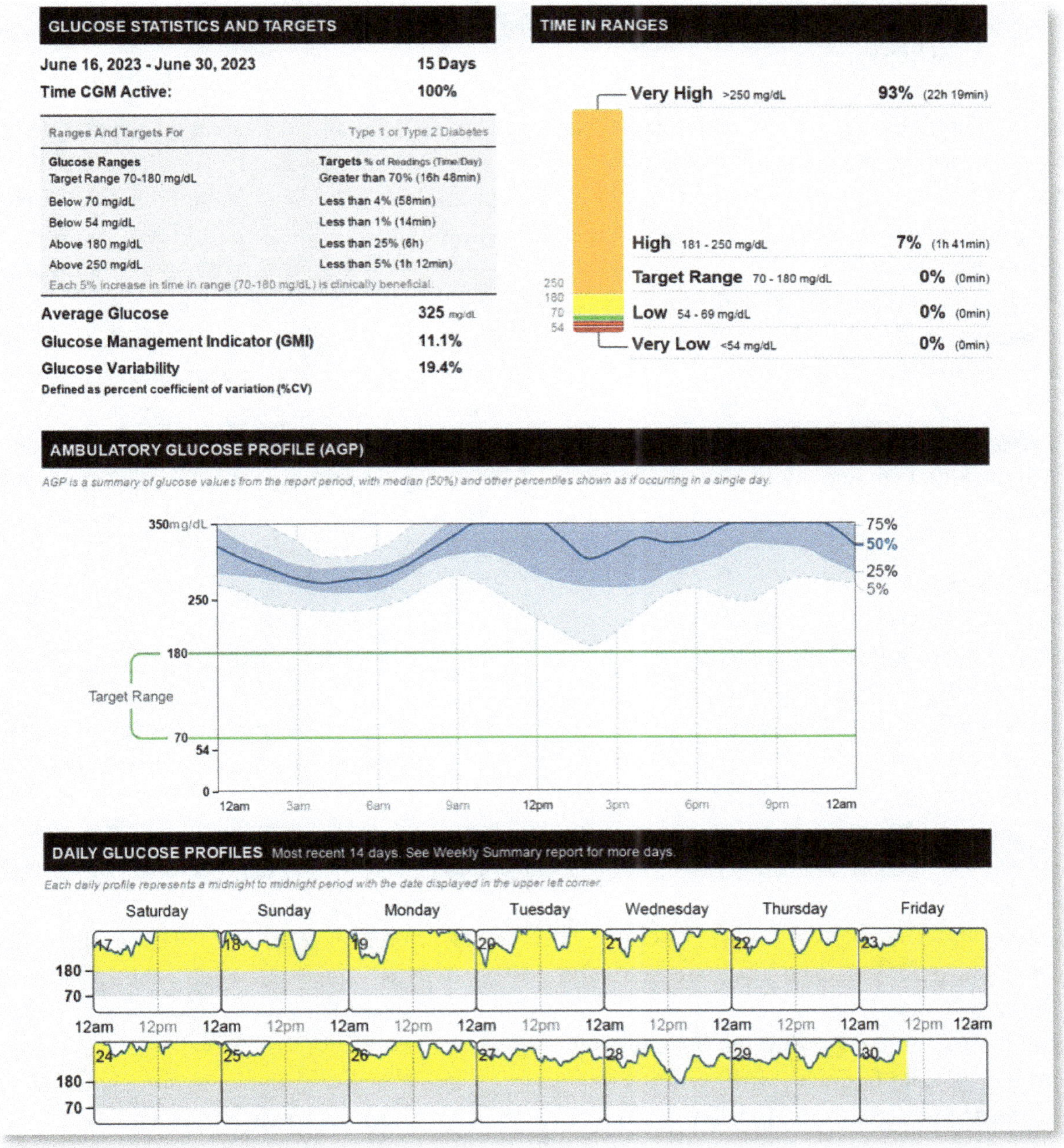

When starting the AID system, which initial glucose target is likely to be safest for this patient in terms of reducing the risk for worsening diabetes complications?

A. 110 mg/dL (6.1 mmol/L)
B. 150 mg/dL (8.3 mmol/L)
C. 180 mg/dL (10.0 mmol/L)
D. 220 mg/dL (12.1 mmol/L)

2 A 45-year-old man has a 20-year history of type 1 diabetes. He recently started having episodes of severe hypoglycemia. His family has access to glucagon in the form of a glucagon kit for which reconstitution is required for injection. His family members have been able to use it successfully, but he has heard that intranasal glucagon might be an easier way to treat his episodes of severe hypoglycemia.

When comparing intranasal glucagon to intramuscular glucagon, the patient should be counseled that intranasal glucagon:

A. Acts more quickly to raise glucose levels
B. Has fewer adverse effects
C. Has no significant difference in the time to a beneficial response
D. Is administered at the same dose

3 A previously healthy 24-year-old woman with diabetic ketoacidosis is admitted to the intensive care unit.

Initial laboratory test results:

Glucose = 546 mg/dL (70-99 mg/dL) (SI: 30.3 mmol/L [3.9-5.5 mmol/L])
Potassium = 3.6 mEq/L (3.5-5.0 mEq/L) (SI: 3.6 mmol/L [3.5-5.0 mmol/L])
pH = 6.8 (7.35-7.45)
Bicarbonate = 7 mEq/L (21-28 mEq/L) (SI: 7 mmol/L [21-28 mmol/L])
Anion gap = 16 mEq/L (3-11 mEq/L) (SI: 16 mmol/L [3-11 mmol/L])
Serum β-hydroxybutyrate = 5.7 mg/dL (<3.0 mg/dL) (SI: 550 μmol/L [<288.2 μmol/L])

She has no history of diabetes but has been feeling increasingly weak and fatigued, with weight loss and frequent urination over the past few weeks.

In the intensive care unit, she is treated with an intravenous insulin drip and intravenous fluids, and she recovers over 24 hours.

Which of the following laboratory measurements would be recommended to show that her diabetic ketoacidosis has resolved?

Answer	Anion gap	Bicarbonate	Plasma/capillary ketones	Venous pH
A.	●	●		
B.	●		●	
C.	●			●
D.		●	●	

4 A 36-year-old woman with type 1 diabetes typically has good glycemic control on a multiple daily insulin injection regimen. She goes on vacation to a wellness spa and returns with glucose values that are 10% to 20% higher than when she left. Her physical activity, diet, and insulin doses have not changed, although she started taking a variety of new supplements while at the spa. She is currently using a continuous glucose monitor (FreeStyle Libre 3).

Which of the following is the most likely high-dosage medication/supplement that this patient began taking?

A. Acetaminophen
B. Biotin
C. Vitamin B_{12} injections
D. Vitamin C

5 A 23-year-old man is interested in starting an automated insulin delivery system.

When discussing his options, which of the following should this patient be told to expect with this change in insulin delivery?

A. Automatic delivery of mealtime bolus doses
B. Basal rates that are set by the user for use during automode
C. Fewer episodes of severe (level 3) hypoglycemia
D. Greater time-in-range with nighttime glucose values than with daytime glucose values

6 A 63-year-old man with type 2 diabetes is currently on a multiple daily insulin injection regimen and uses a continuous glucose monitor. His hemoglobin A_{1c} value is 8.2% (66 mmol/mol), and he wishes to start insulin pump therapy. He has not had success with noninsulin therapies. His BMI is 31 kg/m^2.

Laboratory test results:

C-peptide = 2.7 ng/mL (SI: 0.89 nmol/L)
Glucose = 253 mg/dL (SI: 14.0 mmol/L)

He asks what his C-peptide level signifies about his potential response to insulin pump therapy. This patient's C-peptide concentration:

A. Indicates he should not start insulin pump therapy
B. Is not expected to influence to his response to insulin pump therapy
C. Reduces his risk for hypoglycemia
D. Reduces his risk for complications

7 An 82-year-old woman has a 20-year history of type 2 diabetes. She is lean (BMI = 18.1 kg/m^2). Her current treatment regimen is metformin, 1000 mg twice daily, and insulin glargine, 12 units every morning.

Laboratory test results:

Islet autoantibodies, negative
C-peptide = 1.1 ng/dL (SI: 0.36 nmol/L)
Glucose = 147 mg/dL (SI: 8.16 mmol/L)

She has chronic lymphocytic leukemia and breast cancer, and she recently fractured her pelvis in a fall in a parking lot. Her hemoglobin A_{1c} values have been in the range of 6.0% to 6.6% (42-49 mmol/mol), and her current value is 7.3% (56 mmol/mol). She does not tolerate DPP-4 inhibitors (rash), sulfonylurea agents (hypoglycemia), pioglitazone (edema), or SGLT-2 inhibitors (weight loss and mycotic vaginal infections). She has no diabetes-related complications.

GLUCOSE STATISTICS AND TARGETS

January 23, 2024 - February 5, 2024	14 Days
Time CGM Active:	93%
Ranges And Targets For	Type 1 or Type 2 Diabetes
Glucose Ranges	**Targets** % of Readings (Time/Day)
Target Range 70-180 mg/dL	Greater than 70% (16h 48min)
Below 70 mg/dL	Less than 4% (58min)
Below 54 mg/dL	Less than 1% (14min)
Above 180 mg/dL	Less than 25% (6h)
Above 250 mg/dL	Less than 5% (1h 12min)
Each 5% increase in time in range (70-180 mg/dL) is clinically beneficial.	
Average Glucose	**170** mg/dL
Glucose Management Indicator (GMI)	**7.4%**
Glucose Variability	**28.5%**
Defined as percent coefficient of variation (%CV); target ≤36%	

TIME IN RANGES

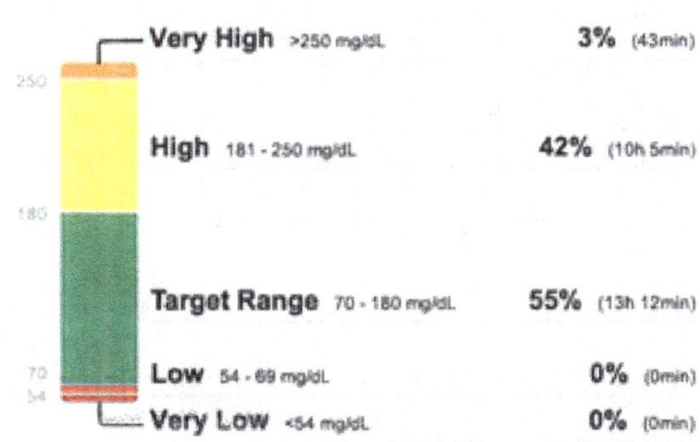

AMBULATORY GLUCOSE PROFILE (AGP)

AGP is a summary of glucose values from the report period, with median (50%) and other percentiles shown as if occurring in a single day.

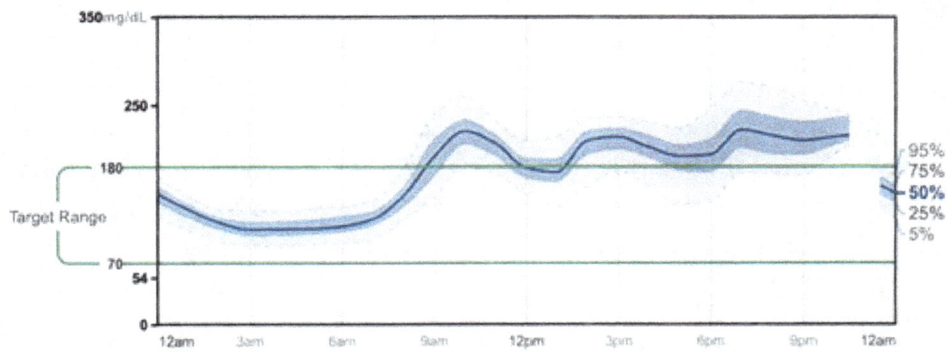

She is very worried that her blood glucose levels are too high, especially after eating, and she wants to discuss adding premeal rapid-acting insulin to her regimen. She has met with a dietitian on multiple occasions and eats an appropriate diet, although she often has trouble finishing her meals or skips meals altogether. She tries to be active, walking during the day, but she has been limited due to her pelvic fractures. Her continuous glucose monitoring data are shown (*see image, previous page*).

Which of the following should be recommended as the safest plan in this situation?

A. Add a GLP-1 receptor agonist
B. Continue her current regimen
C. Increase her morning insulin glargine dose by 2 units
D. Start 2 units of rapid-acting insulin before each meal

8 A 46-year-old woman with type 1 diabetes is treated with a multiple daily insulin injection regimen. Her current hemoglobin A_{1c} value is 6.8% (51 mmol/mol), and BMI is 42 kg/m^2. She has tried to lose weight multiple times with strategies that have included structured programs and nonincretin weight-loss therapies, but she has not been successful. She does not want to have bariatric surgery.

Which of the following is the best recommendation for this patient?

A. Add an SGLT-2 inhibitor
B. Add metformin
C. Add semaglutide or tirzepatide (weight-loss formulation)
D. Switch to automated insulin delivery

9 A 54-year-old man with longstanding type 1 diabetes and peripheral vascular disease is admitted to the intensive care unit with an infected foot ulcer, cellulitis, and septic shock. He weighs 220 lb (100 kg). His condition has stabilized, and he is scheduled to begin eating meals and be transferred to a general surgical unit. He has been receiving continuous intravenous insulin, and glucose values have ranged from 140 to 180 mg/dL (7.8-10.0 mmol/L). He has received 50 units of intravenous regular insulin in the past 24 hours.

It is now 9 AM. Before the intravenous insulin drip is discontinued, basal U100 insulin glargine, 20 units subcutaneously twice daily, is ordered, with the first dose administered now. This insulin glargine dose represents 80% of the total daily insulin dose being delivered via insulin drip—all of which was "basal" insulin because he was not eating. The intravenous insulin infusion is stopped 2 hours after insulin glargine is administered.

In addition to the basal insulin glargine, which of the following orders should also be placed?

A. 10 units of rapid-acting insulin before meals with a correction dose
B. 15 units of rapid-acting insulin before meals
C. 15 units of rapid-acting insulin before meals with a correction dose
D. Rapid-acting insulin every 6 hours based on correction scale

10 A 47-year-old man with a 19-year history of type 1 diabetes has no diabetes-related complications and no specific concerns. He is treated with insulins degludec and aspart. His blood pressure is 129/68 mm Hg, and BMI is 28 kg/m^2.

Laboratory test results:

Hemoglobin A_{1c} = 7.2% (4.0%-5.6%) (55 mmol/mol [20-38 mmol/mol])
Total cholesterol = 173 mg/dL (<200 mg/dL [optimal]) (SI: 4.48 mmol/L [<5.18 mmol/L])
LDL cholesterol = 92 mg/dL (<100 mg/dL [optimal]) (SI: 2.38 mmol/L [<2.59 mmol/L])
HDL cholesterol = 45 mg/dL (>60 mg/dL [optimal]) (SI: 1.17 mmol/L [>1.55 mmol/L])
Triglycerides = 178 mg/dL (<150 mg/dL [optimal]) (SI: 2.01 mmol/L [<1.70 mmol/L])
Serum creatinine = 0.86 mg/dL (0.7-1.3 mg/dL) (SI: 76.0 mmol/L [61.9-114.9 mmol/L])
Urinary albumin-to-creatinine ratio = 19 mg/g creat (<30 mg/g creat)

How should this patient be advised regarding the best course of action to reduce this patient's risk of cardiovascular disease?

A. Intensify his treatment regimen to attain a target hemoglobin A_{1c} value <7.0% (<53 mmol/mol)
B. Refer to a nutritionist for dietary instruction for weight loss
C. Start a statin
D. Start an ACE inhibitor
E. Start aspirin, 81 mg daily

11 A 20-year-old woman with cystic fibrosis affecting her lungs and liver would like to discuss her risk of developing cystic fibrosis–related diabetes (CFRD) and how to screen for it. She has a family history of cystic fibrosis with CFRD. Her cystic fibrosis has been moderately controlled, although she has recurrent infections. Her BMI is 23 kg/m^2.

Which of the following is the best next step to screen this patient for CFRD?

A. Fasting plasma glucose measurement
B. Fructosamine measurement
C. Hemoglobin A_{1c} measurement
D. Oral glucose tolerance test

12 A 43-year-old woman presents for follow-up of type 2 diabetes, which was diagnosed 3 months ago. At diagnosis, her hemoglobin A_{1c} value was 8.7% (72 mmol/mol), and her BMI was 35 kg/m^2. She is enrolled in a commercial weight-loss program with prepackaged meals, she exercises 5 days a week, and she is taking metformin, 1500 mg daily. She has lost 10 lb (4.5 kg).

Laboratory test results from today's visit:

Hemoglobin A_{1c} = 7.9% (4.0%-5.6%) (63 mmol/mol [20-38 mmol/mol])
Fasting blood glucose = 146 mg/dL (70-99 mg/dL) (SI: 8.1 mmol/L [3.9-5.5 mmol/L])

In addition to continuing lifestyle efforts, which of the following is the best next step to improve this patient's glycemic control?

A. Continue metformin at current dosage
B. Continue metformin at current dosage and add dulaglutide
C. Continue metformin at current dosage and add sitagliptin
D. Increase the metformin dosage
E. Stop metformin and start empagliflozin

13 A 52-year-old woman with type 2 diabetes is currently on postoperative day 1 after a surgical procedure. Her home treatment regimen consists of metformin and a GLP-1 receptor agonist. Before surgery, her blood glucose values ranged from 150 to 180 mg/dL (8.3-10.0 mmol/L), and now they range from 185 to 275 mg/dL (10.3-15.3 mmol/L).

On physical examination, her vital signs are unremarkable. She is nauseated and has been unable to eat meals. She remains on nothing-by-mouth status in the surgical unit.

Which of the following is the best diabetes management regimen for this patient?

A. Continuous intravenous insulin infusion
B. Once-daily basal insulin, plus correction insulin dose every 4 to 6 hours
C. Once-daily basal insulin, plus correction insulin dose every 8 to 10 hours
D. Restarting home medications without insulin
E. Sliding-scale insulin regimen administered every 4 to 6 hours

14 A 65-year-old man with a 20-year history of type 2 diabetes and hypertension complicated by nephropathy is referred for help achieving better glycemic control. His regimen consists of premixed NPH/regular insulin, 40 units at breakfast and 30 units at dinner. He performs self-monitoring of blood glucose before meals twice daily, with values ranging between 112 and 140 mg/dL (6.2-7.8 mmol/L). His hemoglobin A_{1c} level has been between 8.5% and 10.0% (69-86 mmol/mol). His medications include ramipril, amlodipine, metoprolol, rosuvastatin, and biotin. His primary care physician recently measured fructosamine to assess his glycemic control.

Laboratory test results:

Hemoglobin A_{1c} = 9.0% (4.0%-5.6%) (75 mmol/mol [20-38 mmol/mol])
Serum creatinine = 2.2 mg/dL (0.7-1.3 mg/dL) (SI: 194.5 μmol/L [61.9-114.9 μmol/L])
Urinary albumin-to-creatinine ratio = 3886 mg/g creat (<30 mg/g creat)
Liver function, normal
TSH = 7.5 mIU/L (0.5-5.0 mIU/L)
Serum fructosamine = 210 μmol/L (200-285 μmol/L)

The discrepancy between this patient's hemoglobin A_{1c} and fructosamine levels is most likely caused by which of the following?

A. Biotin
B. Hemolysis
C. Hypothyroidism
D. Laboratory error
E. Proteinuria

15 A 32-year-old woman with a 7-year history of type 1 diabetes is concerned about her risk for developing nephropathy because her father with type 1 diabetes died of end-stage kidney disease. She is normotensive and has a hemoglobin A_{1c} value of 6.7% (50 mmol/mol), a normal urinary albumin-to-creatinine ratio, mild diabetic retinopathy, a normal LDL-cholesterol concentration, and a low HDL-cholesterol concentration.

Which of the following is the best suggestion to reduce this patient's risk?

A. Continue to control her glucose levels to maintain hemoglobin A_{1c} <7.0% (<53 mmol/mol)
B. Monitor her urinary albumin-to-creatinine ratio semiannually
C. Perform genetic testing to assess the risk of diabetic retinopathy risk
D. Start an ACE inhibitor or angiotensin receptor blocker

16 A 62-year-old man presents for a follow-up visit after kidney transplant 12 months. His hemoglobin A_{1c} value is 7.6% (60 mmol/mol). He has been feeling well and is adherent to his stable posttransplant immunosuppressant regimen, including glucocorticoids. His BMI is 27.4 kg/m^2, and his estimated glomerular filtration rate is 78 mL/min per 1.73 m^2. He has a history of stable cardiovascular disease status post stent placement. He has a family history of type 2 diabetes, but he has not been previously diagnosed with diabetes.

In addition to lifestyle modifications, which of the following options, in conjunction with his transplant team, should be recommended to treat this patient's diabetes?

A. Add a sulfonylurea agent
B. Add a thiazolidinedione
C. Add an SGLT-2 inhibitor
D. Initiate insulin therapy

17 A 68-year-old man with type 2 diabetes describes tingling in his hands and legs over the last 6 months. These sensations are different from his longstanding foot numbness. He also feels unsteady when he gets up at night to void. He eats a well-balanced diet. His treatment regimen consists of metformin, which he has taken since diabetes was diagnosed 11 years ago, an SGLT-2 inhibitor, and insulin glargine (at bedtime).

On physical examination, his blood pressure is 126/74 mm Hg and BMI is 28 kg/m^2. Cranial nerves II through XII are intact, muscle bulk and strength are normal, and coordination in the upper and lower extremities is normal. He has reduced sharp sensation to the knee, decreased vibratory sense in the great toes, and loss of patellar and Achilles reflexes.

Laboratory test results:

Hemoglobin A_{1c} = 7.3% (4.0%-5.6%) (56 mmol/mol [20-38 mmol/mol])
Hematocrit = 40% (41%-51%) (SI: 0.40 [0.41-0.51])
Hemoglobin = 12.3 g/dL (13.8-17.2 g/dL) (SI: 123 g/L [138-172 g/L])

Creatinine = 1.5 mg/dL (0.7-1.3 mg/dL) (SI: 132.6 µmol/L [61.9-114.9 µmol/L])
AST = 55 U/L (20-48 U/L) (SI: 0.92 µkat/L [0.33-0.80 µkat/L])
ALT = 72 U/L (10-40 U/L) (SI: 1.20 µkat/L [0.17-0.67 µkat/L])

Which of the following is the best next step in this patient's management?

A. Measure γ-glutamyltransferase
B. Measure serum vitamin B_6
C. Measure serum vitamin B_{12}
D. Perform MRI of the spine
E. Refer for electromyography and nerve conduction studies

18 A 40-year-old woman with a 25-year history of type 1 diabetes presents with a new skin lesion (*see image*). She describes a nonpainful sore on her anterior left lower extremity that has enlarged over the past 3 months. In addition to the skin lesion, she has diabetic retinopathy and chronic kidney disease with an estimated glomerular filtration rate of 15 mL/min per 1.73 m². She is on the transplant list and is preparing for dialysis.

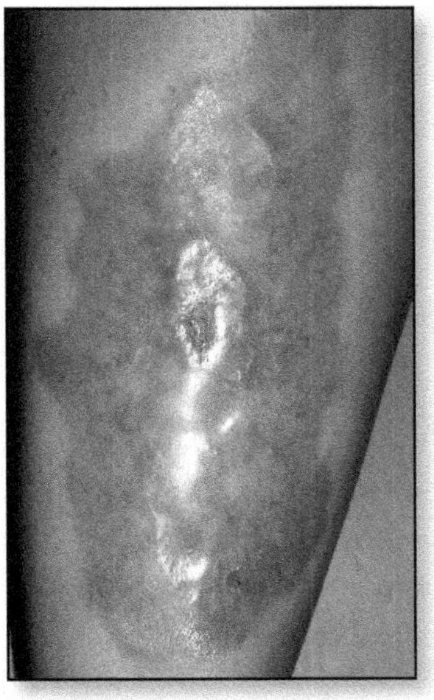

Diabetes-related necrobiosis lipoidica with early ulceration is diagnosed.

Which of the following approaches is most likely to result in complete resolution of this patient's skin lesion?

A. JAK inhibitors
B. Kidney transplant without a pancreas transplant
C. Pancreas transplant with or without a kidney transplant
D. Pentoxifylline
E. Topical calcineurin inhibitors

19 A 32-year-old Asian American man presents to his primary care physician for an annual visit. He feels well and has no concerns. He has no known medical conditions. He does not take any medications. He has no known family history of diabetes and does not smoke cigarettes or drink alcohol.

On physical examination, his blood pressure is 120/70 mm Hg and BMI is 24 kg/m². The rest of his examination findings are unremarkable.

In addition to lifestyle counseling regarding diet and physical activity, when should screening be performed with respect to his prediabetes/diabetes risk?

A. At age 35 years if BMI is greater than 25 kg/m²
B. At age 45 years
C. If symptomatic
D. Now

20 A 25-year-old woman with a 15-year history of type 1 diabetes is considering an isolated pancreas transplant. Her blood glucose values have been highly variable with episodes of level 3 (severe) hypoglycemia at least monthly. Her hemoglobin A_{1c} values have ranged from 8.0% to 10.0% (64-86 mmol/mol), and she has hypoglycemic unawareness despite being on an automated insulin delivery system. She has nephropathy, proliferative retinopathy, gastroparesis, and peripheral neuropathy.

Laboratory test results:

Hemoglobin A_{1c} = 8.8% (4.0%-5.6%) (73 mmol/mol [20-38 mmol/mol])
Creatinine = 1.3 mg/dL (0.6-1.1 mg/dL) (SI: 114.9 µmol/L [53.0-97.2 µmol/L])
Urinary albumin-to-creatinine ratio = 345 mg/g creat (<30 mg/g creat)

Which of the following outcomes can this patient expect within 5 years after a successful pancreas transplant?

A. Recovery of peripheral sensation
B. Regression of gastroparesis
C. Regression of retinopathy
D. Restoration of hypoglycemia awareness

21 A 34-year-old man with type 1 diabetes is in the clinic waiting room. He seems confused when his name is called and is slurring his words. His fingerstick blood glucose value is 39 mg/dL (2.2 mmol/L). After being treated, he reports that despite using a continuous glucose monitor, he has been having episodes of hypoglycemia with blood glucose readings ranging from 40 to 50 mg/dL (2.2-2.8 mmol/L) in the past few months, with no warning symptoms. He has always aimed for tight glycemic control. His hemoglobin A_{1c} value is 5.9% (41 mmol/mol), and he takes multiple daily insulin injections.

Which of the following is the most important advice to give this patient?

A. Begin a regimen of frequent small meals
B. See the diabetes educator to review symptoms and treatment of hypoglycemia
C. Switch to an insulin pump
D. Temporarily relax tight glucose targets

22 A 38-year-old man is referred for evaluation of a 4-year history of low libido and erectile dysfunction. He reports drinking 1 to 2 beers daily.

On physical examination, his BMI is 36 kg/m^2 and blood pressure is 110/60 mm Hg. He has no cushingoid features. He has a mildly enlarged, nontender liver.

Laboratory test results:

Hemoglobin A_{1c} = 6.7% (4.0%-5.6%) (50 mmol/mol [20-38 mmol/mol])
Creatinine = 0.8 mg/dL (0.7-1.3 mg/dL) (SI: 70.7 μmol/L [61.9-114.9 μmol/L])
ALT = 142 U/L (10-40 U/L) (SI: 2.37 μkat/L [0.17-0.67 μkat/L])
Total testosterone = 220 ng/dL (300-900 ng/dL) (SI: 7.6 nmol/L [10.4-31.2 nmol/L])

Which of the following is the best test to determine the etiology of this patient's hypogonadism and diabetes?

A. Glutamic acid decarboxylase antibody titer
B. Liver ultrasonography
C. Pituitary MRI
D. Total iron-binding capacity and serum ferritin measurements

23 A 59-year-old man with suboptimally controlled type 2 diabetes and longstanding hypertension presents to the emergency department because he is worried that he has shingles. He has noticed drooping and pain on the left side of his face and some trouble speaking. He has no other symptoms. He has a history of retinopathy and distal somatosensory neuropathy.

On physical examination, he has a right facial droop and some tenderness in the affected area. There is no rash present. His ear canal and tympanic membrane look normal. The rest of the neurologic examination findings are normal, except for reduced sensation in the lower extremities to the mid-shin.

Laboratory test results:

Hemoglobin A_{1c} = 9.3% (4.0%-5.6%) (78 mmol/mol [20-38 mmol/mol])
Complete blood cell count and chemistries, normal

Findings on head CT without contrast are unremarkable.

Which of the following is the most likely cause of this patient's facial palsy?

A. Diabetes-related radiculopathy
B. Diabetic autonomic neuropathy
C. Herpes zoster
D. Otitis media
E. Stroke

24 An 18-year-old girl is referred for recent diagnosis of diabetes. Her father has confirmed type 1 diabetes and requested that she be screened. A hemoglobin A_{1c} measurement was 6.9% (52 mmol/mol), and a fasting glucose value was 91 mg/dL (5.1 mmol/L). Tests for islet-cell antibodies, insulin autoantibodies, and glutamic acid decarboxylase autoantibodies were negative. The patient began a low-carbohydrate diet and has been exercising regularly for 3 months, but her repeated hemoglobin A_{1c} level is now 7.4% (57 mmol/mol), and many of her postprandial glucose measurements are in the range of 200 to 250 mg/dL (11.1-13.9 mmol/L). She has no symptoms of hyperglycemia.

On physical examination, she has no skin tags or acanthosis nigricans. Her BMI is 23 kg/m^2.

Which of the following should be ordered next?

A. 1,5-Anhydroglucitol measurement
B. Fructosamine measurement
C. Genetic testing for pathogenic variants in the *GCK* gene (glucokinase)
D. Genetic testing for pathogenic variants in the *HNF1A* gene (hepatocyte nuclear factor-1 alpha)
E. Zinc transporter 8 (ZnT8) antibody testing

25 A 62-year-old woman seeks an opinion on how she can prevent diabetes in the future. She has a strong family history of type 2 diabetes. She also has hypertension and dyslipidemia. Her only medications are rosuvastatin and amlodipine.

On physical examination, her BMI is 34 kg/m^2 and blood pressure is 120/60 mm Hg. She has 2+ edema in both lower extremities. Findings are otherwise unremarkable.

Recent laboratory test results:

Hemoglobin A_{1c} = 6.1% (4.0%-5.6%) (43 mmol/mol [20-38 mmol/mol])
Estimated glomerular filtration rate = 76 mL/min per 1.73 m^2 (>60 mL/min per 1.73 m^2)

On the basis of available studies, which of the following is the best treatment option for this patient?

A. Dulaglutide
B. Empagliflozin
C. Lifestyle intervention
D. Metformin
E. Pioglitazone

26 A 68-year-old man with a 22-year history of type 2 diabetes is admitted to the hospital with severe hyperglycemia and change in mental status. The patient lives alone and was found by his neighbor in a confused state.

On physical examination, he is lethargic and unable to answer any questions. His temperature is 100.5°F (38.1°C), blood pressure is 100/60 mm Hg, and pulse rate is 130 beats/min. His weight is 230 lb (104 kg) (BMI = 32 kg/m^2). Skin and mucous membranes are dry. There is no focal neurologic deficit.

Laboratory test results:

Hemoglobin A_{1c} = 10.5% (4.0%-5.6%) (91 mmol/mol [20-38 mmol/mol])
Plasma glucose = 1300 mg/dL (70-99 mg/dL) (SI: 72.2 mmol/L [3.9-5.5 mmol/L])
Serum sodium = 126 mEq/L (136-142 mEq/L) (SI: 126 mmol/L [136-142 mmol/L])
Serum potassium = 4.5 mEq/L (3.5-5.0 mEq/L) (SI: 4.5 mmol/L [3.5-5.0 mmol/L])
Serum bicarbonate = 21 mEq/L (21-28 mEq/L) (SI: 21 mmol/L [21-28 mmol/L])
Serum chloride = 106 mEq/L (96-106 mEq/L) (SI: 106 mmol/L [96-106 mmol/L])
Serum creatinine = 1.2 mg/dL (0.7-1.3 mg/dL) (SI: 106.1 μmol/L [61.9-114.9 μmol/L])
Arterial pH = 7.35 (7.35-7.45)
Serum β-hydroxybutyrate = 2.6 mg/dL (<3.0 mg/dL) (SI: 249.8 μmol/L [<288.2 μmol/L])

Which of the following is the best treatment strategy regarding fluids and intravenous insulin?

Answer	Fluids over 2 to 4 hours	Intravenous insulin
A.	500-1000 mL/h of 0.9% NaCl	Bolus of 10 units, then 10 units/h
B.	500-1000 mL/h of 0.9% NaCl	Bolus of 20 units, then 20 units/h
C.	500-1000 mL/h of 0.9% NaCl	No insulin bolus, start 10 units/h
D.	500-1000 mL/h of 0.45% NaCl	Bolus of 10 units, then 10 units/h
E.	500-1000 mL/h of 0.45% NaCl	No insulin bolus, start 10 units/h

Diabetes Mellitus, Section 2 Board Review

Marie McDonnell, MD

27 A 53-year-old man with a 5-year history of type 2 diabetes, hypercholesterolemia, and high blood pressure presents for evaluation. Six months ago, atorvastatin was discontinued due to elevated transaminase concentrations. Two months ago, without resolution of transaminitis, metformin was also discontinued. Before metformin was stopped, his hemoglobin A_{1c} value was 6.9% (4.0%-5.6%) (52 mmol/mol [20-38 mmol/mol]).

On physical examination, he appears well. His BMI is 34 kg/m^2, and blood pressure is 142/84 mm Hg. There is mild 1+ pitting edema on his ankles bilaterally.

Current medications include metoprolol extended release, 100 mg daily; lisinopril, 10 mg daily; ezetimibe, 10 mg daily; and apixaban, 5 mg twice daily.

Laboratory test results:

- Creatinine = 1.18 mg/dL (0.7-1.3 mg/dL) (SI: 104.3 µmol/L [61.9-114.9 µmol/L])
- Glucose = 180 mg/dL (70-99 mg/dL) (SI: 10.0 mmol/L [3.9-5.5 mmol/L])
- Triglycerides = 320 mg/dL (<150 mg/dL [optimal]) (SI: 3.62 mmol/L [<1.70 mmol/L])
- AST = 51 U/L (20-48 U/L) (SI: 0.85 µkat/L [0.33-0.80 µkat/L])
- ALT = 65 U/L (10-40 U/L) (SI: 1.09 µkat/L [0.17-0.67 µkat/L])
- International normalized ratio = 1.0 (0.8-1.2)
- Platelet count = 151 $10^3/\mu L$ (150-450 × $10^3/\mu L$) (SI: 151 $10^9/L$ [150-450 × $10^9/L$])

With these results, the Fibrosis 4 score is calculated to be 2.22 (low <1.3; intermediate 1.3-2.67; high >2.67).

Vibration-controlled transient elastography is performed, which documents a liver stiffness measurement of 8.2 kPa (low risk: <8kPa; indeterminate risk: 8-12 kPa; high risk: >12kPa).

Which of the following therapies is the best next step to prevent advanced liver disease?

A. Icosapent ethyl
B. Metformin
C. Phentermine
D. Pioglitazone
E. Semaglutide

28 A 48-year-old woman with a 20-year history of cystic fibrosis–related diabetes is undergoing evaluation for pancreas-after-kidney transplant. Diabetes has been complicated by retinopathy and nephropathy. Other relevant history includes mild gastroparesis and anemia of chronic disease.

Six years ago, she received a kidney transplant from a living, related donor, and she has maintained good kidney function. She manages her diabetes with an automated insulin delivery system. Despite achieving time-in-range of 75% to 85%, she reports feeling overwhelmed by the demands of living with diabetes. When access to her continuous glucose monitor is disrupted, she often has severe hypoglycemic episodes and states that "diabetes is controlling my life." Her cystic fibrosis–related lung disease has been in excellent control since she started taking targeted therapy (elexacaftor/tezacaftor/ivacaftor) 6 months ago.

On physical examination, she is alert and appears well. Her BMI is 33 kg/m^2, and blood pressure is 142/78 mm Hg. The rest of her examination findings are unremarkable.

Laboratory test results:

- Hemoglobin A_{1c} = 7.0% (4.0%-5.6%) (53 mmol/mol [20-38 mmol/mol])
- C-peptide = 1.2 ng/mL (0.5-2.0 ng/mL) (SI: 0.40 nmol/L [0.17-0.66 nmol/L])
- Glucose = 182 mg/dL (70-99 mg/dL) (SI: 10.1 nmol/L [3.9-5.5 mmol/L])
- Creatinine = 1.4 mg/dL (0.6-1.1 mg/dL) (SI: 123.8 μmol/L [53.0-97.2 μmol/L])
- Estimated glomerular filtration rate = 48 mL/min per 1.73 m^2 (>60 mL/min per 1.73 m^2)
- Urinary albumin-to-creatinine ratio = 24 mg/g creat (<30 mg/g creat)

Two weeks after her evaluation, the hospital's transplant program committee decides not to make her active on the pancreas-after-kidney transplant list.

Which of the following is the most likely reason for the committee's determination?

A. >5 years since last transplant
B. BMI >30 kg/m^2
C. Cystic fibrosis–related diabetes is not an indication for pancreas transplant
D. Glomerular filtration rate <60 mL/min per 1.73 m^2
E. Hemoglobin A_{1c} <8.0% (<64 mmol/mol)

29 A 62-year-old woman with a 25-year history of type 2 diabetes presents for follow-up. Diabetes was diagnosed in the setting of pregnancy, and her medical history also includes obesity, preeclampsia, dyslipidemia, and hypertension. She had suboptimal glycemic control for many years due to medication nonadherence, but she has been more successful in the last 2 years, consistently achieving hemoglobin A_{1c} values less than 7.0% (<53 mmol/mol). However, over the last few months, she has found self-care to be more difficult because of fatigue, which she attributes to work-related stress.

Her current medications are losartan, 100 mg daily; tirzepatide, 10 mg once weekly; metformin, 500 mg twice daily; and empagliflozin, 25 mg daily.

On physical examination, she appears tired. Her BMI is 28.0 kg/m^2, blood pressure is 136/88 mm Hg, and pulse rate is 92 beats/min. Her lungs are clear to auscultation. Findings on cardiovascular examination are normal, other than previously observed mild pedal edema and diminished dorsalis pedis pulses bilaterally. She has reduced vibration sensation below the knee bilaterally and absent 10-g monofilament sensation on the first 2 metatarsal heads on both feet. There are no visible lesions or ulcerations.

Laboratory test results:

- Hemoglobin A_{1c} = 7.6% (4.0%-5.6%) (60 mmol/mol [20-38 mmol/mol])
- LDL cholesterol = 130 mg/dL (<100 mg/dL [optimal]) (3.37 mmol/L [<2.59 mmol/L])
- Creatinine = 1.4 mg/dL (0.6-1.1 mg/dL) (SI: 123.8 μmol/L [53.0-97.2 μmol/L])
- Urinary albumin-to-creatinine ratio = 1654.7 mg/g (<30 mg/g creat)
- TSH = 0.75 mIU/L (0.5-5.0 mIU/L)
- N-terminal pro-B-type natriuretic peptide = 203 pg/mL (<125 pg/mL)
- Vitamin B_{12} = 456 pg/mL (180-914 pg/mL) (SI: 337 pmol/L [133-674 pmol/L])

Which of the following is the best next step in this patient's management?

A. Add carvedilol, 6.25 mg daily
B. Increase losartan dosage to 150 mg daily
C. Order ankle-brachial index
D. Order echocardiography
E. Switch empagliflozin to sotagliflozin

30 A 73-year-old man with a 16-year history of type 2 diabetes presents for routine follow-up. He has mild nonproliferative retinopathy. Other medical history includes a transient ischemic attack 2 years ago and coronary artery disease status post percutaneous coronary intervention of the left anterior descending artery 6 years ago. Otherwise, he feels well and is active. There is no personal or family history of pancreatic, bladder, or colorectal cancer.

He reports having many problems with medications over the years. While taking empagliflozin, he was hospitalized for euglycemic diabetic ketoacidosis without an apparent underlying cause. During a trial of a GLP-1 receptor agonist, he had severe constipation, 12-lb (5.4-kg) weight loss, and reduced muscle mass. In subsequent discussions, he has declined another trial of drugs in either of these classes. Additionally, he has never been able to consistently take medications more than once daily.

Current medications are aspirin, 81 mg daily; metformin, 1000 mg daily; atorvastatin, 80 mg daily; and ezetimibe, 10 mg daily.

On physical examination, his blood pressure is 142/88 mm Hg and BMI is 25.0 kg/m^2. Findings on cardiovascular and neurologic examinations are unremarkable.

Recent laboratory test results:

- Hemoglobin A_{1c} = 7.8% (4.0%-5.6%) (62 mmol/mol [20-38 mmol/mol])
- Creatinine = 0.78 mg/dL (0.7-1.3 mg/dL) (SI: 69.0 µmol/L [61.9-114.9 µmol/L])
- Estimated glomerular filtration rate = 94 mL/min per 1.73 m^2 (>60 mL/min per 1.73 m^2)
- N-terminal pro-B-type natriuretic peptide = 32 pg/mL (<125 pg/mL)
- LDL cholesterol = 58 mg/dL (<100 mg/dL [optimal]) (SI: 1.50 mmol/L [<2.59 mmol/L])
- Urinary albumin-to-creatinine = 52 mg/g (<30 mg/g creat)

Which of the following treatments would best help this patient achieve his target hemoglobin A_{1c} level?

A. Glyburide
B. Linagliptin
C. Oral semaglutide
D. Pioglitazone
E. Repaglinide

31 A 52-year-old woman presents for evaluation of diabetes management after hospitalization 10 days ago for elective hip replacement for osteoarthritis. During her hospital stay, point-of-care glucose values monitored randomly every 6 hours ranged from 58 to 228 mg/dL (3.2 to 12.7 mmol/L).

She underwent Roux-en-Y gastric bypass 4 years ago and has had occasional difficulty with postmeal hypoglycemia. This was well-controlled on a low-carbohydrate, high-fiber diet rich in lean protein and fats mainly from dairy sources. She was prescribed acarbose in the past, but she was able to discontinue it 6 months ago by carefully adhering to her diet. However, since her hospitalization, she restarted acarbose and is taking it 3 times daily before meals.

Other than some pain, her recovery had been going well until 2 days ago when her husband found her to be confused while watching TV 3 hours after dinner, and emergency medical services were called. Her point-of-care glucose concentration was 38 mg/dL (2.1 mmol/L), and her mental status normalized with ingestion of glucose gel.

Current medications are atorvastatin, 10 mg; lisinopril, 100 mg daily; metformin, 1000 mg at bedtime; acarbose, 50 mg before each meal; tramadol, 50-100 mg 3 times daily; and acetaminophen, 500 mg twice daily.

Which of the following is the best next step in this patient's care?

A. Discontinue acarbose
B. Discontinue acetaminophen
C. Discontinue metformin
D. Discontinue tramadol
E. Reduce intake of dairy fat

32 A 69-year-old woman with type 2 diabetes, hypertension, and history of stroke 2 years ago presents for routine follow-up. She has no specific concerns but reports frustration with her blood pressure remaining uncontrolled despite strict adherence to a 3-drug regimen. She shares a notebook with detailed measurements of blood pressure values, with daily morning systolic pressures ranging from 148 to 162 mm Hg and diastolic pressures ranging from 78 to 82 mm Hg.

Overall, she says she "feels better" than most of her friends. She wakes feeling refreshed most days and follows a daily routine of jogging 20 minutes on a treadmill, taking her medications, and working 8 hours.

On physical examination, her blood pressure is 169/80 mm Hg, pulse rate is 68 beats/min, and BMI is 26 kg/m^2. She appears well, mucus membranes are moist, and extraocular movements are normal. She has mild facial asymmetry (which is unchanged from past visits).

Current medications are semaglutide, 1 mg weekly; nifedipine extended release, 120 mg daily; irbesartan, 300 mg daily; and chlorthalidone, 25 mg daily.

Laboratory test results:

Urinary albumin to creatinine ratio = 135 mg/g creat (<30 mg/g creat)
Hemoglobin A_{1c} = 6.9% (4.0%-5.6%) (52 mmol/mol [20-38 mmol/mol])
Sodium = 142 mEq/L (136-142 mEq/L) (SI: 142 mEq/L [136-142 mmol/L])
Potassium = 3.8 mEq/L (3.5-5.0 mEq/L) (SI: 3.8 mmol/L [3.5-5.0 mmol/L])
Creatinine = 1.2 mg/dL (0.6-1.1 mg/dL) (SI: 106.1 μmol/L [53.0-97.2 μmol/L])
Estimated glomerular filtration rate = 78 mL/min per 1.73 m^2 (>60 mL/min per 1.73 m^2)
Aldosterone = 12 ng/dL (4-21 ng/dL) (SI: 332.9 pmol/L [111.0-582.5 pmol/L])
Renin = 6.2 pg/mL (4-44 pg/mL) (SI: 0.1 pmol/L [0.1-1.0 pmol/L])
Plasma metanephrines, low normal
Renal artery duplex ultrasound, normal

Which of the following is the best next step in this patient's management?

A. Add eplerenone, 25 mg daily
B. Add labetalol, 50 mg twice daily
C. Add sotagliflozin, 200 mg daily
D. Perform adrenal CT
E. Refer for sleep study

33 A 33-year-old woman presents to her primary care physician for an annual visit. She feels well and has no concerns. She had gestational diabetes during a pregnancy 5 years ago. She has no history of hypertension, dyslipidemia, or cardiovascular disease. Her only medication is a daily multivitamin. She has no known family history of diabetes and does not smoke cigarettes or drink alcohol. She exercises regularly.

On physical examination, her blood pressure is 120/70 mm Hg and BMI is 24.0 kg/m^2. The rest of her examination findings are unremarkable.

Her current hemoglobin A_{1c} value is 5.4% (36 mmol/mol).

Regarding lifelong screening with respect to her prediabetes/diabetes risk, in how many years should this patient be advised to have her next hemoglobin A_{1c} measurement?

A. No future testing needed
B. 1 year
C. 3 years
D. 5 years
E. 10 years

34 A 27-year-old man with type 1 diabetes is training for a marathon and presents with his wife to discuss 2 episodes of severe hypoglycemia. Before these episodes, he had not had trouble with hypoglycemia and reports good awareness when his glucose concentration is below 60 mg/dL (<3.3 mmol/L). In both episodes, he required assistance from a family member to identify and administer liquid carbohydrates to treat hypoglycemia. One of the episodes occurred after a correction dose was given for a glucose value of 184 mg/dL (10.2 mmol/L) 1 hour after a training run had ended. The other episode was less expected and happened while he was playing a video game with his daughter. To treat this episode, his wife administered intranasal glucagon before giving him glucose gel.

He uses an automated insulin delivery pump that automatically adjusts basal insulin rates in response to recently measured glucose values from a continuous glucose monitor, but it does not deliver automated correction boluses. He uses the pump's "exercise activity" during his runs, starting it 30 minutes before his run and ending when his run is completed.

Automated insulin delivery pump settings:

Usual glucose target from 12 AM to 12 AM = 100 mg/dL (mmol/L)
Glucose target during exercise = 150 mg/dL (mmol/L)
Insulin-to-carbohydrate ratio from 12 AM to 12 AM = 1:10
Sensitivity factor from 12 AM to 12 AM = 1:40

Continuous glucose monitoring output:

Time-in-range = 77%
Time-above-range = 18%
Time-below-range = 5% (time-very-below-range = 2%)

Which of the following should be recommended to reduce the risk of severe hypoglycemia after his long runs?

A. Change correction factor from 1:40 to 1:20 for 2 hours after completion of a run
B. Increase glucose target to 130 mg/dL (7.2 mmol/L) for 4 hours after a run and take carbohydrate as needed every 30 minutes
C. Ingest a meal with 60 g of carbohydrate without an insulin bolus before a run
D. Ingest gel oral supplement with 30 g of carbohydrate every 15 minutes of exercise, as long as glucose is between 126 and 180 mg/dL (7.0-10.0 mmol/L)
E. Self-administer a mini-dose of glucagon immediately after completion of a run

35 A 26-year-old woman with polycystic ovary syndrome would like to establish care, as her former endocrinologist left the area. She has had irregular menses since menarche, facial hirsutism, and acne. She has had a good clinical response to hormonal contraception and spironolactone. She has no current concerns and no pregnancy plans.

On physical examination, her BMI is 32 kg/m^2 and blood pressure is 110/60 mm Hg. She has acanthosis nigricans on her neck.

Laboratory test results (sample drawn while fasting):

Electrolytes, normal
Creatinine, normal
Glucose = 98 mg/dL (70-99 mg/dL) (SI: 5.4 mmol/L [3.9-5.5 mmol/L])
Complete blood cell count, normal
Hemoglobin A_{1c} = 6.6% (4.0%-5.6%) (49 mmol/mol [20-38 mmol/mol])

Which of the following is the best next step in this patient's care?

A. Diagnose diabetes and refer for medical nutrition therapy
B. Perform a 2-hour oral glucose tolerance test after 2 days of consuming <100 g carbohydrate per day
C. Perform continuous glucose monitoring for 72 hours
D. Repeat fasting glucose measurement
E. Repeat hemoglobin A_{1c} measurement

36 A 33-year-old woman with a 20-year history of type 1 diabetes presents for a follow-up visit. She starts to cry and says she is experiencing major stress due to recent divorce. She reports having intermittent nausea for the last few days. She feels unwell, and she attributes it to stress. She uses insulin pump therapy with insulin aspart at a basal rate of 1.2 units/h, an insulin-to-carbohydrate ratio of 1:15, and a sensitivity factor of 1:40. She has not been doing glucose fingerstick readings at home on a regular basis, but when she does, the values range between 70 and 250 mg/dL (3.9-13.9 mmol/L) without a real pattern. She had declined the use of a continuous glucose monitor in the past. A glucose fingerstick measurement in the office today is 385 mg/dL (21.4 mmol/L).

Laboratory tests from 2 weeks ago show a hemoglobin A_{1c} value of 9.3% (78 mmol/mol) with a normal basic metabolic panel. A pregnancy test is negative.

Which of the following is the best immediate next step?

A. Assessment for ketones
B. Basal rate testing
C. Diabetes education
D. Initiation of a continuous glucose sensor
E. Therapy for stress management

37 An 82-year-old woman with a 22-year history of type 2 diabetes and hypertension is referred for glycemic management following an emergency department visit for severe hypoglycemia with loss of consciousness. Emergency medical technicians report that her initial blood glucose value was 34 mg/dL (1.9 mmol/L).

Her current home diabetes treatment regimen consists of 25 units of insulin glargine at bedtime, 9 units of lispro insulin with meals, and correction doses for blood glucose values greater than 180 mg/dL (>10.0 mmol/L). She does not record the insulin doses taken. She would like to review how and when to take correction insulin doses.

Her home blood glucose measurements are as follows:

Blood glucose values and observations	Fasting	Prelunch	Predinner	Bedtime
Blood glucose values	150-199 mg/dL (SI: 8.3-11.0 mmol/L)	150-199 mg/dL (SI: 8.3-11.0 mmol/L)	100-199 mg/dL (SI: 5.6-11.0 mmol/L)	150-225 mg/dL (SI: 8.3-12.5 mmol/L)
Observations	Occasional values in the range of 68-75 mg/dL (SI: 3.8-4.2 mmol/L) or 211-274 mg/dL (SI: 11.7-15.2 mmol/L)	If lunch is late, values are 90-125 mg/dL (SI: 5.0-6.9 mmol/L)	N/A	Occasional values in the range of 110-130 mg/dL (SI: 6.1-7.2 mmol/L)

On physical examination, her BMI is 19 kg/m^2 and blood pressure is 142/78 mm Hg. She has markedly reduced sensation in both feet. Her mood and affect are normal, and her memory is sharp.

Laboratory test results:

Hemoglobin A_{1c} = 8.7% (4.0%-5.6%) (72 mmol/mol [20-38 mmol/mol]) (estimated average glucose value 203 mg/dL [SI: 11.3 mmol/L])

Estimated glomerular filtration rate = 52 mL/min per 1.73 m^2 (<60 mL/min per 1.73 m^2)

C-peptide = 3.6 ng/mL (0.9-4.3 ng/mL) (SI: 1.2 nmol/L [0.30-1.42 nmol/L])

Which of the following should be recommended to reduce the risk of additional episodes of severe hypoglycemia in this older woman?

A. Reduce glargine to 20 units and keep lispro at 9 units

B. Reduce glargine to 20 units, reduce lispro to 4 units, and start linagliptin

C. Refer to a diabetes educator to help her better understand how to take her insulins

D. Stop basal and mealtime insulins and start repaglinide with meals

38 A 54-year-old woman with a 44-year history of type 1 diabetes is seen for follow-up. Complications include nephropathy, nonproliferative retinopathy, neuropathy, and gastroparesis. She is on a basal-mealtime insulin regimen but is not adherent and misses insulin injections on a regular basis. She has declined insulin pumps and glucose sensors. Her hemoglobin A_{1c} level has ranged between 8.5% and 12.0% (69-108 mmol/mol) in recent years.

Her new concerns are blurred vision, decreased visual acuity, and floaters for the past few months. She has not seen an ophthalmologist in 3 years.

A fundoscopic examination is performed (*see image*).

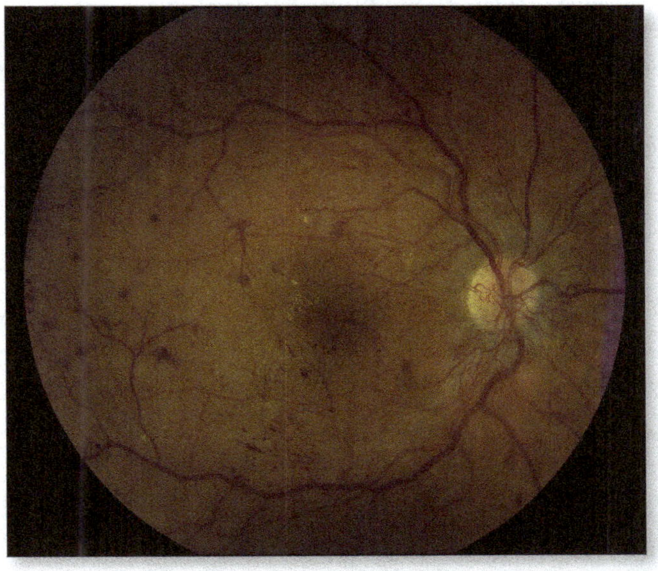

She is immediately referred to ophthalmology.

Based on her nonadherence history and the fundoscopic findings, which of the following is the best next step?

A. Anti-VEGF (vascular endothelial growth factor) agents

B. Focal laser photocoagulation

C. Intravitreal glucocorticoids

D. Panretinal laser photocoagulation

E. Vitrectomy

39 A 46-year-old man with a 10-year history of type 1 diabetes and a BMI of 33 kg/m^2 asks about possible adjunctive treatments that will improve his glycemic control and not increase his weight. He has had reasonable glycemic control, and his most recent hemoglobin A_{1c} measurement is 7.4% (57 mmol/mol). His estimated glomerular filtration rate is 76 mL/min per m^2, and urinary albumin is undetectable. He has no diabetes-related complications.

Which of the following therapies is approved to add to this patient's regimen to lower glucose and body weight?

A. Acarbose
B. Dulaglutide
C. Empagliflozin
D. Metformin
E. Pramlintide

40 A 61-year-old man with type 2 diabetes, nonischemic cardiomyopathy, heart failure with reduced ejection fraction (ejection fraction = 25%-30%), hypertension, obesity, chronic kidney disease, and a venous stasis ulcer has been admitted to the hospital with an acute heart failure exacerbation. His care is being managed by the advanced heart failure team who asks for an endocrine consultation because he has hyperglycemia in the hospital and an estimated glomerular filtration rate of 29 mL/min per 1.73 m^2.

He has had diabetes for 15 years. His most recent insulin regimen at home consisted of insulin glargine, 25 units in the morning, and insulin aspart, 4 units with meals. He reports often missing his mealtime insulin doses and states that he would like to discontinue this part of his regimen permanently.

On physical examination, he has class 2 obesity (BMI = 38.0 kg/m^2), jugular venous distention to the midneck, 2+ to 3+ lower-extremity edema, a left ankle stasis ulcer, and reduced 10-g monofilament sensation below the knee.

Today's laboratory test results:

Sodium = 143 mEq/L (136-142 mEq/L)
(SI: 143 mmol/L [136-142 mmol/L])
Potassium = 4.3 mEq/L (3.5-5.0 mEq/L)
(SI: 4.3 mmol/L [3.5-5.0 mmol/L])
Chloride = 109 mEq/L (96-106 mEq/L)
(SI: 109 mmol/L [96-106 mmol/L])
Bicarbonate = 25 mEq/L (21-28 mEq/L)
(SI: 25 mmol/L [21-28 mmol/L])
Serum urea nitrogen = 25 mg/dL (8-23 mg/dL)
(SI: 8.9 mmol/L [2.9-8.2 mmol/L])
Creatinine = 2.5 mg/dL (0.7-1.3 mg/dL)
(SI: 221 μmol/L [61.9-114.9 μmol/L])
Estimated glomerular filtration rate = 33 mL/min per 1.73 m^2 (>60 mL/min per 1.73 m^2)
Glucose = 154 mg/dL (70-99 mg/dL)
(SI: 8.5 mmol/L [3.9-5.5 mmol/L])
Hemoglobin A_{1c} = 6.8% (4.0%-5.6%)
(SI: 51 mmol/mol [20-38 mmol/mol])
Hematocrit = 39% (41%-51%) (SI: 0.39 [0.41-0.51])

While in the hospital, his treatment regimen consists of insulin glargine, 25 units nightly, and linagliptin, 5 mg daily, plus correction scale as needed, with blood glucose values ranging from 128 to 192 mg/dL (7.1-10.7 mmol/L).

Which of the following is the best agent to use in combination with glargine insulin to achieve optimal disease control upon hospital discharge?

A. Dapagliflozin
B. Dulaglutide
C. Glimepiride
D. Linagliptin
E. Pramlintide

41 A 43-year-old woman is referred for diabetes management. Diabetes was diagnosed at age 22 years, 1 year after she developed dermatomyositis. For a few months, the dermatomyositis was treated with high-dosage steroids, which were then tapered and stopped over a 9-month period. Her diabetes has been difficult to control. Her current treatment regimen consists of 260 units daily of basal and mealtime insulins. She has tried an SGLT-2 inhibitor but could not tolerate it because of recurrent genital mycotic infections. GLP-1 receptor agonists, tried twice, were not effective. Her premeal self-monitoring blood glucose values range between 180 and 300 mg/dL (10.0-16.7 mmol/L).

Her other medical problems include polycystic ovary syndrome, dyslipidemia, hypertension, hypothyroidism, and fatty liver. Her review of systems is notable for some fatigue, mild nocturia, and blurred vision. Her medications include insulin degludec, insulin lispro, metformin, rosuvastatin, fenofibrate, icosapent ethyl, ramipril, levothyroxine, and an oral contraceptive.

On physical examination, her blood pressure is 120/70 mm Hg and BMI is 22 kg/m^2. A photograph of the patient is shown (*see image*).

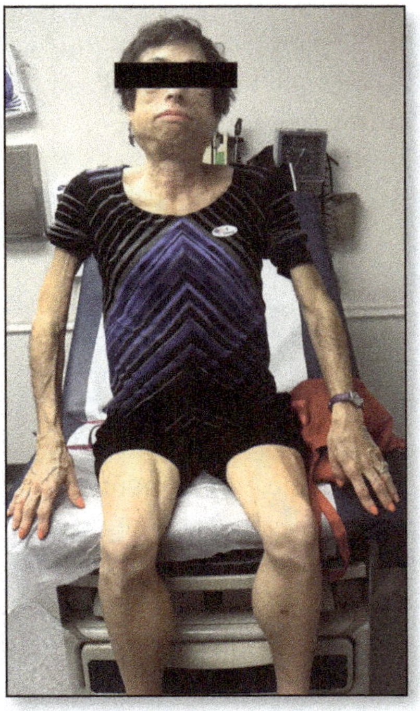

Laboratory test results:

- Hemoglobin A_{1c} = 9.0% (4.0%-5.6%) (75 mmol/mol [20-38 mmol/mol])
- Serum creatinine = 0.9 mg/dL (0.6-1.1 mg/dL) (SI: 79.6 µmol/L [53.0-97.2 µmol/L])
- Total cholesterol = 185 mg/dL (<200 mg/dL [optimal]) (SI: 4.79 mmol/L [<5.18 mmol/L])
- Triglycerides = 550 mg/dL (<150 mg/dL [optimal]) (SI: 6.22 mmol/L [<1.70 mmol/L])
- TSH = 2.5 mIU/L (0.5-5.0 mIU/L)
- TPO antibodies, positive
- ALT = 84 U/L (10-40 U/L) (SI: 1.40 µkat/L [0.17-0.67 µkat/L])
- Urinary albumin-to-creatinine ratio = 240 mg/g creat (<30 mg/g creat)

Which of the following should be ordered next to confirm this patient's diagnosis?

A. Glutamic acid decarboxylase 65 antibody assessment
B. *HNF1A* gene testing
C. Insulin receptor gene testing
D. Leptin measurement
E. Urinary free cortisol excretion

42 A 64-year-old man seeks an opinion on how to prevent diabetes in the future. He has a strong family history of type 2 diabetes and also has hypertension and dyslipidemia, treated with lisinopril and atorvastatin, respectively. Review of systems includes reduced libido, which he attributes to a mildly depressed mood over the past year.

On physical examination, his BMI is 32.0 kg/m^2 and blood pressure is 120/60 mm Hg. Findings are otherwise unremarkable.

Recent laboratory test results:

- Hemoglobin A_{1c} = 6.1% (4.0%-5.6%) (43 mmol/mol [20-38 mmol/mol])
- Estimated glomerular filtration rate = 76 mL/min per 1.73 m^2 (>60 mL/min per 1.73 m^2)
- LDL cholesterol = 110 mg/dL (<100 mg/dL [optimal]) (SI: 2.85 mmol/L [<2.59 mmol/L])
- Total testosterone (measured at 8 AM in the fasting state) = 220 ng/dL (300-900 ng/dL) (SI: nmol/L [10.4-31.2 nmol/L])
- SHBG = 4.5 µg/mL (1.1-6.7 µg/mL) (SI: 40 nmol/L [10-60 nmol/L])

On the basis of available studies, which of the following is the best intervention to prevent diabetes in this patient?

A. Discontinue atorvastatin
B. Exercise 150 minutes per week plus follow a reduced-calorie diet
C. Start empagliflozin
D. Start metformin
E. Start testosterone therapy

43 A 58-year-old man with type 2 diabetes presents for a routine follow-up visit and is accompanied by his wife. His medical history is notable for hypertension, dyslipidemia, and fatty liver. His main concern is fatigue, which he has been experiencing for the past few months. One of his friends told him he should have testing for "adrenal fatigue." He has erectile dysfunction despite normal libido. His medications include metformin, sitagliptin, rosuvastatin, ramipril, and baby aspirin. He does not smoke cigarettes or drink alcohol.

On physical examination, his BMI is 31.0 kg/m^2 and blood pressure is 120/60 mm Hg.

Laboratory test results:

Hemoglobin A_{1c} = 7.2% (4.0%-5.6%) (55 mmol/mol [20-38 mmol/mol])
Hemoglobin = 17.1 g/dL (13.8-17.2 g/dL) (SI: 171 g/L [138-172 g/L])
Serum sodium = 141 mEq/L (136-142 mEq/L) (SI: 141 mmol/L [3.9-5.5 mmol/L])
Serum potassium = 4.0 mEq/L (3.5-5.0 mEq/L) (SI: 4.0 mmol/L [3.5-5.0 mmol/L])
Serum creatinine = 0.6 mg/dL (0.7-1.3 mg/dL) (SI: 53.0 µmol/L [61.9-114.9 µmol/L])
TSH = 1.5 mIU/L (0.5-5.0 mIU/L)
Serum cortisol (8 AM) = 12 µg/dL (5-25 µg/dL) (SI: 331.1 nmol/L [137.9-689.7 nmol/L])
Total testosterone = 275 ng/dL (300-900 ng/dL) (SI: 8.7 nmol/L [10.4-31.2 nmol/L])
LH = 4.0 mIU/mL (1.0-9.0 mIU/mL) (SI: 4.0 IU/L [1.0-9.0 IU/L])
FSH = 6.0 mIU/mL (1.0-13.0 mIU/mL) (SI: 6.0 IU/L [1.0-13.0 IU/L])

Which of the following is the best next step in this patient's management?

A. Discontinue aspirin
B. Perform a cosyntropin-stimulation test
C. Perform pituitary MRI
D. Perform polysomnography
E. Start testosterone

44 An 18-year-old man is referred for management of type 1 diabetes, which was recently diagnosed during a hospital admission for diabetic ketoacidosis. He is taking basal and mealtime insulins. He is currently doing well, with most blood glucose measurements within his target range. He uses a continuous glucose monitor and reports no symptoms or concerns.

Which of the following should be measured as part of screening for other autoimmune diseases?

A. 21-Hydroxylase antibodies
B. Antinuclear antibodies
C. Antiparietal cell antibodies
D. Tissue transglutaminase antibodies
E. TPO antibodies

45 A 25-year-old man with a 7-year history of type 1 diabetes presents for routine follow-up. During the first 3 years after his diagnosis, he struggled to maintain good glycemic control and had an average hemoglobin A_{1c} value of 9.0% (75 mmol/mol). Four years ago, he began using an insulin pump that was integrated with a continuous glucose monitor and has upgraded to the latest version of automated insulin delivery. His average hemoglobin A_{1c} level over the last 4 years is 7.4% (57 mmol/mol). He is pleased to see today's hemoglobin A_{1c} value of 6.8% (51 mmol/mol), consistent with time-in-range (70-180 mg/dL [3.9-10.0 mmol/L]) of 82% on his continuous glucose monitor.

Based on long-term follow-up data, which of the following changes in cardiovascular risk can be expected over the next 15 years from this patient's glycemic control?

Answer	Myocardial Infarction	Stroke	Cardiovascular Death
A.	↓	↓	No change
B.	↓	↑	↓
C.	↓	↓	↓
D.	↓	↓	↑
E.	No change	No change	No change

46 A 58-year-old man with type 2 diabetes has a hemoglobin A_{1c} level of 9.2% (77 mmol/mol) while on a treatment regimen with triple oral agents. Initiation of insulin therapy is recommended. After some discussion, he agrees to start once-daily basal insulin. His job requires frequent travel across time zones, and he wonders if it will be a problem to time the basal insulin injections when he travels to Australia or Latin America. He is concerned about the risk of hypoglycemia while traveling.

Formulary issues aside, which of the following regimens should be recommended for this patient?

A. Insulin degludec; take it at his convenience once daily
B. NPH insulin at bedtime; give at the same time as he would take it at home
C. U100 insulin glargine; give every morning regardless of last injection
D. U300 insulin glargine; give at the same time as he would take it at home

47 A 45-year-old woman presents for evaluation of hypoglycemia. She has had hyperadrenergic symptoms intermittently for 1 year with increasing frequency. In the last 3 months, she has also had episodes of confusion, and 2 weeks ago, she was taken to the hospital after a colleague found her to be slurring her words during a meeting. At that time, her blood glucose concentration measured in the emergency department was 39 mg/dL (2.2 mmol/L). All of her episodes of neuroglycopenia have occurred during the day, and she attributes them to either small meals or meals with large amounts of "sweets." She has not had nocturnal or fasting spells, although she notes that she eats cheese and crackers every night at bedtime. Her symptoms invariably improve with carbohydrate intake. There is a history of heavy alcohol consumption, with associated seizures and withdrawal, but she reports being sober for 6 months. She is currently taking no medications and does not use illicit drugs. She has no family history of diabetes. She lives alone and works fulltime.

On physical examination, her BMI is 28.0 kg/m^2, and she has no other notable features.

The patient returns with a family member for a blood draw after a 12-hour fast. She reports feeling "shaky." Following the blood draw, her symptom is resolved after she consumes 6 oz of juice.

Glucose = 52 mg/dL (70-99 mg/dL)
(SI: 2.9 mmol/L [3.9-5.5 mmol/L])
Insulin = 14 μIU/mL (1.4-14.0 μIU/mL)
(SI: 97.2 pmol/L [9.7-97.2 pmol/L])
C-peptide = 1.5 ng/mL (0.5-2.0 ng/mL)
(SI: 0.5 nmol/L [0.17-0.66 nmol/L])
Cortisol = 21 μg/dL (5-25 μg/dL) (SI: 579.3 nmol/L [137.9-689.7 nmol/L])
TSH = 1.2 mIU/L (0.5-5.0 mIU/L)
IGF-1 = 225 ng/mL (98-261 ng/mL)
(SI: 29.5 nmol/L [12.8-34.2 nmol/L])

An additional blood tube is set aside.

Which of the following additional laboratory tests would be most helpful in making the diagnosis?

A. β-Hydroxybutyrate measurement
B. Blood alcohol level
C. IGF-2 measurement
D. Insulin antibody measurement
E. Sulfonylurea screen

48 A 34-year-old woman delivered a baby 2 years ago. During that pregnancy, she was treated for gestational diabetes with a reduced carbohydrate diet and exercise and was able to maintain her fingerstick blood glucose levels within the target range and her hemoglobin A_{1c} level less than 6.5% (<48 mmol/mol). After delivery, her glycemia normalized. Twelve weeks post partum, her 2-hour plasma glucose concentration during a follow-up oral glucose tolerance test was documented to be 136 mg/dL (7.5 mmol/L). She now presents 6 weeks after her last menstrual period, with a positive pregnancy test confirmed by her obstetrician. She currently has no symptoms of diabetes.

Which of the following approaches is currently recommended to evaluate this woman's glycemic status?

A. Measure hemoglobin A_{1c} now; if normal, perform a 75-g oral glucose tolerance test at 24 to 28 weeks' gestation
B. Measure hemoglobin A_{1c} now; if normal, perform a 100-g oral glucose tolerance test at 24 to 28 weeks' gestation
C. Perform a 50-g oral glucose tolerance test at 24 to 28 weeks' gestation
D. Perform a 75-g oral glucose tolerance test now; if normal, measure hemoglobin A_{1c} at 24 to 28 weeks' gestation

49 A 28-year-old man with type 1 diabetes is concerned about the possibility of future erectile dysfunction. He has had diabetes for 3 years, without any microvascular complications. His treatment regimen consists of basal and mealtime insulins. His most recent hemoglobin A_{1c} measurement is 8.5% (69 mmol/mol). He takes lisinopril for kidney protection.

Which of the following should be recommended to address his main concern?

A. Initiate continuous glucose monitoring
B. Initiate saw palmetto
C. Measure testosterone annually
D. Nothing, his risk is high and will not change with intervention
E. Stop lisinopril

50 A 53-year-old woman with a 13-year history of type 2 diabetes has known chronic kidney disease. Metformin was recently discontinued during a hospitalization for acute kidney injury due to taking high-dosage ibuprofen for gout.

Laboratory test results:

Hemoglobin A_{1c} = 7.2% (4.0%-5.6%) (55 mmol/mol [20-38 mmol/mol])
Estimated glomerular filtration rate: 54 mL/min per 1.73 m^2 (>60 mL/min per 1.73 m^2)
Urinary albumin-to-creatinine ratio = 226 mg/g (<30 mg/g creat)

Empagliflozin is prescribed.

Which of the following correctly describes this therapy's mechanism of action in this patient?

A. Blocks SGLT-2 in the distal renal tubule
B. Down-regulates SGLT-2 transporter in the S1 segment of the distal renal tubule
C. Lowers the renal threshold for glucose excretion to less than 100 mg/dL
D. Lowers the renal threshold for glucose excretion to 180 mg/dL
E. Up-regulates the SGLT-2 transporter in the S3 segment of the proximal renal tubule

51 A 67-year-old woman presents with questions about new treatments for type 2 diabetes. Since her diagnosis 6 years ago, she has been treated with a sulfonylurea because of intolerance to metformin. She is now taking glipizide, 10 mg twice daily, and she documents blood glucose values that are generally less than 150 mg/dL (<8.3 mmol/L) with home glucose monitoring. However, since starting therapy, she has gained 15 lb (6.8 kg) and is frustrated with her inability to lose weight. Findings on hepatic ultrasonography performed last year were consistent with steatosis. She recently saw an ad in a magazine touting empagliflozin and is very interested in a "diabetes pill that causes weight loss." She takes hydrochlorothiazide and lisinopril for hypertension and atorvastatin for elevated cholesterol. She has no history of diabetes-related complications.

On physical examination, her weight is 208 lb (94.5 kg) (BMI = 35.0 kg/m^2), and blood pressure is 136/84 mm Hg. She has no signs of neuropathy.

Laboratory test results (sample drawn while fasting):

Glucose = 166 mg/dL (70-99 mg/dL) (SI: 9.2 mmol/L [3.9-5.5 mmol/L])
Hemoglobin A_{1c} = 8.4% (4.0%-5.6%) (68 mmol/mol [20-38 mmol/mol])
Triglycerides = 217 mg/dL (<150 mg/dL [optimal]) (SI: 2.45 mmol/L [<1.70 mmol/L])
LDL cholesterol = 92 mg/dL (<100 mg/dL [for primary prevention]) (SI: 2.38 mmol/L [<2.59 mmol/L])
Creatinine = 1.9 mg/dL (0.6-1.1 mg/dL) (SI: 168.0 μmol/L [53.0-97.2 μmol/L])

Estimated glomerular filtration rate = 42 mL/min per m^2 (>60 mL/min per 1.73 m^2)
AST = 47 U/L (20-48 U/L) (SI: 0.78 μkat/L [0.33-0.80 μkat/L])
ALT = 41 U/L (10-40 U/L) (SI: 0.68 μkat/L [0.17-0.67 μkat/L])
Albumin = 3.9 (3.5-5.0 g/dL) (SI: 39 g/L [35-50 g/L])
Calcium = 8.9 mg/dL (8.2-10.2 mg/dL) (SI: 2.2 mmol/L [2.1-2.6 mmol/L])
Phosphate = 3.7 mg/dL (2.3-4.7 mg/dL) (SI: 1.2 mmol/L [0.7-1.5 mmol/L])
TSH = 2.3 mIU/L (0.5-5.0 mIU/L)
Urinary albumin-to-creatinine ratio = 110 mg/g creat (<30 mg/g creat)

The patient is eager to start an SGLT-2 inhibitor.

In counseling this patient, which of the following is expected to be a limitation of empagliflozin therapy?

A. Causes only transient weight loss with weight regain in 1 to 2 months
B. Does not sufficiently decrease blood glucose levels
C. Exacerbates hepatic steatosis
D. Improves proteinuria but worsens estimated glomerular filtration in the long term
E. Interferes with the effectiveness of her antihypertensive regimen

52 A 32-year-old woman with a 10-year history of type 1 diabetes attends a follow-up visit. She has no other medical problems. Findings on her last eye examination 6 months ago were normal. Her menses are regular. She is not planning pregnancy soon. She uses an insulin pump with a continuous glucose monitor. Her only medication is insulin aspart.

On physical examination, her BMI is 22.0 kg/m^2 and blood pressure is 110/60 mm Hg. Examination findings are unremarkable.

Laboratory test results:

Measurement	3 Months ago	Current
Hemoglobin A_{1c}	6.4% (46 mmol/mol)	6.9% (52 mmol/mol)
Serum creatinine	0.6 mg/dL (SI: 53.0 μmol/L)	0.6 mg/dL (SI: 53.0 μmol/L)
Electrolytes, TSH, liver enzymes, complete blood cell count	Normal	Normal
Urine albumin-to-creatinine ratio	22 mg/g creat	345 mg/g creat
Pregnancy test	NA	Negative

Which of the following is the best next step in this patient's management?

A. Add canagliflozin
B. Add losartan
C. Add ramipril
D. Lower hemoglobin A_{1c} to less than 6.5% (<48 mmol/mol)
E. Repeat measurement of the urinary albumin-to-creatinine ratio

Female Reproduction Board Review

Margaret Flynn Lippincott, MD

1 A 20-year-old White woman presents for evaluation of patient-important hirsutism. She reports thelarche at age 11 years and menarche at age 15 years. She describes monthly bleeding, with the shortest interval between periods of 20 days. She has about 16 periods a year. She is frustrated by increased hair growth on her chin and abdomen, which she first noted at age 13. The hair growth has been gradually getting worse. She reports that her weight has been stable.

On physical examination, her BMI is 35.0 kg/m^2 and blood pressure is 118/76 mm Hg. She has an increased amount of coarse terminal hair on the upper lip, chin, neck, abdomen, and back. Her modified Ferriman-Gallwey score is 10. She has no clitoromegaly or deepened voice. She has no acanthosis nigricans.

Her primary care physician ordered the following laboratory tests before referring her to endocrinology:

- FSH = 5.0 mIU/mL (2.0-12.0 mIU/mL) (SI: 5.0 IU/L [2.0-12.0 IU/L])
- Estradiol = 45 pg/mL (10-180 pg/mL) (SI:165.2 pmol/L [36.7-660.8 pmol/L])
- Testosterone = 35 ng/dL (8-60 ng/dL) (SI: 1.2 nmol/L [0.3-2.1 nmol/L])
- TSH = 3.0 mIU/L (0.5-5.0 mIU/L)
- Hemoglobin A_{1c} = 5.0% (4.5%-5.6%) (31 mmol/mol [26-38 mmol/mol])
- Prolactin = 7 ng/mL (4-30 ng/mL) (SI: 0.30 nmol/L [0.17-1.30 nmol/L])

Which of the following additional tests is required to confirm this patient's diagnosis?

A. No additional testing needed
B. Serum 17-hydroxyprogesterone measurement
C. Serum free testosterone measurement
D. SHBG measurement
E. Transvaginal ultrasonography

2 A 48-year-old Black transwoman with a history of hypertension and hyperlipidemia presents for annual care. Her regimen consists of leuprolide acetate depot formulation, 11.25 mg every 3 months, and oral estradiol, 2 mg daily. She transitioned 20 years ago, but she was only able to obtain approval for gonadotropin-releasing hormone agonist therapy in the past 5 years. She is happy with her breast growth after having breast augmentation surgery. She has had no health issues in the past year. She recently lost a friend to cancer and is interested in keeping up to date with any cancer screening recommendations.

On physical examination, her BMI is 28 kg/m^2 and blood pressure is 129/76 mm Hg. She has no peripheral edema, and her cardiovascular examination findings are unremarkable. She has Tanner stage 5 breasts. She has a well-estrogenized neo-vagina.

In addition to her gender-affirming hormone therapy, she also takes lisinopril, 10 mg daily, and atorvastatin, 40 mg daily.

Recent laboratory test results:

- Hemoglobin A_{1c} = 5.6% (4.0%-5.6%) (38 mmol/mol [20-38 mmol/mol])
- LDL cholesterol = 105 mg/dL (<100 mg/dL [optimal]) (SI: 2.72 mmol/L [<2.59 mmol/L])
- Total cholesterol = 195 mg/dL (<200 mg/dL [optimal]) (SI: 5.05 mmol/L [<5.18 mmol/L])

Triglycerides = 149 mg/dL (<150 mg/dL [optimal]) (SI: 1.68 mmol/L [<1.70 mmol/L])

Which of the following is the best next step in this patient's care?

A. An increase in the lisinopril dosage to 20 mg daily
B. Mammography
C. Mammography and PSA measurement
D. PSA measurement
E. No additional testing or medication adjustment

3 A 35-year-old woman with polycystic ovary syndrome, class 3 obesity, and a seizure disorder would like to discuss contraceptive options. Her seizures are controlled with carbamazepine. She reports she naturally gets her period every 3 to 4 months.

On physical examination, her BMI is 42 kg/m^2 and blood pressure is 142/78 mm Hg.

Which of the following is the best birth control option for this patient?

A. Copper intrauterine device
B. Ethinyl estradiol, 20 mcg daily/norethindrone acetate, 1 mg daily
C. Etonogestrel/ethinyl estradiol vaginal ring
D. Levonorgestrel-releasing intrauterine device
E. Norethindrone, 0.35 mg daily

4 A 53-year-old Black woman with a medical history of class 3 obesity, hypertension, hyperlipidemia, type 2 diabetes, and polycystic ovary syndrome presents to discuss treatment of her hot flashes. Her last menstrual period was 2 years ago. For the past 3 years, she has struggled with daily hot flashes and night sweats that interfere with her job and sleep. She did not tolerate gabapentin due to drowsiness. She is currently taking citalopram, 20 mg daily, which was increased from a starting dosage of 10 mg daily. She continues to experience daily hot flashes and severe night sweats at least once per week. Additional medications include lisinopril, 20 mg daily; rosuvastatin, 10 mg daily; and metformin, 2000 mg daily.

On physical examination, her BMI is 38 kg/m^2 and blood pressure is 140/89 mm Hg.

Laboratory test results:

Hemoglobin A_{1c} = 7.2% (4.0%-5.6%) (55 mmol/mol [20-38 mmol/mol])
LDL cholesterol = 165 mg/dL (<100 mg/dL [optimal]) (SI: 4.27 mmol/L [<2.59 mmol/L])
Total cholesterol = 235 mg/dL (<200 mg/dL [optimal]) (SI: 6.09 mmol/L [<5.18 mmol/L])
Triglycerides = 149 mg/dL (<150 mg/dL [optimal]) (SI: 1.68 mmol/L [<1.70 mmol/L])
HDL cholesterol = 40 mg/dL (>60 mg/dL [optimal]) (SI: 1.04 mmol/L [>1.55 mmol/L])
AST = 40 U/L (20-48 U/L) (SI: 0.67 μkat/L [0.33-0.80 μkat/L])
ALT = 35 U/L (10-40 U/L) (SI: 0.58 μkat/L [0.17-0.67 μkat/L])

Which of the following is the best next step in this patient's care?

A. Prescribe clonidine patch
B. Prescribe fezolinetant, 45 mg daily
C. Prescribe transdermal estradiol, 25 mcg patch, and oral micronized progesterone, 100 mg nightly
D. Recommend using cooling techniques (eg, fan, looser clothing)
E. Refer for mindfulness-based interventions

5 A 28-year-old woman with polycystic ovary syndrome presents for evaluation of "PMS." Menarche was at age 10 years, and her cycles occur every 30 to 45 days. She describes bloating, breast tenderness, increased irritability, headache, and worsening mood in the week before her periods (most, but not all, periods). She finds these symptoms interfere with her work and personal life, and she has been taking unscheduled vacation days to cope. The symptoms resolve with the onset of her period. She does not feel depressed during other times of the month. Previous workup has demonstrated elevated progesterone concentrations greater than 5 ng/mL (>15.9 nmol/L) when she is symptomatic. She has no family history of clotting disorders. She is satisfied with topical treatments for hirsutism.

Which of the following is the first-line treatment recommendation to address this patient's concern?

A. Cyclic low-dosage oral contraceptive pill
B. GnRH agonist (eg, leuprolide)
C. Norelgestromin, 6.0 mg, and ethinyl estradiol, 0.75 mg patch
D. Norethindrone, 0.35 mg daily
E. Selective serotonin reuptake inhibitor

6 A 20-year-old woman with a 4-year history of functional hypothalamic amenorrhea comes to clinic for follow-up. She has a history of excessive exercise and restricted eating. BMI at her initial visit was 17.5 kg/m^2, and she had low bone mineral density (Z-score at femoral neck, −2.2). She was counseled that her low bone mineral density is related to her nutrition and excessive exercise, as evaluation for secondary causes was negative.

Eighteen months ago, she decided to implement lifestyle changes by moderating her exercise and improving her nutrition. Her weight has increased, and her BMI is now 19 kg/m^2. She is pleased that she has been able to make these changes but is disappointed that her periods have not returned. She wonders whether something else is wrong.

Laboratory test results:

hCG = <3.0 mIU/mL (<3.0 mIU/mL) (SI: <3.0 IU/L [<3.0 IU/L])
TSH = 4.5 mIU/L (0.5-5.0 mIU/L)
Prolactin = 25 ng/mL (4-30 ng/mL) (SI: 1.09 nmol/L [0.17-1.30 nmol/L])
Estradiol = 110 pg/mL (10-180 pg/mL) (SI: 403.8 pmol/L [36.7-660.8 pmol/L])
LH = 2.0 mIU/mL (1.0-18.0 mIU/mL) (SI: 2.0 IU/L [1.0-18.0 IU/L])
FSH = 4.0 mIU/mL (2.0-12.0 mIU/mL) (SI: 4.0 IU/L [2.0-12.0 IU/L])
Progesterone = 3.5 ng/mL (≤1.0 ng/mL) (SI: 11.1 nmol/L [≤3.2 nmol/L])

Which of the following should be recommended now?

A. No treatment
B. Isoflavone supplements
C. Start alendronate, 70 mg weekly
D. Start a low-dosage combined estrogen-progestin oral contraceptive
E. Start transdermal 0.1 mg 17β-estradiol patch with cyclic micronized progesterone, 200 mg

7 A 23-year-old woman presents with irregular menses followed by amenorrhea. Menarche was at age 14 years; her periods were irregular for 18 months, then regular every 28 days. About 2 years ago, her cycle length shortened to 25 days and then to 22 days. She has not had a period in 4 months. She is stressed in her new job. She runs 2 miles 3 times a week. Her BMI is 22 kg/m^2, and she has no evidence of hirsutism or acne.

A pregnancy test is negative. Her TSH value is 4.0 mIU/L (0.5-5.0 mIU/L).

In addition to FSH, which of the following should be measured now?

A. Estradiol and 17-hydroxyprogesterone
B. Estradiol and progesterone
C. Estradiol and prolactin
D. Late-night salivary cortisol
E. LH, testosterone, and DHEA-S

8 A 32-year-old woman is referred for anovulatory infertility. She has a history of irregular periods, acne, hirsutism, and obesity. Polycystic ovary syndrome was diagnosed at age 16 years. She continues to have irregular cycles (32 to 50 days), and she has been trying to conceive for the past 9 months. Metformin was started 3 months ago to induce ovulation. She has had 2 periods since then but has not conceived. Serum hCG is negative.

On physical examination, her blood pressure is 125/80 mm Hg and BMI is 34 kg/m^2.

Which of the following treatments would be the most appropriate next step in this patient's care?

A. Clomiphene citrate
B. Continuation of metformin alone
C. Gonadotropin therapy with recombinant FSH
D. Letrozole
E. Progesterone suppositories

9 A 26-year-old woman presents with a change in her intermenstrual interval. Menarche was at age 11 years, and she had regular menses during high school and college. She took an oral contraceptive pill from age 17 to 22 years. After stopping the oral contraceptive, she initially had 28- to 32-day cycles, but more recently she has been having menses every 22 to 23 days. She exercises for 1 hour 3 times weekly. She has premenstrual acne, no hot flashes, and no galactorrhea. Her BMI is 20 kg/m^2.

Laboratory test results (sample drawn on cycle day 3):

FSH = 40.0 mIU/mL (2.0-12.0 mIU/mL [follicular]) (SI: 40.0 IU/L [2.0-12.0 IU/L])
LH = 35.0 mIU/mL (1.0-18.0 mIU/mL [follicular]) (SI: 35.0 IU/L [1.0-18.0 IU/L])
Estradiol = 70 pg/mL (10-180 pg/mL [follicular]) (SI: 257.0 pmol/L [36.7-660.8 pmol/L])
Antimullerian hormone = 0.9 ng/mL (0.9-9.5 ng/mL) (SI: 6.4 pmol/L [6.4-67.9 pmol/L])
TSH = 4.0 mIU/L (0.5-5.0 mIU/L)
Karyotype = 46,XX
FMR1 gene testing, no premutation detected

Which of the following is most important to measure next?

A. GAD-65 antibodies
B. 21-Hydroxylase antibodies
C. IGF-1
D. Inhibin B
E. Serum ovarian antibodies

10 A 38-year-old woman with a history of premenstrual mood changes and polycystic ovary syndrome (polycystic ovaries on ultrasonography, acne, and mild-moderate hirsutism) presents for evaluation. Her menstrual cycles are usually regular (every 28-34 days). She is currently using topical agents for acne and local measures for hirsutism. She recalls taking a combined estrogen-progestin oral contraceptive briefly as a teenager for acne, but she stopped it during the first cycle because of nausea. The possibility of starting a low-dosage continuous regimen of a combined oral contraceptive (ethinyl estradiol, 20 mcg/norethindrone 1 mg) is discussed, as this would benefit her premenstrual mood changes, hirsutism, and acne. She is willing to try it again; however, she remains very concerned about adverse effects.

On physical examination, her BMI is 29 kg/m^2, she has moderate facial acne, and her modified Ferriman-Gallwey score is 9.

Which of the following symptoms is this patient most likely to experience on the recommended therapy?

A. Depression
B. Hypertension
C. Sexual dysfunction
D. Unscheduled bleeding (breakthrough bleeding)
E. Weight gain

11 A 27-year-old pregnant woman sees her obstetrician for her 25-week visit. She is excited about her pregnancy because it took 18 months to conceive. Before pregnancy, her menstrual cycles occurred every 4 to 6 weeks. She is very concerned about new, rapidly progressing symptoms that began 5 weeks ago, including excess hair, deepening of her voice, and clitoral enlargement. Her only medications are prenatal vitamins and some dietary supplements. Her husband is in good health and takes no medication.

On physical examination, her blood pressure is 105/60 mm Hg. She has facial acne. There are terminal hairs on her upper lip, chin, neck, midsternum, and upper and lower back. A modified Ferriman-Gallwey score is 12 (score >8 = hirsutism). She has clitoromegaly (8 × 5 mm = 40 mm^2 [upper limit of normal = 35 mm^2]), and her voice is deep. There is no increased supraclavicular fullness or dorsocervical fat accumulation. She has lightly pigmented, narrow striae on her lower abdomen and hips.

Total testosterone = 953 ng/dL (8-60 ng/dL)
(SI: 8.7 nmol/L [0.3-2.1 nmol/L])
DHEA-S = 200 µg/dL (44-332 µg/dL)
(SI: 5.42 µmol/L [1.19-9.00 µmol/L])
LH = 5.0 mIU/mL (SI: 5.0 IU/L)
FSH = 2.5 mIU/mL (SI: 2.5 IU/L)

Pelvic ultrasonography shows polycystic ovary morphology and bilateral, solid ovarian masses. The left ovary has a 2 × 7-cm nodular mass with no cystic components, and the right ovary has a 3 × 5-cm nodular mass with no cystic components. A normal-appearing female fetus is visualized (consistent with 25 weeks' gestation).

Which of the following is the most likely cause of this patient's virilization?

A. Dietary supplements
B. Luteomas of pregnancy
C. Nonclassic congenital adrenal hyperplasia due to 21-hydroxylase deficiency
D. Polycystic ovary syndrome
E. Theca lutein cysts

12 A 52-year-old woman presents with concerns of scalp hair loss and facial hair growth. Menarche was at age 12 years, and she had regular menses during her reproductive years. Her final menstrual period was 3 years ago. Over the past 4 to 5 years, she has gained weight and developed acne, hirsutism, and hair loss.

On physical examination, her BMI is 34 kg/m^2 (compared with 29 kg/m^2 4 years ago). Blood pressure is 150/90 mm Hg. She has terminal hairs on her upper lip, chin, and neck, as well as hair on her upper abdomen, lower back, and mid-sternum with a Ferriman-Gallwey score of 12. She has thinning hair over the frontal scalp and vertex of the scalp. She has acanthosis nigricans in the axillae and on the neck and elbows. Her clitoris measures 11 mm × 5 mm (upper normal limit for clitoral index is 35 mm^2).

Laboratory test results:
Testosterone = 200 ng/dL (8-60 ng/dL)
(SI: 6.9 nmol/L [0.3-2.1 nmol/L])
DHEA-S = 120 µg/dL (15-200 µg/dL)
(SI: 3.25 µmol/L [0.41-5.42 µmol/L])
FSH = 19.0 mIU/mL (>30.0 mIU/mL [postmenopausal]) (SI: 19.0 IU/L [>30.0 IU/L])
LH = 12.0 mIU/mL (>30.0 mIU/mL [postmenopausal]) (SI: 12.0 IU/L [>30.0 IU/L])

Which of the following is the best next test to evaluate this patient?

A. Adrenal CT
B. 1-mg Dexamethasone-suppression test
C. Serum 17-hydroxyprogesterone measurement
D. Serum inhibin measurement
E. Transvaginal ultrasonography

13 A 42-year-old woman seeks advice on the treatment of menopausal symptoms. Six months ago, she underwent a total abdominal hysterectomy and bilateral salpingo-oophorectomy for a history of leiomyomata. Since her surgery, she has had intractable hot flashes (both at night and during the day). She is otherwise in excellent health and has no contraindications to hormone therapy.

Which of the following should be suggested for her hot flashes?

A. Estradiol, 50 mcg patch twice weekly, and micronized progesterone, 100 mg daily
B. Gabapentin, 300 to 900 mg daily
C. Micronized progesterone, 100 mg nightly
D. Oral 17β-estradiol, 2 mg daily
E. Venlafaxine, 75 mg daily

14 A 38-year-old woman seeks evaluation of hormonal symptoms that are becoming increasingly difficult to manage. She has always had minor mood changes before her periods. However, for the past 2 years, she has experienced premenstrual anger, irritability, and tearfulness that start approximately 6 days before menses and continue until day 2 or 3 of menses. These symptoms are accompanied by bloating, night sweats, and fatigue, and she has difficulty functioning at work. The patient's menstrual cycles occur approximately once monthly.

On physical examination, her BMI is 24 kg/m^2, pulse rate is 88 beats/min, and blood pressure is 130/80 mm Hg.

Which of the following is the best next step to confirm her diagnosis?

A. Daily prospective symptom diary for 2 cycles
B. Day 3 serum FSH measurement
C. Depression screening
D. Serum antimullerian hormone measurement
E. Serum TSH measurement

15 A 17-year-old woman requests evaluation for primary amenorrhea. She reports a healthy childhood. Pubic hair appeared at age 10 years and breast development started at age 12 years, but she has never menstruated. She is sexually active.

On physical examination, her height is 65 in (165 cm) and weight is 132 lb (60 kg) (BMI = 22 kg/m^2). Mild acne is noted on her face and back. Several dark hairs are present on her upper lip and chest. The patient has Tanner stage 5 breasts and stage 5 pubic hair.

Laboratory test results:

Serum LH = 5.0 mIU/L (1.0-18.0 mIU/L)
(SI: 5.0 IU/L [1.0-18.0 IU/L])
FSH = 4.0 mIU/mL (2.0-12.0 mIU/mL)
(SI: 4.0 IU/L [2.0-12.0 IU/L])
Serum prolactin = 15 ng/mL (4-23 ng/mL)
(SI: 0.65 nmol/L [0.17-1.00 nmol/L])
Serum estradiol = 35 pg/mL (10-180 pg/mL)
(SI: 128.5 pmol/L [36.7-660.8 pmol/L])
Serum testosterone = 29 ng/dL (8-60 ng/dL)
(SI: 1.0 nmol/L [0.3-2.1 nmol/L])

Pelvic ultrasonography reveals the absence of a uterus.

Which of the following is this patient's most likely karyotype?

A. 45,X
B. 46,XX
C. 46,XY
D. 45,X/46,XX
E. 47,XXY

16 A 24-year-old transgender woman is referred to discuss hormone therapy. Preferred pronouns are female (she/her/hers). She has disclosed her gender dysphoria to family and close friends and is seeing a therapist, who recommended that she seek information about gender-affirming hormone therapy. For the past year, she has experimented with wearing make-up and dressing in feminine clothes on the weekends. She uses gender-neutral bathrooms at work. Her medical history is notable for heterozygosity for a factor V Leiden pathogenic variant identified on screening after her mother had an unprovoked pulmonary embolism. She does not smoke cigarettes and takes no medications.

On physical examination, her BMI is 22 kg/m^2 and blood pressure is 110/70 mm Hg.

Which of the following would be the most appropriate initial hormone regimen for this patient?

A. Leuprolide, 3.75 mg intramuscularly, plus estradiol, 2 mg orally
B. Leuprolide, 3.75 mg intramuscularly, plus estradiol, 50 mcg by transdermal patch
C. Low-dosage birth control pill containing 20 mcg of ethinyl estradiol and drospirenone plus spironolactone, 100 mg orally
D. Spironolactone, 100 mg, and finasteride, 5 mg orally
E. Spironolactone, 200 mg, plus estradiol, 1 mg orally

Male Reproduction Board Review

Stephanie Page, MD, PhD

1 A 69-year-old man is referred for evaluation and treatment of suspected hypogonadism. He describes decreased libido, increased fatigue, and gradual weight gain over the last 10 years. He has type 2 diabetes managed without insulin, hypertension, hypercholesterolemia, and a history of COVID-19 infection for which he was hospitalized for 4 days (3 months ago). He and his wife have 3 grown children in their 30s.

Medications:

Metformin, 1000 mg twice daily
Empaglifozin, 10 mg daily
Lisinopril, 10 mg daily
Atorvastatin, 40 mg daily

His primary care physician obtained the following laboratory results at his post discharge visit, 1 week following his hospitalization:

Comprehensive metabolic panel, normal
Liver function, normal
Creatinine = 1.4 mg/dL (0.7-1.3 mg/dL) (SI: 123.8 µmol/L [61.9-114.9 µmol/L])
Hemoglobin = 15.8 g/dL (13.8-17.2 g/dL) (SI: 158 g/L [138-172 g/L])
Hematocrit = 49% (41%-51%) (SI: 0.49 [0.41-0.51])
Hemoglobin A_{1c} = 7.7% (4.0%-5.6%) (61 mmol/mol [20-38 mmol/mol])
Total testosterone = 170 ng/dL (300-900 ng/dL) (SI: 5.9 nmol/L [10.4-31.2 nmol/L])
Free testosterone = 7.5 ng/dL (9.0-30.0 ng/dL) (SI: 0.26 nmol/L [0.31-1.04 nmol/L])
COVID 19, PCR negative

On physical examination, his blood pressure is 142/91 mm Hg and pulse rate is 82 beats/min. His weight is 260 lb (117.9 kg) (BMI = 32.0 kg/m^2), and he has central adiposity. He has normal male-pattern hair and no gynecomastia. On genitourinary examination, he has 20-cc testes bilaterally and a normal phallus.

Laboratory test results (sample drawn while fasting at 8 AM):

Total testosterone = 240 ng/dL (300-900 ng/dL) (SI: 8.33 nmol/L [10.4-31.2 nmol/L])
Free testosterone = 8.5 ng/dL (9.0-30.0 ng/dL) (SI: 0.29 nmol/L [0.31-1.04 nmol/L])

Which of the following is the best next step in this patient's care?

A. Initiate daily testosterone transdermal gel after appropriate counseling regarding risks and benefits of testosterone therapy
B. Initiate intramuscular testosterone enanthate, 150 mg every 2 weeks, after appropriate counseling regarding risks and benefits of testosterone therapy
C. Refer for nutritional counseling and encourage him to exercise for 30 minutes 3 to 4 times weekly
D. Repeat morning fasting total and free testosterone measurement with concomitant LH and FSH in 1 month
E. Screen for depression with a Patient Health Questionnaire 9

2 A 66-year-old man is referred for consideration of testosterone therapy. His concerns include decreased libido, erectile dysfunction, depressed mood, mental "fogginess," fatigue, gradual weight gain of approximately 15 lb (6.8 kg), and decreased stamina on daily walks with his wife (45 minutes) and at his regular weekly tennis game. His symptoms have gotten worse since he retired 2 years ago. He is a nonsmoker and has no history of diabetes, cardiovascular disease, or pulmonary disease. His only medications are hydrochlorothiazide for hypertension and atorvastatin, 40 mg daily, for hypercholesterolemia.

Findings on physical examination, including genitourinary examination, are unremarkable. His blood pressure is 128/78 mm Hg, pulse rate is 72 beats/min, and weight is 221 lb (100.2 kg) (BMI = 28 kg/m^2).

Laboratory test results (sample drawn while fasting at 8 AM):

Total testosterone = 239 ng/dL (300-900 ng/dL) (SI: 8.4 nmol/L [10.4-31.2 nmol/L])
Free testosterone = 7.5 ng/dL (9.0-30.0 ng/dL) (SI: 0.26 nmol/L [0.31-1.04 nmol/L])
Hemoglobin = 13.1 g/dL (13.8-17.2 g/dL) (SI: 131 g/L [138-172 g/L])
Hematocrit = 39% (41%-51%) (SI: 0.39 [0.41-0.51])
Complete blood cell count, normal
Comprehensive metabolic panel, normal
Liver function, normal
Total cholesterol = 212 mg/dL (<200 mg/dL [optimal]) (SI: 5.49 mmol/L [<5.18 mmol/L])
LDL cholesterol = 120 mg/dL (<100 mg/dL [optimal]) (SI: 3.11 mmol/L [<2.59 mmol/L])
HDL cholesterol = 45 mg/dL (>60 mg/dL [optimal]) (SI: 1.17 mmol/L [>1.55 mmol/L])
Triglycerides = 100 mg/dL (<150 mg/dL [optimal]) (SI: 1.13 mmol/L [<1.70 mmol/L])

Repeat morning laboratory test results 3 weeks later:

Total testosterone = 247 ng/dL (SI: 8.6 nmol/L)
Free testosterone = 8.1 ng/dL (SI: 0.28 nmol/L)
FSH = 4.4 mIU/mL (1.0-13.0 mIU/mL) (SI: 4.4 IU/L [1.0-13.0 IU/L])
LH = 5.1 mIU/mL (1.0-9.0 mIU/mL) (SI: 6.1 IU/L [1.0-9.0 IU/L])
PSA = 1.4 ng/mL (<5.3 ng/mL) (SI: 1.4 μg/L [<5.3 μg/L])

Testosterone therapy with transdermal testosterone gel is recommended.

In counseling this patient regarding possible risks and benefits of testosterone therapy, evidence from large, randomized controlled trials supports that testosterone therapy is most likely to do which of the following?

A. Improve his anemia
B. Improve his cognition and "mental fogginess"
C. Increase his risk of myocardial infarction or stroke
D. Reduce his risk of hip fracture
E. Significantly lower his LDL cholesterol

3 A 54-year-old transgender man is referred for initiation of gender-affirming hormone therapy. He has been living as a man for more than a year and has a mental health provider who affirms ongoing care. He does not smoke cigarettes. He takes lisinopril for hypertension and sertraline for depression and anxiety. His father has prostate cancer, and his youngest sister had breast cancer at age 39 years. He exercises regularly and had cessation of menses approximately 1 year ago and is no longer bothered by hot flashes.

On physical examination, his blood pressure is 135/92 mm Hg, weight is 165 lb (74.8 kg), BMI is 27 kg/m^2, and pulse rate is 72 beats/min.

Laboratory test results:

Hemoglobin = 15.1 g/dL (13.8-17.2 g/dL) (SI: 151 g/L [138-172 g/L])
Hematocrit = 45% (41%-51%) (SI: 0.45 [0.41-0.51])
Comprehensive metabolic panel, normal
Liver function, normal

Testosterone enanthate, 200 mg intramuscularly every 2 weeks, is prescribed. At a follow-up appointment 3 months later, he is pleased that he has experienced some facial hair growth.

Physical examination findings are remarkable for significantly increased facial and axillary hair: blood pressure is 155/85 mm Hg, weight is 169 lb (76.7 kg), BMI is 27.5 kg/m^2, and pulse rate is 82 beats/min.

Laboratory test results (sample drawn midweek through his injection interval):

Total testosterone = 550 ng/dL (300-900 ng/dL) (SI: 19.1 nmol/L [10.4-31.2 nmol/L])
Hemoglobin = 16.5 g/dL (13.8-17.2 g/dL) (SI: 165 g/L [138-172 g/L])
Hematocrit = 48% (41%-51%) (SI: 0.48 [0.41-0.51])

Which of the following is the best next step in his care:

A. Change the testosterone enanthate dosing to 100 mg every week
B. Decrease the testosterone enanthate dosage to 175 mg every 2 weeks
C. Ensure that he is up-to-date with mammography
D. Measure PSA
E. Refer for oophorectomy

4 A 44-year-old man is referred for evaluation of low libido. He is recently divorced with 2 children and is interested in beginning online dating but is concerned that he has little sexual interest and diminished morning erections. He is otherwise healthy with the exception of chronic low back pain treated with physical therapy, nonsteroidal anti-inflammatory agents, and occasional doses of hydrocodone with pain flares.

On physical examination, his BMI is 23 kg/m^2. He has normal secondary sexual characteristics and normal testicular size. His neurologic examination reveals no focal deficits.

Laboratory test results (sample drawn while fasting at 8 AM):

Total testosterone = 110 ng/dL (300-900 ng/dL) (SI: 3.8 nmol/L [10.4-31.2 nmol/L])
LH = 1.0 mIU/mL (1.0-9.0 mIU/mL) (SI: 1.0 IU/L [1.0-9.0 IU/L])
FSH = 1.2 mIU/mL (1.0-13.0 mIU/mL) (SI: 1.2 IU/L [1.0-11.0 IU/L])

Repeated morning testosterone evaluation and additional laboratory test results:

Total testosterone = 130 ng/dL (SI: 4.5 nmol/L)
TSH = 1.2 mIU/L (0.5-5.0 mIU/L)
Free T_4 = 1.1 ng/dL (0.8-1.8 ng/dL) (SI: 14.2 nmol/L [0.31-1.04 nmol/L])
Prolactin= 10 ng/mL (0.43 nmol/L) (4-23 ng/mL (SI: 0.43 nmol/L [0.17-1.00 nmol/L])
Complete blood cell count, normal
Ferritin, normal
Transferrin saturation, normal

Which of the following is the most appropriate next step in this patient's management?

A. Perform pituitary MRI
B. Start a phosphodiesterase-5 inhibitor
C. Start hCG
D. Start testosterone replacement
E. Urge him to work with his primary care provider to eliminate narcotics used to treat back pain and measure testosterone in 6 months

5 A 32-year-old man presents with erectile dysfunction. He and his wife have been trying to have their third child for the last year. He sometimes cannot maintain an erection for sexual intercourse and climax, and his libido is not what it was 10 years ago. They currently have 2 biological children, ages 4 and 6 years. He underwent normal puberty. He exercises multiple days per week, is a nonsmoker, and takes no medications. He has had no testicular trauma, and he states that he does not use androgens. His 30-year-old wife has regular menstrual cycles.

On physical examination, the patient is normally virilized. His blood pressure is 110/70 mm Hg, and BMI is 26 kg/m^2. He has no gynecomastia. He has no striae or ecchymoses. His phallus is normal, and testicular volume is 20 cc bilaterally.

Laboratory test results (sample drawn while fasting at 8 AM):

Total testosterone (8 AM) (by liquid chromatography tandem mass spectrometry) = 290 ng/dL (300-900 ng/dL) (SI: 10.1 nmol/L [10.4-31.2 nmol/L])
LH = 4.0 mIU/mL (1.0-9.0 mIU/mL) (SI: 4.0 IU/L [1.0-9.0 IU/L])
FSH = 2.0 mIU/mL (1.0-13.0 mIU/mL) (SI: 2.0 IU/L [1.0-13.0 IU/L])
TSH = 2.2 mIU/L (0.5-5.0 mIU/L)
Free T_4 = 1.0 ng/dL (0.8-1.8 ng/dL) (SI: 12.87 pmol/L [10.30-23.17 pmol/L])

Repeat laboratory test results (sample drawn while fasting at 8 AM):

Total testosterone (8 AM) (by liquid chromatography tandem mass spectrometry) = 360 ng/dL (SI: 12.5 nmol/L)
Free testosterone = 10.1 ng/dL (9.0-30.0 ng/dL) (SI: 0.35 nmol/L [0.31-1.04 nmol/L])
Prolactin = 5 ng/mL (4-23 ng/mL) (SI: 0.22 pmol/L [0.17-1.00 nmol/L])
Seminal fluid analysis, normal

Which of the following is the best next step in this patient's care?

A. Perform pituitary MRI
B. Refer for assisted reproductive services
C. Start a phosphodiesterase inhibitor
D. Start hCG therapy, 1000 international units 3 times weekly
E. Start hCG therapy, 1000 international units 3 times weekly, and a phosphodiesterase inhibitor

6 An 18-year-old man is accompanied by both parents to discuss his recent diagnosis of Klinefelter syndrome. He was noted to have small testes during a routine physical examination by his pediatrician and was found to have a 47,XXY karyotype.

On physical examination, his height is 72 in (182.9 cm). He has mild gynecomastia and has normal facial, axillary, and pubic hair. His testes measure 4 cc bilaterally.

Laboratory test results:

Total testosterone = 306 ng/dL (300-900 ng/dL) (SI: 10.6 nmol/L [10.4-31.2 nmol/L])
Free testosterone = 4.2 ng/dL (9.0-30.0 ng/dL) (SI: 0.15 nmol/L [0.31-1.04 nmol/L])
LH = 33.7 mIU/mL (1.0-9.0 mIU/mL) (SI: 33.7 IU/L [1.0-9.0 IU/L])
FSH = 58.1 mIU/mL (1.0-13.0 mIU/mL) (SI: 58.1 IU/L [1.0-13.0 IU/L])

He asks whether the diagnosis of Klinefelter syndrome means that he can never father a child.

Which of the following options is most likely to help this patient achieve biologic paternity?

A. Clomiphene citrate
B. hCG injections, 1000 international units 3 times weekly
C. He is unable to father a child and he should be counseled regarding donor sperm
D. Microdissection testicular sperm extraction followed by intracytoplasmic sperm injection
E. No treatment is needed because he has a high likelihood of having sperm in his ejaculate

7 A 28-year-old man is concerned about recent-onset breast tenderness and swelling associated with weight loss, irritability, and insomnia. His only medication is extended-release methylphenidate, 75 mg daily, which he takes for attention-deficit disorder. He reports no use of anabolic steroids or recreational drugs. He has a sedentary job.

On physical examination, his BMI is 23 kg/m^2 and pulse rate is 100 beats/min. He has normal facial, axillary, and pubic hair. He has 1-cm bilateral breast enlargement that is tender to palpation. Testicular volume is 20 cc bilaterally, and there are no palpable masses.

Laboratory test results:

TSH = <0.01 mIU/L (0.5-5.0 mIU/L)
Free T_4 = 4.6 ng/dL (0.8-1.8 ng/dL) (SI: 59.21 pmol/L [10.30-23.17 pmol/L])
Total T_3 = 410 ng/dL (70-200 ng/dL) (SI: 6.31 nmol/L [1.08-3.08 nmol/L])

Which of the following hormone profiles would be expected in this patient?

	Total testosterone	Free testosterone	Estradiol	LH
A.	Low	Low	Low	Low
B.	High or high-normal	Low or low-normal	High	Normal
C.	Normal	Normal	High	Low
D.	High	High	High	High

8 A 32-year-old man is referred for concerns about future fertility. He has type 2 diabetes diagnosed 8 months ago. He was originally treated with metformin, initiated at a dosage of 1000 mg twice daily. His hemoglobin A_{1c} value is 8.2% (66 mmol/mol). He has a sedentary job and does not exercise. He drinks 4 beers per week, and he takes cannabis edibles twice a month.

He has recently married and has no concerns regarding sexual function and libido. The couple does not desire children for a few years, but the patient did a home sperm kit, and his sperm count was "below normal." He is concerned about future fertility.

On physical examination, his blood pressure is 132/86 mm Hg and BMI is 34 kg/m^2. He has normal male-pattern body hair and no gynecomastia. He has central adiposity. Testicular volume is 20 cc bilaterally, and his testes have no palpable nodules.

Laboratory test results:

Total testosterone = 260 ng/dL (300-900 ng/dL) (SI: 9.0 nmol/L [10.4-31.2 nmol/L])
LH = 3.0 mIU/mL (1.0-9.0 mIU/mL) (SI: 3.0 IU/L [1.0-9.0 IU/L])
FSH = 5.0 mIU/mL (1.0-13.0 mIU/mL) (SI: 5.0 IU/L [1.0-13.0 IU/L])
Semen analysis = 14 million sperm/mL

Additional laboratory test results (sample drawn at 8 AM while fasting):

Total testosterone = 280 ng/dL (300-900 ng/dL) (SI: 9.7 nmol/L [10.4-31.2 nmol/L])
Free testosterone (calculated) = 16 ng/dL (9-30 ng/dL) (SI: 0.56 nmol/L [0.31-1.04 nmol/L])
Semen analysis = 18 million sperm/mL; motility and morphology are normal

Which of the following is the best next step in this patient's management to optimize his future fertility?

A. Counsel him to stop using edibles because cannabis decreases sperm numbers
B. Start clomiphene citrate, 25 mg daily
C. Start a GLP-1 receptor agonist, refer to a nutritionist, and encourage lifestyle modifications, including weight-loss goals
D. Start hCG therapy, 1500 international units 3 times weekly
E. Start testosterone enanthate, 200 mg intramuscularly every 2 weeks

9 A 28-year-old man presents for evaluation of a 5-month history of tender gynecomastia. He is otherwise well with normal energy levels and sexual function. He and his wife have a 2-month-old baby. His medical history is remarkable for hepatitis C. He takes finasteride, 1 mg daily, to prevent male-pattern alopecia.

On physical examination, his BMI is 26 kg/m^2 and pulse rate is 80 beats/min. His thyroid gland is not enlarged. He has tender bilateral gynecomastia. His phallus is normal, and testes are 20 cc bilaterally with no palpable masses.

Laboratory test results:

Total testosterone = 780 ng/dL (300-900 ng/dL) (SI: 27.1 nmol/L [10.4-31.2 nmol/L])
Free testosterone (calculated) = 35 ng/dL (9.0-30.0 ng/dL) (SI: 1.21 nmol/L [0.31-1.04 nmol/L])
Estradiol = 70 pg/mL (10-40 pg/mL) (SI: 257.0 pmol/L [36.7-146.8 pmol/L])
FSH = 0.5 mIU/mL (1.0-13.0 mIU/mL) (SI: 0.5 IU/L [1.0-13.0 IU/L])
LH = 0.5 mIU/mL (1.0-9.0 mIU/mL) (SI: 0.5 IU/L [1.0-9.0 IU/L])

Which of the following most likely explains this patient's hormone profile?

A. Decreased 5α-reductase activity due to finasteride
B. Elevated SHBG due to hepatitis C
C. Estrogen-secreting testicular tumor
D. hCG use
E. Synthetic anabolic steroid use

10 A 49-year-old man who has been HIV positive for 15 years is referred for unintentional weight loss. He has had considerable difficulty maintaining his weight over the last year and has lost approximately 10 lb (4.5 kg) in the last 6 months despite a robust appetite.

CD4 cell count has been within the normal range for more than 10 years while on highly active antiretroviral therapy (dolutegravir, abacavir, and lamivudine). He has hypertension treated with 2 medications. He has no concerns regarding sexual function and shaves daily. He has had no febrile illnesses, and findings from gastrointestinal workup, including evaluation for celiac sprue, are normal.

Laboratory test results (sample drawn at 8 AM while fasting):

- Hematocrit = 39% (41%-51%) (SI: 0.39 [0.41-0.51])
- TSH = 2.0 mIU/L (0.5-5.0 mIU/L)
- Hemoglobin A_{1c} = 5.7% (4.0%-5.6%) (39 mmol/mol [20-38 mmol/mol])
- Total testosterone = 390 ng/dL (300-900 ng/dL) (SI: 13.5 nmol/L [10.4-31.2 nmol/L])
- Free testosterone = 7.9 ng/dL (9-30 ng/dL) (SI: 0.27 nmol/L [0.31-1.04 nmol/L])

On physical examination, he is a thin man with normal male-pattern body hair. His blood pressure is 155/92 mm Hg, and pulse rate is 75 beats/min. His weight is 165 lb (74.8 kg) (BMI = 18.0 kg/m^2). Testicular volume is 20 cc bilaterally.

Additional laboratory test results (ordered 1 week later, sample drawn at 8 AM):

- Total testosterone = 370 ng/dL (300-900 ng/dL) (SI: 12.8 nmol/L [10.4-31.2 nmol/L])
- Free testosterone = 7.7 ng/dL (9-30 ng/dL) (SI: 0.27 nmol/L [0.31-1.04 nmol/L])
- LH = 5.2 mIU/mL (1.0-9.0 mIU/mL) (SI: 5.2 IU/L [1.0-9.0 IU/L])
- PSA = 2.0 ng/mL (<2.8 ng/mL) (SI: 2.0 μg/L [<2.8 μg/L])
- Cortisol = 24 μg/dL (5-25 μg/dL) (SI: 662.1 nmol/L [137.9-689.7 nmol/L])

Which of the following is the best recommendation to address this patient's weight loss?

A. Initiate finasteride, 5 mg daily
B. Initiate megestrol acetate therapy, 800 mg daily
C. Initiate oral testosterone undecanoate therapy, 237 mg twice daily
D. Initiate transdermal testosterone therapy
E. Refer to a nutritionist for counseling and instructions on keeping a food diary

11 A 36-year-old man presents for evaluation of infertility. His wife, age 33, has normal findings on fertility evaluation, has normal menstrual cycles, and had a previous pregnancy. They are having regular intercourse. The patient completed normal spontaneous puberty at age 15 years and reports normal libido and erectile function. He had a pituitary macroadenoma removed at age 24 years and is treated with daily transdermal testosterone gel, hydrocortisone, and levothyroxine.

On physical examination, he is normally virilized. His weight is 180 lb (81.6 kg) (BMI = 28.0 kg/m^2). His blood pressure is 135/88 mm Hg, and pulse rate is 80 beats/min. He has normal male-pattern hair, including a beard. Testicular volume is 20 cc bilaterally.

Initial laboratory test results:

- LH = 0.8 mIU/mL (1.0-9.0 mIU/mL) (SI: 0.7 IU/L [1.0-9.0 IU/L])
- FSH = 0.9 mIU/mL (1.0-13.0 mIU/mL) (SI: 0.8 IU/L [1.0-13.0 IU/L])
- Total testosterone = 450 ng/dL (300-900 ng/dL) (SI: 15.6 nmol/L [10.4-31.2 nmol/L])
- Free T_4 = 1.0 ng/dL (0.8-1.8 ng/dL) (SI: 12.87 pmol/L [10.3-23.17 pmol/L)
- Semen analysis = 0.0 million sperm/mL

Transdermal testosterone gel is discontinued, and hCG injections, 750 international units 3 times weekly, are initiated.

He returns for follow-up in 2 months and reports that he and his wife have not achieved pregnancy. He feels a bit run down and reports some decrease in libido. Weight and vital signs are stable.

Laboratory test results:

- LH = 0.3 mIU/mL (1.0-9.0 mIU/mL) (SI: 0.3 IU/L [1.0-9.0 IU/L])
- FSH = 1.0 IU/mL (1.0-13.0 mIU/mL) (SI: 1.0 IU/L [1.0-13.0 IU/L])
- Testosterone = 200 ng/dL (300-900 ng/dL) (SI: 6.9 nmol/L [10.4-31.2 nmol/L])

Which of the following is the most appropriate next step in this patient's care?

A. Add clomiphene citrate
B. Add recombinant FSH, 75 international units daily
C. Increase the hCG dosage to 1500 international units 3 times weekly
D. Obtain a seminal fluid analysis
E. Wait another 3 months before altering the current regimen

12 A 38-year-old man is found to have a low testosterone concentration during an extensive laboratory evaluation performed as part of health insurance screening. He reports normal energy levels and sexual function and has no history of headaches or vision problems. He describes decreased sense of smell that he attributes to a recent viral infection. He goes to the gym regularly, drinks 1 to 2 cocktails per night, and follows a ketogenic diet.

On physical examination, his BMI is 28 kg/m^2. He has no gynecomastia. He has normal facial, axillary, and pubic hair. Testicular volume is 10 cc bilaterally, and he has a normal phallus.

Laboratory test results:

- Testosterone = 51 ng/dL (300-900 ng/dL) (SI: 1.8 nmol/L [10.4-31.2 nmol/L])
- LH = <1.0 mIU/mL (1.0-9.0 mIU/mL) (SI: <1.0 IU/L [1.0-9.0 IU/L])
- FSH = <1.0 mIU/mL (1.0-13.0 mIU/mL) (SI: <1.0 IU/L [1.0-13.0 IU/L])
- Hematocrit = 52% (41%-51%) (SI: 0.52 [0.41-0.51])
- Prolactin = 24 ng/mL (4-23 ng/mL) (SI: 1.04 nmol/L [0.17-1.00 nmol/L])

Pituitary MRI shows a 5-mm hypoenhancing lesion.

Which of the following is this patient's most likely diagnosis?

A. Anabolic steroid use
B. Hereditary hemochromatosis
C. Kallmann syndrome
D. Opioid use
E. Prolactinoma

13 A 22-year-old man is referred by his oncologist to discuss options for fertility preservation after a recent diagnosis of Hodgkin lymphoma, which will require treatment with alkylating agents. The patient is currently single but may wish to have children in the future.

On physical examination, testicular volume is 25 cc bilaterally.

Laboratory test results:

- Total testosterone = 280 ng/dL (300-900 ng/dL) (SI: 9.7 nmol/L [10.4-31.2 nmol/L])
- LH = 2.0 mIU/mL (1.0-9.0 mIU/mL) (SI: 2.0 IU/L [1.0-9.0 IU/L])
- Semen analysis = 11 million sperm/mL, normal motility and morphology

Which of the following is the most reliable option for optimizing his potential to father children in the future?

A. Combination of testosterone and progestin to suppress spermatogenesis during chemotherapy
B. Cryopreservation of spermatogonial stem cells before chemotherapy for future transplant
C. Sperm cryopreservation before chemotherapy
D. Treatment with a GnRH agonist to suppress spermatogenesis during chemotherapy
E. Treatment with hCG before cryopreservation

14 An 18-year-old man is referred for further evaluation of congenital hypogonadotropic hypogonadism. He has no sense of smell, which was confirmed by quantitative smell testing. There is no history of deafness. There is no family history of anosmia, delayed puberty, or hypogonadism.

On physical examination, his height is 67 in (170.2 cm) (BMI = 22.0 kg/m^2), and arm span is 70 in (177.8 cm). He has slight axillary hair and Tanner stage 2 pubic hair but no facial or chest hair. He has a normal phallus, and testicular volume is 2 cc bilaterally. There is no evidence of synkinesia. Musculoskeletal examination shows fusion (syndactyly) of 2 fingers and toes. The patient notes he has 4 missing teeth (he was born with this condition).

Laboratory test results:

- Total testosterone = 52 ng/dL (300-900 ng/dL) (SI: 1.8 nmol/L [10.4-31.2 nmol/L]
- Gonadotropins, undetectable
- IGF-1, low
- Prolactin, normal
- TSH, normal
- Free T_4, normal
- ACTH, normal

Pituitary MRI shows no structural abnormality.

A pathogenic variant in which of the following genes most likely underlies this patient's presentation?

A. *ANOS1*
B. *CHD7*
C. *FGFR1*
D. *GNRHR*
E. *NR0B1*

15 A 32-year-old man is referred for evaluation of azoospermia noted during workup for primary infertility. He and his wife have had unprotected intercourse for the past 2 years without a confirmed pregnancy. The patient underwent normal puberty and reports normal libido and erections. His wife is 30 years old, and her infertility workup is normal.

On physical examination, his BMI is 25.5 kg/m^2. He is well virilized and has no gynecomastia. Testicular volume is 15 cc bilaterally.

Laboratory test results:

- Total testosterone = 500 ng/dL (300-900 ng/dL) (SI: 17.4 nmol/L [10.4-31.2 nmol/L])
- FSH = 21.5 mIU/mL (1.0-13.0 mIU/mL) (SI: 21.5 IU/L [1.0-13.0 IU/L])
- LH = 5.0 mIU/mL (1.0-9.0 mIU/mL) (SI: 5.0 IU/L [1.0-9.0 IU/L])
- Karyotype = 46,XY

A second semen analysis documents a pH of 7.5 (normal >7.2) and volume of 3 mL (normal ≥1.5 mL) and confirms azoospermia.

Which of the following genetic conditions does this patient most likely have?

A. Congenital bilateral absence of the vas deferens
B. Kallmann syndrome
C. Mosaic Klinefelter syndrome
D. Retrograde ejaculation
E. Y-Chromosome microdeletion

16 A 52-year-old man is found to have a low serum testosterone concentration during workup of decreased energy levels and libido. He is otherwise healthy and takes no medications.

On physical examination, his BMI is 24.0 kg/m^2 and blood pressure is 118/77 mm Hg. He is well virilized and has no gynecomastia. He has no ecchymoses or striae. His testicular volume is 20 cc bilaterally. He has no difficulty rising from a squatting position. His visual fields are grossly intact.

Laboratory test results (morning AM, fasting):

- Total testosterone = 180 ng/dL (300-900 ng/dL) (SI: 6.2 nmol/L [10.4-31.2 nmol/L])
- Calculated free testosterone = 4.5 ng/dL (9.0-30.0 ng/dL) (SI: 0.16 nmol/L [0.31-1.04 nmol/L])
- LH = 2.8 mIU/mL (1.0-9.0 mIU/mL) (SI: 2.8 IU/L [1.0-9.0 IU/L])
- FSH = 3.5 mIU/mL (1.0-13.0 mIU/mL) (SI: 3.5 IU/L [1.0-13.0 IU/L])

Repeated tests (morning AM, fasting):

- Total testosterone = 210 ng/dL (300-900 ng/dL) (SI: 7.2 nmol/L [10.4-31.2 nmol/L])
- Calculated free testosterone = 6.0 ng/dL (9.0-30.0 ng/dL) (SI: 0.21 nmol/L [0.31-1.04 nmol/L])
- TSH = 1.2 mIU/L (0.5-5.0 mIU/L)
- Free T_4 = 0.9 ng/dL (0.8-1.8 ng/dL) (SI: 11.58 pmol/L [10.30-23.17 pmol/L])

Which of the following is the most appropriate next test?

A. Karyotype analysis
B. Late-night salivary cortisol measurement
C. Pituitary MRI
D. Serum prolactin measurement
E. Testicular ultrasonography

Lipids & Obesity Board Review

Sangeeta Kashyap, MD

1 A 62-year-old White woman is referred by her primary care clinician to discuss potential statin initiation. Her medical history is notable for treated hypertension and longstanding rheumatoid arthritis.

Recent laboratory test results:

- Complete blood cell count, normal
- Basic metabolic panel, normal
- Hemoglobin A_{1c} = 5.5% (4.0%-5.6%) (37 mmol/mol [20-38 mmol/mol])
- Total cholesterol = 220 mg/dL (<200 mg/dL) (SI: 5.70 mmol/L [<5.18 mmol/L])
- Triglycerides = 117 mg/dL (<150 mg/dL) (SI: 1.32 mmol/L [<1.70 mmol/L])
- HDL cholesterol = 40 mg/dL (>60 mg/dL) (SI: 1.04 mmol/L [>1.55 mmol/L])
- LDL cholesterol = 146 mg/dL (<100 mg/dL) (SI: 3.78 mmol/L [<2.59 mmol/L])

Her 10-year estimated risk of atherosclerotic cardiovascular disease is calculated to be 9% using the pooled cohort risk equation. Statin therapy is recommended after discussing the risks and benefits. However, she is hesitant given what she has read about possible adverse effects and asks about the strength of this recommendation.

Which of the following is the best next step?

A. Obtain a coronary artery calcium score
B. Start evolocumab instead of a statin
C. Start ezetimibe instead of a statin
D. Start red yeast rice
E. Strongly recommend starting a statin

2 A 65-year-old man of East Asian ancestry who has hypothyroidism (taking levothyroxine; TSH = 1.9 mIU/L) seeks a second opinion regarding statin therapy. His primary care physician recommended lifestyle modification and prescribed simvastatin, 40 mg daily, 5 years ago for isolated hyperlipidemia and an elevated 10-year atherosclerotic cardiovascular disease (ASCVD) risk of 9%. The patient discontinued simvastatin after 1 month because of mild muscle aches that he noted while participating in fitness classes. His primary care physician did not diagnose any muscle weakness at the time. He subsequently tried daily atorvastatin, 20 mg daily, but stopped it after 2 weeks because of similar mild symptoms.

He has not taken any lipid-lowering therapy for 2 years but has continued to engage in vigorous cardio exercise training.

Recent lipid profile:

- Total cholesterol = 202 mg/dL (<200 mg/dL) (SI: 5.23 mmol/L [<5.18 mmol/L])
- Triglycerides = 155 mg/dL (<150 mg/dL) (SI: 1.75 mmol/L [<1.70 mmol/L])
- HDL cholesterol = 50 mg/dL (>60 mg/dL) (SI: 1.30 mmol/L [>1.55 mmol/L])
- LDL cholesterol = 121 mg/dL (<100 mg/dL) (SI: 3.13 mmol/L [<2.59 mmol/L])

He has no history of heart disease, hypertension, diabetes, or chronic kidney disease. He is a lifelong nonsmoker. He has no family history of ASCVD, although his sister is taking statin therapy for hyperlipidemia. His current 10-year ASCVD risk is calculated to be 10%.

Which of the following is the best next step in this patient's care?

A. Avoid daily exercise to prevent future muscle aches
B. Measure creatine kinase before restarting statin therapy
C. Challenge with another more potent statin such as rosuvastatin
D. Recommend coenzyme Q10 supplements with a statin to prevent muscle symptoms

3 A 45-year-old man has premature coronary disease and is treated with rosuvastatin, 40 mg daily, for an LDL-cholesterol concentration of 260 mg/dL (6.73 mmol/L). He has a family history of hypercholesterolemia, and his father sustained a myocardial infarction in his early 40s. He has infrequent muscle aches, usually noted after strenuous workouts. Currently, his LDL-cholesterol concentration is 150 mg/dL (3.89 mmol/L), and his HDL-cholesterol concentration is 28 mg/dL (0.73 mmol/L). He wants to know what else he can do to reduce his risk of cardiovascular events.

He is subsequently started on ezetimibe, which further lowers his LDL-cholesterol concentration to 130 mg/dL (3.37 mmol/L) but not to the targeted goal of less than 100 mg/dL (<2.59 mmol/L). He does not tolerate evolocumab or alirocumab as second-line therapy because of severe rash. He recently developed carpal tunnel syndrome with hand weakness that limits him from administering self-injection therapies.

He is counseled about his genetic hypercholesterolemia and the importance of family screening.

In addition to referring him to trusted sources of information about familial hypercholesterolemia, which of the following actions would be most appropriate?

A. Add inclisiran
B. Add niacin
C. Continue rosuvastatin, 40 mg daily, and add colesevelam
D. Recommend LDL apheresis
E. Reduce rosuvastatin to 10 mg daily and add fenofibrate

4 A 50-year-old man with chronic kidney disease and a creatinine clearance of 45 mL/min per 1.73 m^2 presents to a weight management clinic. He has been told he must lose weight to become eligible for future kidney transplant. The patient has a history of metabolic syndrome (hypertension, hyperlipidemia, type 2 diabetes). His BMI is 46.3 kg/m^2, and he has been unsuccessful with hypocaloric diet alone, as he lost less than 5% of his body weight. Medications are discussed in detail.

Which of the following would be the most appropriate and effective treatment to start now?

A. Cellulose and citric acid hydrogel
B. Naltrexone/bupropion ER
C. Orlistat
D. Phentermine/topiramate ER
E. Semaglutide

5 A 44-year-old woman with class 2 obesity and no comorbidities consumes more than 50% of her calories after her evening meal. In the morning, she is not hungry and often skips breakfast. She notes weight gain of 10 lb (4.5 kg) in the past 4 months.

Which additional finding is most likely present?

A. Excessive sleep
B. Increased caffeine intake during the day
C. Increased dietary carbohydrate-to-protein ratio
D. Purging behaviors after eating episodes
E. Sense of lack of control with overeating throughout the day

6 A 39-year-old woman presents to a family practice clinic with concerns of brittle hair and cold intolerance. She has a history of hypothyroidism. Although she has been on a stable levothyroxine dosage for 3 years, her most recent TSH measurement is 12.0 mIU/L. She has been to a weight-loss clinic and takes an antiobesity medication.

Which of the following weight-loss medications best explains her presenting symptoms?

A. Bupropion ER
B. Naltrexone
C. Orlistat
D. Phentermine

7 A 38-year-old woman is found to have modest elevation of liver transaminases and a subsequent elevated FIB-4 score of 2.1 (intermediate). She has diet-controlled type 2 diabetes (current hemoglobin A_{1c} = 8.4% [68 mmol/mol]) on metformin), class 1 obesity (BMI = 32 kg/m^2), obstructive sleep apnea treated with continuous positive airway pressure, hypertension treated with lisinopril, and history of premature menopause treated with daily estrogen/progesterone therapy. Rather than undergo a liver biopsy, she elects to have liver elastography for liver stiffness measurement. The result is a reading of 14 kPa and CAP 330 (positive for fibrosis). Liver biopsy shows advanced stages of cirrhosis.

Which of the following in the patient's clinical presentation is her strongest risk factor for metabolic dysfunction-associated steatohepatitis?

A. Age
B. Class 1 obesity
C. Menopause status
D. Obstructive sleep apnea
E. Type 2 diabetes

8 A patient with class 1 obesity who is addicted to soda has recently started topiramate to help with soda aversion (as it alters carbonic anhydrase on the tongue) and facilitate weight loss.

Which of the following describes this medication's mechanism of action for weight loss?

A. Agonist of GLP-1 receptor
B. Enhancement of GABA activity and sodium channels
C. Neuronal reuptake inhibition of norepinephrine and dopamine
D. Stimulation of the hypothalamus to release norepinephrine

9 A 50-year-old woman with class 3 obesity, gastroesophageal reflux disease, prediabetes, metabolic dysfunction-associated steatotic liver disease (MASLD), asthma, and depression returns to the weight management clinic with the concern of marked weight regain 4 years after Roux-en-Y gastric bypass. Her initial body weight was 389 lb (176.8 kg) (BMI = 65 kg/m^2), and her nadir weight after surgery was 183 lb (83.2 kg) (BMI = 30.5 kg/m^2), which represents a total body weight loss of 53%. During the initial 2 years after surgery, she experienced multiple life stressors related to divorce, becoming an empty nester, and moving to a new home. A psychiatrist treated her with venlafaxine for mild depression, and she did not have time to attend bariatric support groups. During this time, she started to notice increased hunger and regained 25 lb (11.4 kg). Over the next 2 years, she gained another 20 lb (9.1 kg) for a total of 45 lb (20.5 kg) above nadir despite counseling on lifestyle modifications.

Upon further questioning, the patient reports increasing nighttime cravings and consumption of alcohol (vodka, wine, and beer; >20 drinks per week for the past 2 years). Her laboratory profile shows elevated fasting glucose (106 mg/dL [5.9 mmol/L]), elevated γ-glutamyltransferase, and iron deficiency anemia. She regularly misses doses of postbariatric vitamins and minerals.

In addition to advising her to attend Alcoholics Anonymous meetings and rejoin a bariatric support group, which of the following is the best next step in this patient's management of alcohol use?

A. Determine standard addiction score for shopping and gambling addictions
B. Refer her to a social worker to address alcohol use disorder
C. Start calcium citrate, magnesium, and vitamin D supplementation
D. Start naltrexone, bupropion, or a GLP-1 receptor agonist

10 A 78-year-old woman would like to discuss treatment of hyperlipidemia. She had a myocardial infarction at age 75 years and started taking atorvastatin, 40 mg daily. She describes feeling terrible on atorvastatin and "hurting all over." She then tried low-dosage rosuvastatin and simvastatin with the same symptom of diffuse muscle aches. Ezetimibe is recommended as a next step, but she would also like an opinion about supplements that could lower cholesterol.

Given her statin intolerance, which of the following supplements should she avoid taking?

A. Berberine
B. Coenzyme Q10
C. Folate
D. Red yeast rice
E. Vitamin D

11 A 55-year-old woman is concerned about high cholesterol. Menopause occurred 3 years ago. She does not have diabetes or cardiovascular disease. However, she is concerned because her father had a myocardial infarction at age 45 years.

Measurements of TSH and fasting glucose are normal. Her 10-year cardiovascular disease risk is estimated to be 6.3%. She does not want to take a statin. She undergoes CT to determine her coronary artery calcium score, which returns as "0." She elects to follow a vegan diet rich in olive oil and low in saturated fat. Six months later, her LDL-cholesterol value is 123 mg/dL (3.19 mmol/L).

Fasting lipid profile:

Analyte	Baseline	After change to vegan diet	Reference ranges
Total cholesterol	252 mg/dL (SI: 6.53 mmol/L)	239 mg/dL (SI: 6.19 mmol/L)	<200 mg/dL (SI: <5.18 mmol/L)
LDL cholesterol	169 mg/dL (SI: 4.38 mmol/L)	123 mg/dL (SI: 3.19 mmol/L)	<100 mg/dL (SI: <2.59 mmol/L)
HDL cholesterol	47 mg/dL (SI: 1.22 mmol/L)	41 mg/dL (SI: 1.06 mmol/L)	>60 mg/dL (SI: >1.55 mmol/L)
Triglycerides	214 mg/dL (SI: 2.42 mmol/L)	374 mg/dL (SI: 4.23 mmol/L)	<150 mg/dL (SI: <1.70 mmol/L)

Which of the following is the best next test to assess her risk of cardiovascular disease?

A. Apolipoprotein B measurement
B. Chylomicron measurement
C. Lipoprotein (a) measurement
D. Non–HDL-cholesterol measurement
E. Nuclear magnetic resonance spectroscopy

12 A 39-year-old woman who recently moved to the area seeks assistance to manage low cholesterol. She was diagnosed with low cholesterol as an infant when she presented with failure to thrive. She was on parenteral nutrition until age 12 years and, since then, she has been treated with daily high-dosage vitamin supplements A, D, E, and K and with intravenous lipid infusions 3 times weekly. She has a history and osteoporosis for which she takes alendronate and anemia. Both of her parents have normal cholesterol concentrations. Baseline blood tests are ordered, and she is referred to ophthalmology and neurology.

On physical examination, her blood pressure is 111/81 mm Hg and weight is 105.5 lb (48 kg) (BMI = 21 kg/m^2).

Laboratory test results:

Total cholesterol = 22 mg/dL (<200 mg/dL) (SI: 0.57 mmol/L [<5.18 mmol/L])
HDL cholesterol = 16 mg/dL (>60 mg/dL) (SI: 0.41 mmol/L [>1.55 mmol/L])
Triglycerides = 12 mg/dL (<150 mg/dL) (SI: 0.14 mmol/L [<1.70 mmol/L])
LDL cholesterol = <10 mg/dL (<100 mg/dL) (SI: <0.26 mmol/L [<2.59 mmol/L])
Apolipoprotein B = <3 mg/dL (50-110 mg/dL) (SI: 0.03 g/L [0.5-1.1 g/L])
Hemoglobin = 14.0 g/dL (12.1-15.1 g/dL) (SI: 140 g/L [121-151 g/L])
Hematocrit = 42% (35%-45%) (SI: 0.42 [0.35-0.45])
ALT = 29 U/L (10-40 U/L) (SI: 0.48 µkat/L [0.17-0.67 µkat/L])
AST = 44 U/L (20-48 U/L) (SI: 0.73 µkat/L [0.33-0.80 µkat/L])

This patient most likely has a pathogenic variant in which of the following genes?

A. Apolipoprotein A1 (*APOA1*)
B. Apolipoprotein CII (*APOC2*)
C. Cholesterol ester transfer protein (*CETP*)
D. Lipoprotein lipase (*LPL*)
E. Microsomal triglyceride transfer protein (*MTTP*)

13 A 31-year-old woman is referred by her obstetrician-gynecologist because of very high cholesterol. She has no history of cardiovascular disease but notes that multiple family members have been diagnosed with coronary artery disease in their 40s and 50s. She has never been on lipid-lowering therapy. Her only medical problems are infertility and abnormal uterine bleeding. She delivered a healthy baby 5 months ago and is currently breastfeeding.

Measurement	Prepregnancy	Current
Total cholesterol	361 mg/dL (SI: 9.35 mmol/L)	364 mg/dL (SI: 9.43 mmol/L)
LDL cholesterol	300 mg/dL (SI: 7.77 mmol/L)	301 mg/dL (SI: 7.80 mmol/L)
HDL cholesterol	41 mg/dL (SI: 1.06 mmol/L)	53 mg/dL (SI: 1.37 mmol/L)
Triglycerides	99 mg/dL (SI: 1.12 mmol/L)	49 mg/dL (SI: 0.55 mmol/L)
TSH	0.72 mIU/L	...
Free T_4	0.83 ng/dL (SI: 10.7 pmol/L)	...
Fasting glucose	100 mg/dL (SI: 5.55 mmol/L)	...

Which of the following should be added as the best next step in this patient's management?

A. Atorvastatin
B. Colesevelam
C. Evolocumab
D. Pitavastatin
E. Simvastatin

14 On the basis of the clinical characteristics shown in the table, which of the listed patients with type 2 diabetes and a BMI of 44 kg/m² would be expected to achieve remission of diabetes (hemoglobin A_{1c} <5.7% [<39 mmol/mol] without the need for any diabetes medication) following bariatric surgery?

Answer	Patient age	Current hemoglobin A_{1c}	Duration of diabetes	Diabetes medication	Type of bariatric procedure
A.	38 years	8.2% (66 mmol/mol)	11 years	Basal insulin, 70 units; sitagliptin; metformin	Roux-en-Y gastric bypass
B.	48 years	7.0% (53 mmol/mol)	4 years	Metformin	Roux-en-Y gastric bypass
C.	55 years	6.2% (44 mmol/mol)	10 years	Basal insulin, 20 units	Sleeve gastrectomy
D.	32 years	7.0% (53 mmol/mol)	8 years	Metformin, glimepiride	Laparoscopic gastric banding

15 A 35-year-old woman with class 1 obesity (BMI = 31 kg/m²) and obstructive sleep apnea has lost 20 lb (9.1 kg) in 4 months by adhering to a Mediterranean meal plan of 1800 calories per day with 15% saturated fat intake and regular cardio training 5 times per week. However, her weight has now plateaued, and in the past 2 weeks she has started to regain weight despite no changes to her caloric intake (which she monitors with an app) or exercise program.

In addition to reduced satiety and increased hunger, which of the following metabolic adaptations are present with diet-induced weight loss that promote weight regain?

Answer	Total daily expenditure	Resting metabolic rate	Exercise energy expenditure
A.	Reduced	Reduced	Reduced
B.	Increased	Reduced	Increased
C.	Stable	Reduced	Increased
D.	Reduced	Increased	Increased

16 A 32-year-old woman with class 1 obesity (BMI = 34 kg/m²) complicated by hypertriglyceridemia and hypertension presents for a follow-up appointment. She has been adhering to a regimen of alternate-day fasting. She consumes only 25% of her calories on fast days and 125% of her calories on feast days. After 2 months following this meal plan, the patient has lost 6% of her total body weight.

Compared with daily caloric restriction, which of the following should this patient expect after 6 months of alternate-day fasting?

Answer	Dietary adherence	Weight loss	Triglycerides	Blood pressure
A.	Improved	Increased	Decreased	Decreased
B.	Worsened	No difference	No difference	No difference
C.	Improved	No difference	No difference	No difference
D.	Improved	No difference	Increased	Decreased

17 A 48-year-old woman presents with dyslipidemia and elevated LDL-cholesterol concentrations. She has a history of diet-controlled hypertension, myocardial infarction, and ischemic stroke and no history of diabetes. Her fasting glucose concentration is 115 mg/dL (6.4 mmol/L), and hemoglobin A_{1c} level is 5.9% (41 mmol/mol). She has optimized her cardiofitness and lifestyle intervention with nutrition therapy and a personal exercise trainer. There is a paternal family history of coronary artery disease. Her primary care physician wants to initiate a statin, but the patient is worried that her blood glucose will get worse.

Which of the following regimens should be started as the best next step in this patient's management?

A. Both metformin, 750 mg twice daily, and pravastatin, 10 mg daily
B. Metformin, 750 mg twice daily, and in 3 months add rosuvastatin, 10 mg daily
C. Pravastatin, 10 mg daily, and reevaluate in 3 months
D. Rosuvastatin, 10 mg daily, and reevaluate in 3 months

18 A 54-year-old woman with class 1 obesity (BMI = 32 kg/m^2) and type 2 diabetes is interested in pursuing an intensive lifestyle modification program with meal replacement shakes and regular exercise training for weight loss to lower her cardiovascular risk. She has a history of metabolic syndrome with elevated triglyceride levels and hypertension and is taking atorvastatin and losartan. Her father had a myocardial infarction at age 60 years.

Based on data from randomized controlled trials evaluating the effect of intensive lifestyle modification vs standard care on cardiovascular risk in patients with type 2 diabetes, which of the following benefits can this patient expect over time?

A. Diabetes remission with normalization of hemoglobin A_{1c} levels and withdrawal of antidiabetes medications
B. Significant reduction in cardiovascular disease mortality
C. Significant and sustained reduction in visceral fat levels
D. Significant improvement in quality of life, depression, and sleep apnea
E. Substantial weight loss that peaks within the first year and is durable over 5 years

19 A 44-year-old woman with dyslipidemia and class 3 obesity (BMI = 42 kg/m^2) is diagnosed with metabolic dysfunction-associated steototic liver disease based on elevated liver transaminase levels and liver ultrasonography that shows steatosis. Transient elastography of the liver shows some evidence of fibrosis, and a subsequent liver biopsy demonstrates ballooning and lobular inflammation. Her hemoglobin A_{1c} level is 5.2% (33 mmol/mol), and her fasting plasma glucose concentration is 88 mg/dL (4.9 mmol/L).

Which of the following therapies would be best for managing this patient's steatotic liver disease?

A. Atorvastatin, 40 mg daily
B. Metformin, 1500 mg daily
C. Pioglitazone, 30 mg daily
D. Vitamin D, 4000 international units daily
E. Vitamin E, 800 international units daily

20 A 42-year-old, well-appearing woman with a history of type 2 diabetes controlled with diet and metformin (hemoglobin A_{1c} = 7.2% [55 mmol/mol]) underwent a Roux-en-Y gastric bypass 3 years ago. Her BMI was

45 kg/m^2 before surgery. She had an uneventful recovery and lost 130 lb (60 kg) in 6 months. Her diabetes resolved immediately after surgery. Her current hemoglobin A_{1c} level is 5.3% (34 mmol/mol). She no longer takes metformin.

One year ago, she started having episodes of diaphoresis, heart pounding, and shakiness. She has not lost consciousness but recently began having difficulty speaking and thinking, which has been interfering with her professional life. These episodes occur 2 to 3 times per week during the day. She does not recall having any symptoms at night. She has gained 30 lb (13.6 kg) over the last year, and she notes that her carbohydrate intake has increased.

Findings on physical examination are normal.

She undergoes a mixed-meal study following unrestricted carbohydrate ingestion for 3 days. Ninety minutes into the study, she develops palpitations, weakness, drowsiness, and blurred vision. Her plasma glucose concentration is 50 mg/dL (2.8 mmol/L).

Her symptoms improve several minutes after glucose ingestion.

Which of the following initial treatment options should be offered before discharge?

A. Dietary modification and acarbose
B. Ketogenic diet
C. Liraglutide
D. Propranolol
E. Reversal of gastric bypass

21 A 40-year-old woman with a history of hyperlipidemia, prediabetes, and obesity (BMI = 33 kg/m^2) comes for a follow-up appointment. Several months ago, she had a bout of major depression after the anniversary of her son's death. Despite engaging in psychotherapy, she began having suicidal thoughts and was referred to psychiatry. Her psychiatrist prescribed a medication, and within 8 weeks of initiating this therapy, she noted a 12-lb (5.4-kg) weight gain and increased hunger. She is concerned that she will become diabetic if she continues to gain weight at this pace. She takes atorvastatin for hyperlipidemia.

Which of the following antidepressant drugs is most likely responsible for her initial weight gain?

A. Amitriptyline
B. Bupropion
C. Fluoxetine
D. Paroxetine
E. Venlafaxine

22 A 22-year-old woman with class 3 obesity complicated by obstructive sleep apnea, impaired glucose tolerance, and polycystic ovary syndrome underwent gastric bypass surgery 9 months ago. She can tolerate small low-carbohydrate meals and has lost more than 50 lb (22.6 kg). Her current BMI is 36 kg/m^2, which is down from 45 kg/m^2 before surgery. Her menses are now regular, and she and her husband are interested in pregnancy. She is adherent to her regimen of daily replacement supplements, including a prepregnancy vitamin, folic acid, sublingual vitamin B_{12}, calcium citrate, vitamin D_3, and iron daily.

Which of the following is the most appropriate clinical advice for this patient regarding pregnancy planning?

A. Avoid pregnancy (with use of an intrauterine device) until she is weight stable
B. Avoid pregnancy (with use of an oral contraceptive pill) until she is weight stable
C. Proceed with pregnancy as long as her hemoglobin A_{1c} level is in the normal range (ie, <5.7% [<39 mmol/mol])
D. Proceed with pregnancy as long as she increases vitamin supplementation dosages to those recommended during pregnancy
E. Proceed with pregnancy but advise her that breastfeeding after gastric bypass is contraindicated

23 A 64-year-old man with no clinical atherosclerotic cardiovascular disease seeks evaluation regarding his lipid panel. He has chronic atrial fibrillation, hyperlipidemia, and hypertension. Medications include metoprolol and atorvastatin, 80 mg daily. He drinks 10 to 12 alcoholic beverages per week and does not follow any specific meal plan. He eats at fast-food restaurants once or twice weekly.

His BMI is 33 kg/m^2, and blood pressure is 135/80 mm Hg.

Laboratory test results (8 AM, fasting):

- Hemoglobin A_{1c} = 5.7% (4.0%-5.6%) (39 mmol/mol [20-38 mmol/mol])
- Total cholesterol = 170 mg/dL (<200 mg/dL) (SI: 5.90 mmol/L [<5.18 mmol/L])
- Triglycerides = 385 mg/dL (<150 mg/dL) (SI: 4.35 mmol/L [<1.70 mmol/L])
- HDL cholesterol = 36 mg/dL (>60 mg/dL) (SI: 1.25 mmol/L [>1.55 mmol/L])
- LDL cholesterol = 57 mg/dL (<100 mg/dL) (SI: 1.98 mmol/L [<2.59 mmol/L])
- Non-HDL cholesterol = 134 mg/dL (<130 mg/dL) (SI: 4.65 mmol/L [<3.37 mmol/L])
- TSH = 1.7 mIU/L (0.5-5.0 mIU/L)

Which of the following is the best next step in treating this patient's hyperlipidemia?

A. Change atorvastatin, 80 mg daily, to rosuvastatin, 40 mg daily, after measurement of apolipoprotein B
B. Refer him for nutritional counseling to reduce his intake of saturated fat and alcohol
C. Start colesevalam, 625 mg daily
D. Start fenofibrate, 145 mg once daily
E. Start niacin, 1000 mg twice daily

24 A 52-year-old man with a history of coronary artery disease status post stent of the right coronary artery seeks consultation for lipid management. His father had coronary artery disease in his late 40s. He has a history of atrial fibrillation, hypertension, and prediabetes and quit cigarette smoking 10 years ago. Following stent placement, he was prescribed atorvastatin, 80 mg daily, but was only able to tolerate 40 mg daily because of myalgias. Ezetimibe was subsequently prescribed to achieve target LDL-cholesterol levels.

His 6-month follow-up LDL-cholesterol measurement is 120 mg/dL (3.11 mmol/L). He has been intolerant of evolocumab and alirocumab due to severe injection site inflammation/swelling.

Which of the following steps would be expected to lower this patient's LDL cholesterol to target for secondary prevention?

A. Change atorvastatin to rosuvastatin, 20 mg daily
B. Start bempedoic acid
C. Start fenofibrate
D. Start niacin
E. Start omega-3 fatty acids, 4 g daily

25 A 35-year-old woman with a history of gastroesophageal reflux disease, dyslipidemia, mild liver steatosis, and polycystic ovary syndrome presents for weight management. Her BMI is 42 kg/m^2. She lost 15 lb (6.8 kg) with protein-sparing modified fasting and an aerobic exercise program, but she regained the weight within 2 years. She is interested in taking a medication that would help reduce weight, cardiovascular risk, and liver fat levels. She currently takes atorvastatin. She has a strong family history of coronary artery disease; her father had a myocardial infarction at age 55 years. She is concerned about her weight and cardiometabolic risk.

Which of the following agents would be most effective in achieving this patient's goals?

A. Bupropion
B. Orlistat
C. Phentermine
D. Semaglutide
E. Tirzepatide

26 A 44-year-old man with a history of type 2 diabetes, dyslipidemia, hypertension, and a BMI of 38 kg/m^2 presents for counseling regarding his weight and related conditions. He reports reduced energy and low-back pain but is otherwise asymptomatic. He does not use tobacco or drink alcohol. His medications include metformin; atorvastatin, 40 mg daily; and lisinopril, 10 mg daily.

Laboratory test results:

- Hemoglobin A_{1c} = 7.2% (4.0%-5.6%) (55 mmol/mol [20-38 mmol/mol])
- LDL cholesterol = 95 mg/dL (<100 mg/dL) (SI: 2.46 mmol/L [<2.59 mmol/L])
- Triglycerides = 320 mg/dL (<150 mg/dL) (SI: 3.62 mmol/L [<1.70 mmol/L])
- ALT, normal
- AST, normal

Which of the following is the best initial approach to evaluate for metabolic dysfunction-associated steatohepatitis in this patient

A. Assess for secondary causes of liver fibrosis, including alcohol history, hepatitis, and medications that can cause liver steatosis

B. Calculate FIB-4 score and consider liver elastography

C. Perform liver ultrasonography and prescribe vitamin E

D. Recommend no further evaluation for metabolic dysfunction-associated steatohepatitis

Pituitary Board Review

John David Carmichael, MD

1 A 32-year-old woman presents for follow-up of thyroid hormone replacement therapy. She had surgery to remove a pituitary macroadenoma 5 years ago and stereotactic radiosurgery for residual tumor 3 years ago. She has been tested routinely for pituitary deficiency. Two years ago, GH deficiency was diagnosed, and she began GH replacement. When she developed amenorrhea 1 year ago, she started an estrogen-containing oral contraceptive pill. Recently, central hypothyroidism was diagnosed after the following laboratory values were documented:

TSH = 0.85 mIU/L (0.5-5.0 mIU/L)
Free T_4 = 0.48 ng/dL (0.8-1.8 ng/dL)
(SI: 6.17 pmol/L [10.30-23.17 pmol/L])
Total T_4 = 5.6 μg/dL (5.5-12.5 μg/dL)
(SI: 72.07 nmol/L [70.79-160.88 nmol/L])

Levothyroxine was initiated at a dosage of 112 mcg daily, based on her weight. Before starting levothyroxine, a corticotropin-stimulation test result was documented to be normal.

Now, 3 months after starting levothyroxine, she presents for titration of replacement therapy. She is asymptomatic.

Current laboratory test results (drawn before her morning dose of levothyroxine):

TSH = 0.27 mIU/L (0.5-5.0 mIU/L)
Free T_4 = 0.93 ng/dL (0.8-1.8 ng/dL)
(SI: 11.97 pmol/L [10.30-23.17 pmol/L])
Total T_4 = 9.0 μg/dL (5.5-12.5 μg/dL)
(SI: 115.83 nmol/L [70.79-160.88 nmol/L])
Cortisol (8 AM) = 16.1 μg/dL (5-25 μg/dL)
(SI: 444.1 nmol/L [137.9-689.7 nmol/L])

Which of the following is the best modification and corresponding rationale to change her thyroid treatment regimen?

A. Continue levothyroxine at 112 mcg daily because the free T_4 concentration is in the reference range
B. Decrease levothyroxine to 100 mcg daily because the TSH concentration is below the reference range
C. Decrease levothyroxine to 100 mcg daily because the use of an estrogen-containing contraceptive pill is artifactually lowering the free T_4 concentration
D. Increase levothyroxine to 125 mcg daily because the free T_4 concentration is in the lower half of the reference range
E. Increase levothyroxine to 125 mcg daily because the TSH concentration is not at target (<0.1 mIU/L)

2 A 32-year-old man is referred after an emergency department visit resulting from a pedestrian vs motor vehicle accident. CT demonstrated a sellar mass, and follow-up MRI describes a 1.2-cm, nonenhancing lesion centered in the sella on T1-weighted images with contrast. There is no cavernous sinus invasion noted, but there is suprasellar extension with mild compression of the optic chiasm. T2-weighted images do not demonstrate any cystic component of the mass. He reports no symptoms. He takes no medications.

On physical examination, there are no signs of acromegaly or hypercortisolism. Extraocular muscles are intact, and visual fields are full to confrontation testing. There is no gynecomastia or testicular atrophy.

Laboratory test results:

Serum IGF-1, normal
Free and total testosterone, normal
Free T_4, normal
TSH, normal
Cortisol (8 AM) = 18.3 μg/dL (5-25 μg/dL) (SI: 504.8 nmol/L [137.9-689.7 nmol/L])

Prolactin was mildly elevated when a sample was drawn in the emergency department, but a recent measurement is at the upper normal limit (15.1 ng/mL [0.65 nmol/L]).

Which of the following is the best next step in this patient's management?

A. 1-mg overnight dexamethasone-suppression testing
B. Formal testing of visual fields by an ophthalmologist
C. Referral for transsphenoidal surgical resection of the mass
D. Repeat MRI in 6 months
E. Repeat prolactin measurement with specific request to the lab for serial dilutions

3 A 26-year-old woman underwent brain MRI for a research study as a healthy volunteer. She has no notable medical history and takes no medications. She has never been pregnant or taken birth control medications. Menstrual periods are regular, and the laboratory testing she had done for the study revealed normal serum concentrations of TSH and free T_4. MRI shows an enlarged sellar mass extending superiorly, with suprasellar convexity, abutting the optic chiasm (*see image*). The T1-weighted images with contrast show uniform enhancement throughout the mass. There is no discrete hypoenhancing lesion noted. T2-weighted images do not show any cystic changes and demonstrate homogeneous tissue throughout the mass. The posterior pituitary bright spot is noted on the sagittal noncontrast T1-weighted images.

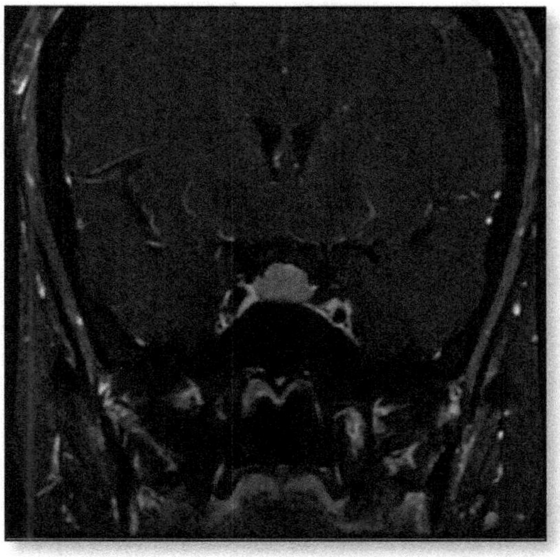

Which of the following is the most likely cause of this patient's sellar mass?

A. Lymphocytic hypophysitis
B. Parasellar meningioma
C. Pituitary hyperplasia
D. Pituitary macroadenoma
E. Rathke cleft cyst

4 A 21-year-old man with GH deficiency is transferring care from his pediatric endocrinologist. He is currently treated with daily GH injections; testosterone enanthate, 200 mg intramuscularly every 2 weeks; and levothyroxine, 125 mcg daily. In childhood, the patient had short stature secondary to GH deficiency (with confirmatory testing). Shortly after beginning GH treatment, central hypothyroidism was diagnosed, and levothyroxine was initiated. Testosterone was started when puberty was delayed. He is tolerating his medications well, and recent testing confirms normal concentrations of IGF-1, testosterone, and levothyroxine. His serum prolactin concentration is low. He reports no polydipsia or polyuria. He does not recall if his previous doctors did any genetic testing or GH testing.

In addition to routine monitoring of GH, testosterone, and thyroid hormone replacement, which of the following is the best treatment plan for this patient?

A. Assessment for adrenal insufficiency now and then annually with stimulation testing (likely *PROP1* pathogenic variant)
B. Assessment for adrenal insufficiency now (likely *TPIT* pathogenic variant)
C. Discontinuation of GH for 1 month followed by GH-stimulation testing
D. Empiric treatment with hydrocortisone, with instructions for sick-day dosing and safety precautions
E. No screening of adrenal insufficiency is needed (likely *POU1F1* pathogenic variant)

5 A 34-year-old woman presents to the emergency department with worsening of chronic headache. There are no other neurological signs. She reports intermittent headache for 10 years since the birth of her youngest child. Review of systems is notable for chronic constipation and several years of amenorrhea.

On physical examination, her blood pressure is 110/68 mm Hg, pulse rate is 62 beats/min, temperature is 95.4°F (35.2°C), and BMI is 24.6 kg/m^2. Her skin is cool and dry, and she has periorbital edema. Deep tendon reflexes are delayed. Head CT suggests the presence of fluid in the sella but no other abnormal findings. MRI demonstrates a normal-sized but empty sella; no normal pituitary tissue is noted, and no pituitary tumor is visible.

Laboratory test results:

TSH = 0.68 mIU/L (0.5-5.0 mIU/L)
LH and FSH, undetectable
IGF-1 = 52 ng/mL (113-297 ng/mL)
(SI: 6.8 nmol/L [14.8-38.9 nmol/L])
Prolactin = 35.4 ng/mL (4-23 ng/mL)
(SI: 1.54 nmol/L [0.17-1.00 nmol/L])
Serum cortisol (4 PM) = 0.8 μg/dL (2-14 μg/dL)
(SI: 22.1 nmol/L [55.2-386.2 nmol/L])

Which of the following is the most likely etiology of this patient's empty sella?

A. Pituitary apoplexy from a nonfunctioning adenoma
B. *PROP1* pathogenic variant
C. Pseudotumor cerebri due to increased intracranial pressure
D. Ruptured Rathke cleft cyst
E. Sheehan syndrome with infarction of normal pituitary during childbirth

6 A 30-year-old woman presents for evaluation of oligomenorrhea. She has no significant galactorrhea and no other relevant medical history. She describes mild facial hirsutism, which she treats with cosmetic electrolysis. She reports getting 6 menstrual periods over the last year, with some skipped periods, and the interval between periods otherwise being 45 days.

Laboratory test results:

Basic metabolic panel, normal
Plasma glucose = 95 mg/dL (70-99 mg/dL)
(SI: 5.3 mmol/L [3.9-5.5 mmol/L])
Prolactin = 82 ng/mL (4-23 ng/mL)
(SI: 3.56 nmol/L [0.17-1.00 nmol/L])
LH and FSH, normal
Total testosterone = 52 ng/dL (8-60 ng/dL)
(SI: 1.8 nmol/L [0.3-2.1 nmol/L])
Serum TSH = 5.2 mIU/L (0.5-5.0 mIU/L)
Free T_4 = 1.1 ng/dL (0.8-1.8 ng/dL)
(SI: 14.16 pmol/L [10.30-23.17 pmol/L])

Pituitary MRI shows no evidence of tumor, cyst, or other abnormality.

Which of the following is the best next laboratory test in this patient's evaluation?

A. DHEA-S
B. IGF-1
C. Macroprolactin
D. Prolactin with serial dilutions
E. TPO antibodies

7 A 42-year-old man with headaches is evaluated with MRI and is found to have a 2.6-cm sellar mass that extends into the left cavernous sinus. His headaches have been worsening over the past 2 months. He describes normal vision. In retrospect, he has had reduced libido over the preceding 6 months, along with progressive erectile dysfunction. He has also noted more fatigue and poor short-term memory.

On physical examination, he is a tired-appearing man. His blood pressure is 96/66 mm Hg, pulse rate is 96 beats/min, and BMI is 31.1 kg/m^2. Examination findings are unremarkable except for increased abdominal girth.

Laboratory results demonstrate hypopituitarism, with hypogonadotropic hypogonadism, low IGF-1, central hypothyroidism, low serum cortisol, and elevated prolactin (142 ng/mL [SI: 6.17 nmol/L]).

Transsphenoidal surgery with an experienced neurosurgeon reveals an SF-1 staining pituitary adenoma. Postoperative MRI shows residual tumor in the left cavernous sinus. Repeated MRI 6 months later shows growth of the cavernous sinus tumor.

Which of the following treatments is the best choice now to manage the residual tumor and control tumor growth?

A. Another surgery
B. Bromocriptine
C. Cabergoline
D. Octreotide long-acting release
E. Stereotactic radiotherapy

8 A 41-year-old woman presents with acromegaly. She previously underwent transsphenoidal surgery for a macroadenoma, and she has residual disease in the left cavernous sinus. Her postoperative IGF-1 concentration was 932 ng/mL (98-261 ng/mL) (SI: 122.1 nmol/L [12.8-34.2 nmol/L]). Octreotide long-acting release, 20 mg monthly, was initiated, which lowered her IGF-1 concentration to 850 ng/mL (111.4 nmol/L). The octreotide dosage was increased to 30 mg monthly, but her IGF-1 concentration remains unchanged, and the tumor is slightly larger on MRI.

Which of the following interventions would best reduce this patient's tumor size and IGF-1 levels in the next 6 months?

A. Add cabergoline
B. Add pegvisomant
C. Perform stereotactic radiotherapy
D. Switch to pasireotide
E. Switch to the oral octreotide capsule

9 A 27-year-old woman (G0) presents for evaluation after her gynecologist noted hyperprolactinemia. She had menarche at age 12 years and has always had normal menses. In the past 8 months, she has had scant, bilateral nipple discharge, but this does not bother her. She is considering starting a family, although not for a few years. She has no headaches, hirsutism, or acne.

On physical examination, she appears comfortable. Her blood pressure is 96/68 mm Hg, and pulse rate is 74 beats/min. There are no physical stigmata of acromegaly or Cushing disease. She has scant bilateral nipple discharge on palpation. Her breast examination findings are otherwise normal.

Laboratory test results:

Prolactin = 54 ng/mL (4-30 ng/mL)
(SI: 2.35 nmol/L [0.17-1.30 nmol/L])
IGF-1 = 185 ng/mL (117-321 ng/mL)
(SI: 24.2 nmol/L [15.3-42.1 nmol/L])
TSH = 2.5 mIU/L (0.5-5.0 mIU/L)
Free T_4 = 1.3 ng/dL (0.8-1.8 ng/dL)
(SI:16.73 pmol/L [10.30-23.17 pmol/L])

MRI reveals a 7-mm hypoenhancing abnormality in the left side of the sella, with mild deviation of the stalk to the right.

Which of the following is the most appropriate next step in this patient's management?

A. Another pituitary MRI in 6 months
B. Cabergoline therapy
C. Prolactin measurement with serial dilution
D. Repeated clinical assessment and laboratory monitoring in 6 months
E. Stereotactic radiotherapy

10 A 64-year-old man is found to have a 2.3-cm sellar mass abutting the optic chiasm after his ophthalmologist identified a left eye visual field defect. MRI shows a relatively normal-sized sella with a large cystic mass extending in a suprasellar fashion. In retrospect, he has had headaches, poor energy, frequent urination, increased thirst, and a 46-lb (20.9-kg) weight gain over the past 2 years.

Laboratory test results:

Complete blood cell count, normal
Hematocrit = 32% (41%-51%) (SI: 0.32 [0.41-0.51])
Fasting blood glucose = 78 mg/dL (70-99 mg/dL) (SI: 7.3 mmol/L [3.9-5.5 mmol/L])
TSH = 0.5 mIU/L (0.5-5.0 mIU/L)
Free T_4 = 0.6 ng/dL (0.8-1.8 ng/dL) (SI: 7.72 pmol/L [10.30-23.17 pmol/L])
Prolactin = 42.7 ng/mL (4-23 ng/mL) (SI: 1.86 nmol/L [0.17-1.00 nmol/L])
Cortisol (8 AM) = 6 µg/dL (5-25 µg/dL) (SI: 165.5 nmol/L [137.9-689.7 nmol/L])
Total testosterone (8 AM) = 115 ng/dL (300-900 ng/dL) (SI: 4.0 nmol/L [10.4-31.2 nmol/L])
IGF-1 = 76 ng/mL (72-207 ng/mL) (SI: 10.0 nmol/L [9.4-27.1 nmol/L])
Sodium = 154 mEq/L (136-142 mEq/L) (SI: 154 mmol/L [136-142 mmol/L])
Potassium = 3.9 mEq/L (3.5-5.0 mEq/L) (SI: 3.9 mmol/L [3.5-5.0 mmol/L])

Which of the following is the most likely diagnosis?

A. Craniopharyngioma
B. Gonadotroph adenoma
C. Langerhans cell histiocytosis
D. Prolactinoma
E. Silent corticotroph adenoma

11 The parents of an 18-year-old man ask if he should continue taking GH when he goes to college. Isolated idiopathic GH deficiency was diagnosed at age 9 years, and the patient experienced a substantial increase in height when he started GH treatment. His growth rate slowed to less than 1 cm/y for the past 2 years.

Which of the following is the best recommendation for this patient?

A. Continue GH therapy but decrease the dosage to a more typical adult dosage
B. Discontinue GH therapy because growth has been completed
C. Measure IGF-1 one month after stopping GH
D. Measure morning GH one month after stopping GH
E. Perform a GH-stimulation test one month after stopping GH

12 A 37-year-old woman with ACTH-dependent Cushing syndrome has an MRI finding of a 4-mm left-sided sellar lesion, adjacent to the cavernous sinus. Her ACTH concentration is 58 pg/mL (12.8 pmol/L). Inferior petrosal sinus catheterization shows central ACTH hypersecretion, and there is lateralization to the left side. The patient undergoes transsphenoidal surgery, and the left-sided lesion is determined to be an adenoma, subsequently staining positive for ACTH. The adjacent dura has tumor involvement as well. Postoperatively, serum cortisol fails to normalize. Reoperation with left hemihypophysectomy does not lower cortisol any further, and no tumor is detected.

Laboratory test results:

Hemoglobin A_{1c} = 7.5% (4.0%-5.6%) (58 mmol/mol [20-38 mmol/mol])
ACTH = 28 pg/mL (10-60 pg/mL) (SI: 6.2 pmol/L [2.2-13.2 pmol/L])
Cortisol = 26.4 µg/dL (5-25 µg/dL) (SI: 728.3 nmol/L [137.9-689.7 nmol/L])

Medical therapy is initiated, and over the subsequent weeks her cushingoid features improve and her plasma glucose concentration normalizes. Her current plasma ACTH concentration is 42 pg/mL (9.2 pmol/L), and her morning cortisol concentration is 11.5 µg/dL (317.3 mmol/L). However, a few months later she notes bothersome hair growth on her face and periareolar area.

Which of the following medications is she most likely receiving?

A. Ketoconazole
B. Mifepristone
C. Mitotane
D. Osilodrostat
E. Pasireotide

13 A 39-year-old man presents with acromegaly. He previously underwent transsphenoidal surgery for a macroadenoma, and he has residual disease in the left cavernous sinus. His postoperative IGF-1 concentration was 932 ng/mL (106-277 ng/mL) (SI: 122.1 nmol/L [13.9-36.3 nmol/L]). He was started on lanreotide depot, 90 mg monthly, which normalized his IGF-1 level. He asks whether he may be a candidate for the oral octreotide capsule.

Which of the following outcomes is most likely if he switches to the oral octreotide capsule?

A. Increased gastrointestinal symptoms
B. Increased GH levels
C. Increased glucose levels
D. Increased IGF-1 levels
E. Maintenance of normal IGF-1 levels

14 A 44-year-old man is evaluated for persistent fatigue. He was previously diagnosed with a seizure disorder and pituitary adenoma, and he underwent transsphenoidal surgery followed by fractionated radiation therapy 2 years ago. He developed partial hypopituitarism, and he has been taking levothyroxine, 88 mcg orally daily, and testosterone gel (1.62%), 40.5 mg daily. He notes difficulty with short-term memory and has been unable to function at work due to poor attention span. Family history and personal medical history are unremarkable (aside from his pituitary adenoma).

On physical examination, he appears fatigued and slightly depressed. His blood pressure is 115/84 mm Hg, pulse rate is 84 beats/min, and BMI is 29 kg/m^2. He has increased abdominal girth, but examination findings are otherwise normal.

Laboratory test results:

Cortisol (8 AM) = 19.1 μg/dL (5-25 μg/dL)
(SI: 526.9 nmol/L [137.9-689.7 nmol/L])
Free T_4 = 1.6 ng/dL (0.8-1.8 ng/dL)
(SI: 20.6 pmol/L [10.30-23.17 pmol/L])
Prolactin = 7.6 ng/mL (4-23 ng/mL)
(SI: 0.33 nmol/L [0.17-1.00 nmol/L])
Total testosterone = 320 ng/dL (300-900 ng/dL)
(SI: 11.1 nmol/L [10.4-31.2 nmol/L])
IGF-1 = 115 ng/dL (98-261 ng/mL)
(SI: 15.1 nmol/L [12.8-34.2 nmol/L])
Comprehensive chemistry panel, normal
Complete blood cell count, normal

Which of the following is the best next step in his endocrine management?

A. Measure random GH level
B. Perform a glucagon-stimulation test to assess GH levels
C. Perform an insulin tolerance test
D. Provide him with information regarding an active lifestyle with diet and exercise modification
E. Refer to a psychiatrist for management of depression

15 A 43-year-old woman presents with weight loss, tremor, palpitations, and sweating. She has mild frontal headaches, irregular menses, and atrial fibrillation.

Laboratory test results:

Free T_4 = 2.3 ng/dL (0.8-1.8 ng/dL)
(SI: 29.60 pmol/L [10.30-23.17 pmol/L])
Total T_3 = 386 ng/dL (70-200 ng/dL)
(SI: 5.94 nmol/L [1.08-3.08 nmol/L])
TSH = 2.8 mIU/L (0.5-5.0 mIU/L)
Prolactin = 33 ng/mL (4-30 ng/mL)
(SI: 1.43 nmol/L [0.17-1.30 nmol/L])

A radioiodine scan reveals 55% uptake in a homogeneous pattern in the thyroid gland. Brain MRI reveals a 2.1-cm pituitary adenoma invading the cavernous sinus.

She is caring for her elderly parents and cannot take time off for surgery.

Which of the following is the best next step for managing both the hyperthyroidism and the pituitary adenoma?

A. Cabergoline
B. Methimazole
C. Octreotide long-acting release
D. Radiation therapy
E. Radioactive iodine

16 Cushing disease is diagnosed in a 48-year-old woman.

Preoperative laboratory test results:
Cortisol (8 AM) = 26.7 μg/dL (5-25 μg/dL) (SI: 736.6 nmol/L [137.9-689.7 nmol/L])
ACTH (8 AM) = 109 pg/mL (10-60 pg/mL) (SI: 24.0 pmol/L [2.2-13.2 pmol/L])

MRI shows a 4-mm pituitary lesion. Glucocorticoids are withheld after surgery. Twenty-four hours after transsphenoidal surgery, her morning cortisol concentration is 11 μg/dL (303.5 nmol/L). Seventy-two hours after surgery, her morning cortisol and ACTH concentrations are 10.2 μg/dL (281.4 nmol/L) and 31 pg/mL (6.8 pmol/L), respectively, and she is discharged home. Two weeks postoperatively, her morning cortisol concentration is 13 μg/dL (358.6 nmol/L). She feels weak and tired.

Which of the following is the best management recommendation?

A. Another transsphenoidal surgery
B. Cosyntropin-stimulation test to determine whether maintenance hydrocortisone treatment is needed
C. Empiric hydrocortisone daily
D. Medical therapy with mitotane
E. Stereotactic radiosurgery

17 A 41-year-old woman presents with amenorrhea and galactorrhea and is found to have a prolactin concentration of 152 ng/mL (4-30 ng/mL) (SI: 6.61 nmol/L [0.17-1.30 nmol/L]). MRI documents a 2.4-cm pituitary adenoma that abuts the optic chiasm. Findings on formal visual field testing are normal. While taking bromocriptine, 2.5 mg daily, her prolactin concentration decreases to 18 ng/mL (0.78 nmol/L), menses return but are irregular, and galactorrhea resolves. Follow-up MRI in 3 months shows no change in adenoma size. She asks whether this management is sufficient for long-term care.

Which of the following is the best next step in this patient's care?

A. Administer octreotide long-acting release
B. Discuss surgery
C. Increase the bromocriptine dosage
D. Perform pituitary-directed MRI in 6 months
E. Switch bromocriptine to cabergoline

18 A 29-year-old man underwent surgical removal of a nonfunctioning pituitary macroadenoma 3 years ago. He has hypopituitarism and is currently taking hormone replacement with levothyroxine, hydrocortisone, GH, and injectable testosterone ester. He has normal libido and erectile function. He is interested in fertility.

On physical examination, he is well virilized with 18-cc testes bilaterally that have normal consistency.

Which of the following is the best next step in this patient's management?

A. Stop testosterone and obtain a semen analysis
B. Suggest he consider adoption
C. Switch from testosterone to clomiphene citrate
D. Switch from testosterone to hCG injections, 3 times weekly
E. Switch from testosterone to hCG injections, 3 times weekly, and FSH injections, twice weekly

19 A 24-year-old woman is referred for endocrine evaluation. Her parents report that she received GH injections since age 1 year for growth failure and GH deficiency. Her growth rate was appropriate while on treatment. At age 9 years, she developed fatigue and weight gain, and laboratory tests revealed the following:

TSH = 0.2 mIU/L (0.5-5.0 mIU/L)
Free T_4 = 0.3 ng/dL (0.8-1.8 ng/dL)
(SI: 3.86 pmol/L [10.30-23.17 pmol/L])

Levothyroxine was initiated at that time. Menarche occurred at age 11 years, and her periods have always been regular. At age 15 years, she was in a bike accident and had brief loss of consciousness. Concussion was subsequently diagnosed. She stopped taking GH when she completed growth at age 18 years. She has no polyuria or polydipsia.

Laboratory test results (ordered by the referring physician):

Prolactin = 2 ng/mL (4-30 ng/mL) (SI: 0.09 nmol/L [0.17-1.30 nmol/L])
Free T_4 = 1.3 ng/dL (SI: 16.7 pmol/L)
LH = 13.0 mIU/mL (1.0-18.0 mIU/L [follicular]) (SI: 13.0 IU/L [1.0-18.0 IU/L])
FSH = 9.0 mIU/mL (2.0-12.0 mIU/L [follicular]) (SI: 9.0 IU/L [1.0-13.0 IU/L])

A 250-mcg intravenous cosyntropin-stimulation test results in a 60-minute serum cortisol value of 23 µg/dL (635 nmol/L). Brain MRI reveals a slight reduction in sellar contents.

On physical examination, she has normal vital signs and appears euthyroid.

Which of the following is the most likely cause of these biochemical findings?

A. Hypopituitarism following brain injury
B. Langerhans cell histiocytosis
C. Pathogenic variant in the *POU1F1* gene
D. Pathogenic variant in the *PROP1* gene
E. Pathogenic variant in the *TBX19(TPIT)* gene

20 A 37-year-old woman with amenorrhea and galactorrhea is found to have a prolactin concentration of 1593 ng/mL (69.3 nmol/L) and a 2.6-cm pituitary macroadenoma on MRI. With cabergoline, 0.5 mg twice weekly, prolactin levels normalize and the tumor size decreases to 7 mm. Over the next 18 months (while taking her medication regularly), her prolactin concentration increases to 284 ng/mL (12.3 nmol/L) and her tumor grows to 1.4 cm. Despite a gradual increase in the cabergoline dosage to 2 mg daily over the next year, her prolactin concentration rises to 4513 ng/mL (196.2 nmol/L) and her tumor grows to 3.2 cm and involves the local parenchyma. She subsequently undergoes a 2-stage transsphenoidal/transcranial near-total resection and stereotactic radiosurgery. Over the ensuing 8 months, the tumor continues to grow into the temporal and frontal lobes.

Which of the following treatments is the best choice now?

A. Another craniotomy
B. Conventional radiotherapy
C. Octreotide long-acting release
D. Pasireotide
E. Temozolomide

21 A 19-year-old woman has hypopituitarism and arginine vasopressin deficiency due to Langerhans cell histiocytosis involving her hypothalamus and pituitary stalk. She was just admitted to the hospital following head trauma from a motor vehicle crash and is now in a drug-induced coma. She is being treated with stress-dose steroids and has continued desmopressin, as well as D5W (5% dextrose in water) at a rate of 100 mL/h. Endocrinology is consulted when her morning serum sodium concentration is documented to be 112 mEq/L (112 mmol/L).

In addition to holding the desmopressin, which of the following is the best treatment plan?

A. Change the D5W to half-normal saline and measure serum sodium every 2 to 4 hours
B. Change the D5W to normal saline and measure serum sodium in 2 to 4 hours
C. Change the D5W to normal saline and measure serum sodium in 12 hours
D. Give hypertonic saline to raise the serum sodium by 6 mEq/L (6 mmol/L) over 6 hours
E. Give hypertonic saline to raise the serum sodium by 2 mEq/L (2 mmol/L) over 12 hours

22 A 23-year-old woman has developed headaches and mild weakness in her third trimester of pregnancy. She was previously well and had regular menses. After discontinuing barrier contraception, she became pregnant within 2 months. Her pregnancy has gone well, aside from recent symptoms.

On physical examination, she is an ill-appearing woman. Her blood pressure is 96/68 mm Hg, and pulse rate is 74 beats/min. Her uterus is appropriately sized for 36 weeks' gestation.

Laboratory test results:

Free T_4 = 0.9 ng/dL (0.8-1.8 ng/dL)
(SI: 11.6 pmol/L [10.3-23.2 pmol/L])
TSH = 1.3 mIU/L (0.5-5.0 mIU/L)
Prolactin = 198 ng/mL (4-30 ng/mL)
(SI: 8.61 nmol/L [0.17-1.30 nmol/L])

Noncontrast MRI shows diffusely enlarged sellar contents extending above the sella and impinging the optic chiasm (*see image*). The craniocaudal diameter is 18 mm. A Goldmann visual field examination shows a small degree of bilateral superior and temporal visual field defects.

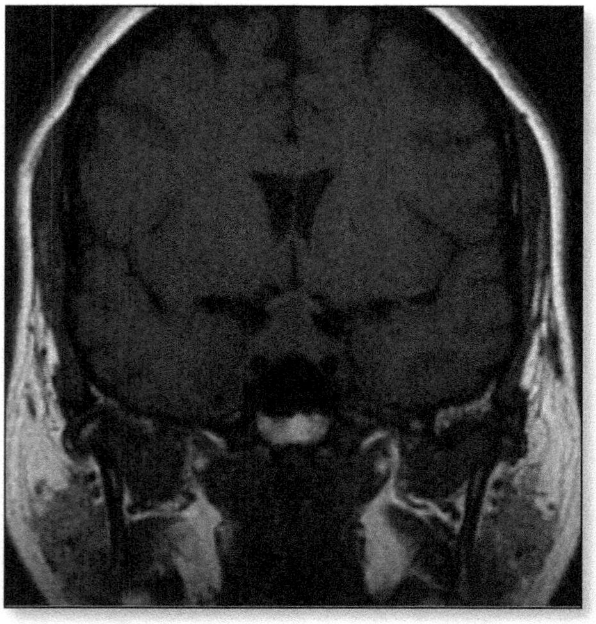

Courtesy of William Young.

Which of the following is the most likely diagnosis?

A. Clinically nonfunctioning pituitary adenoma
B. Craniopharyngioma
C. Lymphocytic hypophysitis
D. Pituitary hyperplasia of pregnancy
E. Prolactinoma

Thyroid, Section 1 Board Review

Jacqueline Jonklaas, MD, PhD, MPH

1 A 58-year-old woman has been treated with atorvastatin, 40 mg daily, for hyperlipidemia for 5 years. She has been adherent to her statin therapy and has never reported any adverse effects. At today's visit, she feels tired and notes new constipation, muscle pain, stiffness, and cramping.

On physical examination, she has proximal muscle weakness and has difficulty rising from a seated position. She has decreased patellar reflexes.

Laboratory test results:

LDL cholesterol = 80 mg/dL (<100 mg/dL) (SI: 2.07 mmol/L [<2.59 mmol/L])
Creatine kinase = 2300 U/L (50-200 U/L) (SI: 38.41 µkat/L [0.84-3.34 µkat/L])

Which of the following additional diagnostic assessments would be helpful in determining what precipitated the patient's myopathy?

A. Aldolase measurement
B. Electromyography
C. Erythrocyte sedimentation rate measurement
D. MRI of the lower extremities
E. TSH measurement

2 A 29-year-old pregnant woman with postsurgical hypothyroidism was taking levothyroxine, 88 mcg daily, before pregnancy. Her levothyroxine dosage was increased to 112 mcg daily early in the first trimester. She then required a further increase to 125 mcg daily and has been maintained at that dosage throughout the pregnancy. Her TSH concentration has remained in a good range (<2.5 mIU/L). The patient has gained 26.5 lb (12 kg) during her pregnancy. She is approaching her estimated due date. She asks what levothyroxine dosage she should start taking when she returns home after delivery. She is planning to breastfeed her baby.

Which of the following is the best recommendation for an appropriate levothyroxine dosage after delivery?

A. Alternate 112 mcg daily and 125 mcg daily
B. Continue 125 mcg daily
C. Decrease to early first-trimester dosage of 112 mcg daily
D. Decrease to prepregnancy dosage of 88 mcg daily
E. Hold the decision about her levothyroxine dosage until her weight is assessed at 6 weeks post partum

3 A 30-year-old body builder was preparing for a major competition for which he wished to improve his muscle definition. He was taking multiple supplements for this purpose. Before a competitive event last year, he developed atrial fibrillation that subsequently resolved. He has been referred to endocrinology for tachycardia (reportedly 130 beats/min). The patient is vague about the drug regimen that he uses as part of his training, but he does share that he uses multiple agents in a cyclic pattern.

On physical examination, he appears lean and muscular. His heart rate is currently 99 beats/min.

Initial laboratory test results:

Hematocrit = 57% (41%-51%) (SI: 0.57 [0.41-0.51])
Testosterone = 1000 ng/dL (300-900 ng/dL) (SI: 34.7 nmol/L [10.4-31.2 nmol/L])
LH = <0.1 mIU/mL (1.0-9.0 mIU/mL) (SI: <0.1 IU/L [1.0-9.0 IU/L])
SHBG = 10.5 µg/mL (1.1-6.7 µg/mL) (SI: 93.4 nmol/L [10-60 nmol/L])
TSH = <0.01 mIU/L (0.5-5.0 mIU/L)

Free T_4 = 0.6 ng/dL (0.8-1.8 ng/dL) (SI: 7.7 pmol/L [10.30-23.17 pmol/L])
Total T_3 = 180 ng/dL (70-200 ng/dL) (SI: 2.8 nmol/L [1.08-3.08 nmol/L])
TRAb = ≤1.75 IU/L (≤1.75 IU/L)

The endocrinologist believes that the patient is using thyroid hormone as part of his drug cocktail.

Which of the following is the best diagnostic approach to confirm recent use of thyroid hormone?

A. Free T_3 measurement
B. hCG measurement
C. ^{123}I thyroid scan and uptake
D. Measurement of free T_4 using a different immunoassay
E. Thyroid ultrasonography

4 A 25-year-old transgender woman had a previous diagnosis of primary hypothyroidism before her transition. She is adherent to levothyroxine therapy and has maintained a normal TSH concentration over the years. She recently started a feminizing hormonal regimen, and the following effects on her thyroid function are observed:

Thyroid analyte	1 Month before hormonal regimen	3 Months after hormonal regimen initiated	Reference range
TSH	1.08 mIU/L	7.16 mIU/L	0.5-5.0 mIU/L
Free T_4	1.57 ng/dL (SI: 20.21 pmol/L)	1.05 ng/dL (SI: 13.51 pmol/L)	0.8-1.8 ng/dL (SI: 10.30-23.17 pmol/L)
Total T_4	9.1 μg/dL (SI: 117.12 nmol/L)	11.4 μg/dL (SI: 146.72 nmol/L)	5.5-12.5 μg/dL (SI: 70.79-160.88 nmol/L)

Based on the changes in the thyroid function, what is the most likely therapy that the patient has started?

A. Cyproterone acetate
B. Estrogen gel
C. Estrogen patch
D. Oral conjugated estrogens
E. Progesterone

5 A 23-year-old man was diagnosed with Graves disease and initially treated with methimazole. He elected to undergo thyroidectomy due to difficulty titrating his methimazole dosage. Following thyroidectomy, he was treated with levothyroxine and attained consistent euthyroidism. He transitioned care to his primary care physician but then returned 12 years later with concerns of recurrent hyperthyroidism. His primary care physician had reduced his levothyroxine dosage from 125 mcg to 25 mcg daily.

At today's visit, the patient appears thyrotoxic, agitated, and restless. Physical examination shows no palpable tissue in the thyroid bed. However, a midline mass is noted at the level of the hyoid bone.

Laboratory test results:
TSH = <0.01 mIU/L (0.5-5.0 mIU/L)
Free T_4 = 3.1 ng/dL (0.8-1.8 ng/dL) (SI: 39.90 pmol/L [10.30-23.17 pmol/L])
Total T_3 = 376 ng/dL (70-200 ng/dL) (SI: 5.79 nmol/L [1.08-3.08 nmol/L])
Thyroid-stimulating immunoglobulin = 230% (≤120% of basal activity)

Which additional evaluation would be most helpful?

A. Further questioning about over-the-counter and dietary supplements
B. ^{123}I thyroid scan and uptake
C. Measurement of hCG
D. Serum thyroglobulin
E. Whole-body ^{123}I iodine scan

6 A 36-year-old woman presents with new weight gain (14-lb [4.5-kg]), constipation, irregular menses, and cold intolerance. She gets up very early in the morning for her job as a school bus driver and reports that she is exhausted by the early afternoon.

Laboratory test results (sample collected while fasting):
TSH = 134.0 mIU/L (0.5-5.0 mIU/L)
Free T_4 = 0.2 ng/dL (0.8-1.8 ng/dL) (SI: 2.57 pmol/L [10.30-23.17 pmol/L])
TPO antibodies = 466 IU/mL (<2.0 IU/mL) (SI: 466 kIU/L [<2.0 kIU/L])

LDL cholesterol = 201 mg/dL (<100 mg/dL [optimal]) (SI: 5.21 mmol/L [<2.59 mmol/L])
Total cholesterol = 300 mg/dL (<200 mg/dL [optimal]) (SI: 7.77 mmol/L [<5.18 mmol/L])
HDL cholesterol = 52 mg/dL (>60 mg/dL [optimal]) (SI: 1.35 mmol/L [>1.55 mmol/L])
Triglycerides = 195 mg/dL (<150 mg/dL [optimal]) (SI: 2.20 mmol/L [<1.70 mmol/L])
Homocysteine = 2.97 mg/L (≤1.76 mg/L) (SI: 22 µmol/L [≤13 µmol/L])

Levothyroxine is started.

Once she is euthyroid, which of the following effects should the patient anticipate as a result of levothyroxine therapy?

A. Decreased total cholesterol and increased HDL cholesterol
B. Increased serum homocysteine
C. Restoration of ovulatory menstrual cycles
D. Significant loss of fat mass
E. Unaltered braking time when driving

7 A 28-year-old pregnant woman with Graves disease treated with an antithyroid drug is referred for medication adjustment. She is in her 18th week of pregnancy.

Which of the following sets of laboratory results is within recommended targets for this patient?

Answer	TSH	Free T_4	Total T_3
A.	0.05 mIU/L	2.30 ng/dL (SI: 29.60 pmol/L)	400 ng/dL (SI: 6.16 nmol/L)
B.	0.1 mIU/L	1.85 ng/dL (SI: 23.81 pmol/L)	350 ng/dL (SI: 5.39 nmol/L)
C.	1.5 mIU/L	1.10 ng/dL (SI: 14.16 pmol/L)	330 ng/dL (SI: 5.08 nmol/L)
D.	2.5 mIU/L	1.00 ng/dL (SI: 12.87 pmol/L)	280 ng/dL (SI: 4.31 nmol/L)
E.	3.5 mIU/L	0.90 ng/dL (SI: 11.58 pmol/L)	210 ng/dL (SI: 3.23 nmol/L)

Reference ranges: TSH, 0.5-5.0 mIU/L; free T_4, 0.8-1.8 ng/dL (10.30-23.17 pmol/L); total T_3, 70-200 ng/dL (1.08-3.08 nmol/L).

8 A 52-year-old woman with weight gain and fatigue is documented to have an elevated serum TSH level, which is confirmed on repeat testing. Her primary care physician prescribes levothyroxine, but the patient's symptoms do not resolve. Her physician is concerned about her unanticipated lack of biochemical response to treatment and refers the patient for management of levothyroxine therapy. In addition to levothyroxine, she takes calcium and a multivitamin with iron.

On physical examination, her pulse rate is 80 beats/min. She has no goiter or thyroidectomy scar, and her deep tendon reflexes are normal. Serial thyroid function test results and levothyroxine dosing are shown (*see table*).

Date	TSH	Free T_4	Levothyroxine dosage
January	11.9 mIU/L	1.3 ng/dL (SI: 16.73 pmol/L)	None
March	10.2 mIU/L	1.8 ng/dL (SI: 23.17 pmol/L)	75 mcg daily
May	10.7 mIU/L	2.1 ng/dL (SI: 27.03 pmol/L)	112 mcg daily

Reference ranges: TSH, 0.5-5.0 mIU/L; free T_4, 0.8-1.8 ng/dL (10.30-23.17 pmol/L).

Which of the following is the most likely explanation for these findings?

A. Heterophilic antibody interference with the TSH assay
B. Poor absorption of levothyroxine
C. Poor adherence to levothyroxine therapy
D. Resistance to thyroid hormone
E. TSH-secreting pituitary adenoma

9 A 47-year-old man starts a regimen of interferon alfa for chronic hepatitis C. Three months later, he reports palpitations and a 5-lb (2.3-kg) weight loss. He has no eye discomfort, vision problems, or neck pain.

On physical examination, his pulse rate is 95 beats/min, and his thyroid gland is 25 g without tenderness, nodules, or bruit.

Laboratory test results:

TSH = <0.01 mIU/L (0.5-5.0 mIU/L)

Free T_4 = 2.4 ng/dL (0.8-1.8 ng/dL)
(SI: 30.89 pmol/L [10.30-23.17 pmol/L])

TPO antibody titer = 230 IU/mL (<2.0 IU/mL)
(SI: 180 kIU/L [<2.0 kIU/L])

Radioactive iodine uptake at 24 hours = 0.4%

His hepatologist stops the interferon alfa.

Which of the following should be recommended now?

A. Atenolol
B. Intravenous immunoglobulin
C. Methimazole
D. Prednisone
E. Propylthiouracil

10 A 62-year-old woman with hypothyroidism is admitted to the surgical intensive care unit with acute necrotizing pancreatitis. Her serum TSH concentration 1 month before admission was 1.8 mIU/L. Her outpatient levothyroxine dosage is 100 mcg daily, which she has been taking in the morning on an empty stomach. Her surgical team is concerned about poor levothyroxine absorption due to bowel edema and would like to change to parenteral thyroid hormone therapy.

Which of the following regimens would be most appropriate?

A. Levothyroxine, 70 mcg intravenously once daily
B. Levothyroxine, 100 mcg intravenously once daily
C. Levothyroxine, 150 mcg intravenously once daily
D. Levothyroxine, 1000 mcg intramuscularly once weekly
E. Liothyronine, 25 mcg intravenously twice daily

11 A 37-year-old woman who is having difficulty losing weight is referred for abnormal thyroid function test results. She is otherwise asymptomatic and takes no medications. Her mother has hypothyroidism.

On physical examination, her pulse rate is 86 beats/min. Her thyroid is slightly enlarged without nodules or bruit, there is no tremor, and deep tendon reflexes are normal.

Laboratory test results:

TSH = 0.12 mIU/L (0.5-5.0 mIU/L)

Free T_4 = 1.7 ng/dL (0.8-1.8 ng/mL)
(SI: 21.88 pmol/L [10.30-23.17 pmol/L])

Total T_3 = 154 ng/dL (70-200 ng/dL)
(SI: 2.37 nmol/L [1.08-3.08 nmol/L])

Thyroid-stimulating immunoglobulin = 135%
(normal ≤120%)

Which of the following is the best next step in this patient's management?

A. Repeat laboratory tests in 3 months
B. Start an iodine-containing multivitamin
C. Start atenolol, 50 mg daily
D. Start methimazole, 20 mg daily
E. Treat with radioactive iodine

12 A 27-year-old woman with Graves hyperthyroidism has been treated with methimazole, 10 mg daily, for 14 months. On palpation, her thyroid gland is at the upper limit of normal size. There is no bruit. She does not smoke cigarettes. She would like to stop methimazole if possible.

Current laboratory test results:

TSH = 0.7 mIU/L (0.5-5.0 mIU/L)

Total T_3 = 166 ng/dL (70-200 ng/dL)
(SI: 2.56 nmol/L [1.08-3.08 nmol/L])

Free T_4 = 1.6 ng/dL (0.8-1.8 ng/dL)
(SI: 20.59 pmol/L [10.30-23.17 pmol/L])

TPO antibodies = 594 IU/mL (<2.0 IU/mL)
(SI: 594 kIU/L [<2.0 kIU/L])

Thyroid-stimulating immunoglobulin = 396%
(≤120% of basal activity)

Which of the following characteristics of this patient predicts a greater likelihood that Graves hyperthyroidism will recur if methimazole is stopped?

A. Age
B. Cigarette smoking status
C. Thyroid size
D. Thyroid-stimulating immunoglobulin level
E. TPO antibody titer

13 A 63-year-old man with metastatic renal cell carcinoma is prescribed sunitinib therapy. The patient has no history of thyroid dysfunction, and baseline thyroid function is normal.

Which of the following thyroid abnormalities is most likely to occur in this patient after starting sunitinib?

A. "Euthyroid sick" syndrome
B. Primary hyperthyroidism
C. Primary hypothyroidism
D. Secondary hyperthyroidism
E. Secondary hypothyroidism

14 A 57-year-old man with Graves disease develops agranulocytosis while taking methimazole. Methimazole is stopped and his white blood cell count recovers, but he develops nausea and vomiting and presents to the emergency department.

On physical examination, his temperature is 103°F (39.4°C), pulse rate is 140 beats/min and irregular, and crackles are heard to the mid lung fields. Free T_4 and T_3 concentrations are 3 times the upper normal limit. He is admitted to the intensive care unit and receives antipyretics, intravenous propranolol, hydrocortisone, and oral potassium iodide therapy. His condition continues to deteriorate and urgent thyroidectomy is planned.

Which additional measure could be considered for this patient before thyroidectomy?

A. Cholestyramine therapy
B. Intravenous immunoglobulin therapy
C. Hemodialysis
D. Plasmapheresis
E. Replacement of propranolol with atenolol

15 A 52-year-old man presents with palpitations. His weight has recently decreased from 237 to 211 lb (107.7 to 95.9 kg). He has otherwise been healthy and has had no recent illnesses. He states that he takes no medications or supplements.

On physical examination, his thyroid gland is nontender and there is no goiter. He has a fine tremor of his outstretched hands, and his pulse rate is 97 beats/min. He has no stigmata of Graves disease.

Laboratory test results:

TSH = <0.01 mIU/L (0.5-5.0 mIU/L)
Free T_4 = 4.3 ng/dL (0.8-1.8 ng/dL)
(SI: 55.35 pmol/L [10.30-23.17 pmol/L])
Total T_3 = 290 ng/dL (70-200 ng/dL)
(SI: 4.47 nmol/L [1.08-3.08 nmol/L])
Radioactive iodine uptake = <1% at 24 hours (15%-30%)

A spot urinary iodine concentration on the day of the radioactive iodine uptake test is not elevated.

Which of the following tests is most likely to provide further confirmation of this patient's diagnosis?

A. Assessment of serum erythrocyte sedimentation rate
B. A repeat radioactive iodine uptake/scan after a low-iodine diet
C. Serum thyroglobulin measurement
D. Thyroid-stimulating immunoglobulin measurement
E. Thyroid ultrasonography with color Doppler

16 A 75-year-old woman with longstanding subclinical hyperthyroidism takes methimazole, 7.5 mg daily. At the time of diagnosis, she expressed concern about exposure to radioactive materials and desired to proceed with medical therapy. She takes her current medications regularly. She has recently developed fatigue and is worried about this symptom.

On physical examination, her pulse rate is 64 beats/min and her thyroid gland is enlarged and nodular.

Laboratory test results:

TSH = 8.9 mIU/L (0.5-5.0 mIU/L)
Free T_4 = 0.75 ng/dL (0.8-1.8 ng/dL)
(SI: 9.65 pmol/L [10.30-23.17 pmol/L])

Thyroid scan from 2 years earlier is shown (*see image*).

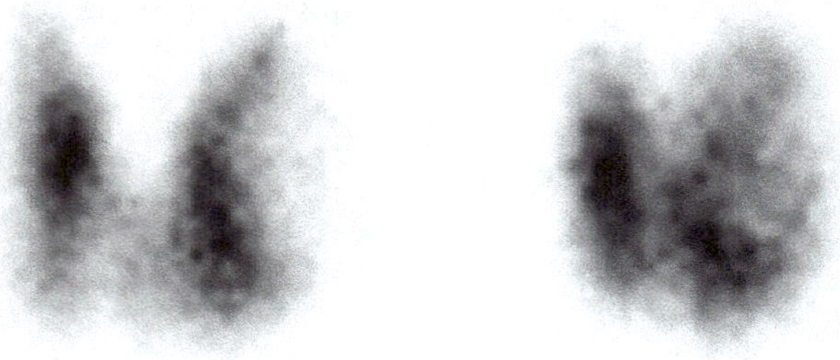

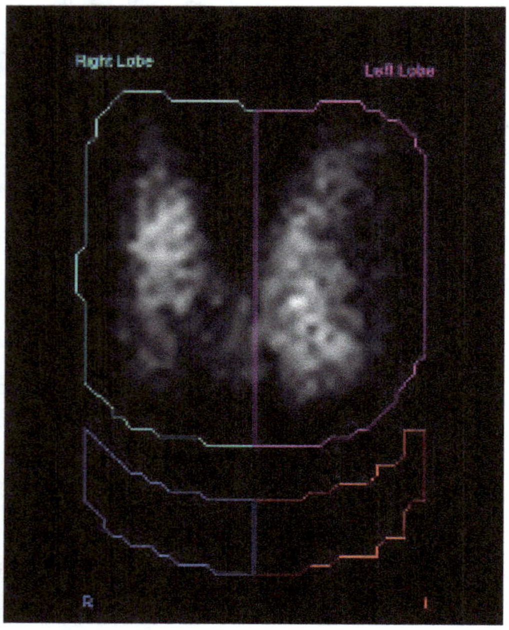

Which of the following is the most important next step in this patient's management?

A. Discontinue methimazole
B. Discontinue methimazole and start levothyroxine therapy
C. Perform the thyroid scan again with radioactive iodine uptake
D. Reduce the methimazole dosage
E. Treat the patient with ^{131}I based on the uptake from her prior scan

Thyroid, Section 2 Board Review

Kaniksha Desai, MD

17 A 76-year-old man presents for evaluation of an enlarged thyroid gland. He has hypertension, hyperlipidemia, suboptimally controlled type 2 diabetes (hemoglobin A_{1c} = 11.1% [98 mmol/mol]), and coronary artery disease with a recent myocardial infarction. He reports that he is having some dysphagia and a choking sensation when lying flat at night. Thyroid ultrasonography shows a 4.1-cm, left-sided thyroid nodule. Findings on FNA biopsy are consistent with a Bethesda category II benign thyroid nodule. His TSH concentration is 2.1 mIU/L (0.5-5.0 mIU/L).

Which of the following is the best next step in this patient's care?

A. Observation with repeat ultrasonography in 6 to 12 months
B. Radioactive iodine
C. Radiofrequency ablation
D. Thyroid lobectomy
E. Total thyroidectomy

18 A 53-year-old woman presents for evaluation of newly diagnosed thyroid cancer. Final pathology on surgery shows a 4.1-cm classic papillary thyroid cancer with negative margins and no extrathyroidal extension. She had 14/17 positive lymph nodes in level IV and VI on the left side with the largest lymph node being 4.2 cm with no extranodal extension. The pathology report states that her TNM staging is T3aN1bM0.

Which of the following is her American Joint Committee on Cancer staging and her American Thyroid Association risk status?

A. Stage 1 high risk
B. Stage 1 intermediate risk
C. Stage 2 high risk
D. Stage 2 intermediate risk
E. Stage 3 high risk

19 A 47-year-old woman with thyroid cancer recently had total thyroidectomy completed at an outside institution. Pathology showed a 2.7-cm follicular thyroid cancer with 3/15 positive lymph nodes (with the largest lymph node being 1.2 cm) in the left lateral neck. She was treated with 75 mCi of radioactive iodine. Her 1-year follow-up after radioactive iodine treatment includes a thyroglobulin concentration of 0.3 ng/mL (0.3 μg/L). Neck ultrasonography shows a 0.3-cm hypoechoic nodule in the left thyroid bed.

Which of the following classifies her current response to treatment?

A. Biochemical incomplete response
B. Excellent response
C. Indeterminate response
D. Structural incomplete response
E. Unable to determine current response to treatment

20 A 33-year-old woman is referred for a new diagnosis of papillary thyroid cancer. Thyroid ultrasonography shows a 1.7-cm hypoechoic nodule with jagged borders and punctate echogenic foci in the mid right thyroid lobe. On ultrasonography, her left thyroid lobe has no nodules, and there are no abnormal lymph nodes in the neck.

Laboratory test results:

Serum TSH = 1.95 mIU/L (0.5-5.0 mIU/L)

TPO antibodies = 121.0 IU/mL (<2.0 IU/mL) (SI: 121.0 kIU/L [<2.0 kIU/L])

She is not currently taking thyroid hormone replacement. Her surgeon has recommended right lobectomy to treat her thyroid cancer. She would like to know whether she should have a total thyroidectomy and asks about the likelihood that she will require thyroid hormone replacement after surgery.

Which of the following is the best recommendation for surgery and the most accurate counseling regarding possible thyroid hormone replacement?

A. Lobectomy; >50% chance of requiring thyroid hormone replacement
B. Lobectomy; <20% chance of requiring thyroid hormone replacement
C. Lobectomy; unable to determine risk of hypothyroidism until after surgery
D. Total thyroidectomy because she has positive TPO antibodies; 100% chance of requiring thyroid hormone replacement

21

A 47-year-old man presents to the emergency department with shortness of breath. Chest CT shows a large 6-cm thyroid nodule. Ultrasonography shows a 5.4-cm isoechoic solid nodule that is taller than wide with a smooth border. A comet tail artifact is also noted on the radiology report. The nodule is scored as TI-RADS 4, and FNA biopsy is recommended.

Which of the following ultrasound characteristics of this thyroid nodule is most likely to be associated with malignancy?

A. Composition
B. Echogenic foci
C. Echogenicity
D. Shape
E. Size

22

A 76-year-old Hispanic man undergoing evaluation for headaches by his primary care physician is referred to endocrinology for abnormalities identified on thyroid function testing. He has hypertension and takes hydrochlorothiazide.

On physical examination, his pulse rate is 92 beats/min and he has a normal thyroid gland. He has a fine tremor, but normal deep tendon reflexes.

Thyroid function test results:

Total T_4 = 16.8 µg/dL (5.5-12.5 µg/dL) (SI: 216.22 nmol/L [70.79-160.88 nmol/L])

Free T_4 = 1.7 ng/dL (0.8-1.8 ng/dL) (SI: 21.88 pmol/L [10.30-23.17 pmol/L])

Total T_3 = 170 ng/dL (70-200 ng/dL) (SI: 2.62 nmol/L [1.08-3.08 nmol/L])

Free T_3 = 3.2 pg/mL (2.3-4.2 pg/mL) (SI: 4.92 pmol/L [3.53-6.45 pmol/L])

TSH = 2.1 mIU/L (0.5-5.0 mIU/L)

Which of the following is this patient's most likely diagnosis?

A. Familial dysalbuminemic hyperthyroxinemia
B. Familial thyroxine-binding globulin excess
C. Selenium deficiency
D. Thyroid hormone resistance
E. TSH-secreting pituitary adenoma

23

A 61-year-old woman seeks a second opinion regarding management of papillary thyroid carcinoma. Four months ago, a thyroid nodule was incidentally noted during carotid ultrasonography. Subsequent thyroid ultrasonography revealed a solitary hypoechoic, 0.9-cm, right-sided nodule with microcalcifications located in the mid lobe, not adjacent to the thyroid capsule. Ultrasonography did not identify other thyroid abnormalities or abnormal cervical lymph nodes. FNA biopsy of the nodule was interpreted as Bethesda VI (papillary carcinoma). The serum TSH concentration was 1.52 mIU/L. Neither TPO nor thyroglobulin antibodies have been detected.

She lives close to the hospital and has a good history of attending medical visits. High-quality neck ultrasonography is available at the center. The patient has read about active surveillance strategies and strongly wishes to avoid thyroid surgery.

During active surveillance of this patient, which of the following circumstances would prompt surgery?

A. Increase in serum thyroglobulin of at least 0.3 ng/mL
B. Increase in serum thyroglobulin of at least 30%
C. Tumor size increase of at least 3 mm
D. Tumor volume increase of 100%

24 A 58-year-old man with widely metastatic papillary thyroid carcinoma returns for follow-up. He underwent total thyroidectomy 8 years ago. He has subsequently been treated 3 times with radioactive iodine (cumulative dose 470 mCi). There was no uptake on his posttreatment scans after his third treatment. On recent PET-CT imaging, he had diffuse lung metastases throughout both lobes and widespread mediastinal lymphadenopathy, which has been increasing over the past year. His largest lung nodule is now 1.5 cm.

On physical examination, his blood pressure is 122/74 mm Hg, and pulse rate is 74 beats/min. His weight is 142 lb (64.5 kg). He has been experiencing rapidly worsening exertional dyspnea.

Laboratory test results:

Serum TSH = 0.1 mIU/L (0.5-5.0 mIU/L)
Serum thyroglobulin = 1245 ng/mL (3-42 ng/mL) (SI: 1245 µg/L [3-42 µg/L]) (substantially increased from his last measurement 6 months ago)
Thyroglobulin antibodies, negative

Which of the following is the best next step in his treatment?

A. Cytotoxic chemotherapy with doxorubicin and cisplatin
B. Ipilimumab
C. Lenvatinib
D. Sorafenib
E. Vandetanib

25 A 25-year-old man is referred for a 2.5-cm right thyroid nodule. His father had thyroid cancer. The patient has been in good health. Physical examination confirms the right thyroid nodule and reveals no cervical adenopathy. The rest of the examination findings are unremarkable, with the exception of an erythematous patch of skin on the upper back (*see image*) that the patient notes to be highly pruritic and present since childhood. Biopsy of this lesion demonstrates thickened epidermis, increased melanin granules in the basal layer, and accumulation of amyloid in the dermal papillae.

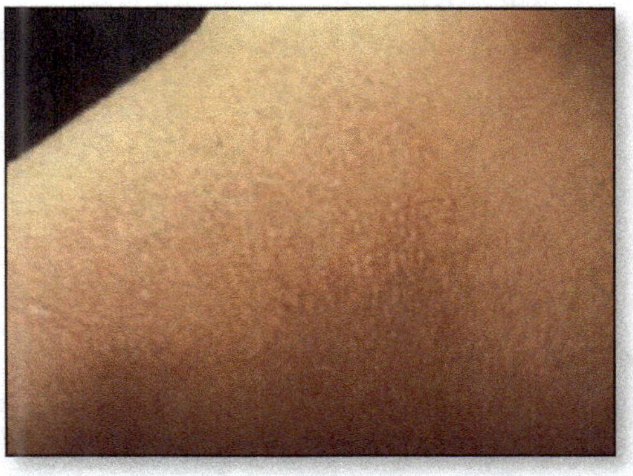

Which of the following is this patient's most likely diagnosis?

A. Amyloidosis
B. Hashimoto thyroiditis
C. Medullary thyroid cancer
D. Metastatic disease to the thyroid
E. Papillary thyroid cancer

26 An 82-year-old man is referred by his pulmonologist before a planned surgery for stage IIIa non–small cell lung cancer. As part of his workup for lung cancer, FDG-PET is performed, which shows focal FDG uptake in the left lobe of the thyroid. No other uptake is seen in the surrounding neck area. Subsequent thyroid ultrasonography shows a 1.2-cm thyroid nodule that is TI-RADS level 5. Suspicious features include punctate echogenic foci, irregular margins, and hypoechogenicity. No extrathyroidal extension or cervical adenopathy is appreciated. His serum TSH concentration is normal. The patient has hypertension and diabetes.

He states that immune checkpoint inhibitors, chemotherapy, and radiation are all being considered following his surgery. The pulmonologist has requested an opinion regarding further workup for the incidentally found thyroid nodule.

Which of the following is the best initial approach regarding the patient's thyroid nodule?

A. Measure free T_4
B. Measure serum thyroglobulin
C. Perform FNA biopsy after surgery and chemotherapy
D. Perform FNA biopsy before surgery
E. Stain lung biopsy specimen for thyroglobulin

27 A 35-year-old man presents with a new palpable, 2-cm thyroid nodule. Thyroid ultrasonography demonstrates the following finding in the right thyroid lobe (*see image, arrow*).

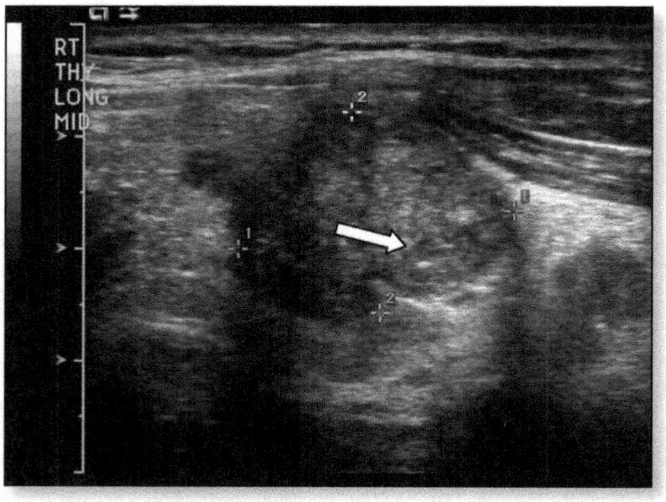

On the basis of the ultrasound pattern observed, what is the likelihood of thyroid cancer?

A. <3%
B. 10%-20%
C. 20%-40%
D. 70%-90%
E. Ultrasonographic patterns do not predict thyroid cancer risk

28 A 67-year-old man with refractory atrial fibrillation is prescribed amiodarone. Baseline thyroid function is normal. Three months later, the patient is referred to endocrinology for further evaluation after the following laboratory test results are documented:

Total T_4 = 13.7 µg/dL (5.5-12.5 µg/dL)
(SI: 176.3 nmol/L [70.79-160.88 nmol/L])
Free T_4 = 1.9 ng/dL (0.8-1.8 ng/dL)
(SI: 24.5 pmol/L [10.30-23.17 pmol/L])
Total T_3 = 61 ng/dL (70-200 ng/dL)
(SI: 0.94 nmol/L [1.08-3.08 nmol/L])
TSH = 4.8 mIU/L (0.5-5.0 mIU/L)

Which of the following is the most likely explanation for these findings?

A. Amiodarone-induced hypothyroidism
B. Assay interference by amiodarone metabolites
C. Euthyroid sick syndrome
D. Expected changes in euthyroid patients on amiodarone
E. Type 1 amiodarone-induced thyrotoxicosis

29 A 26-year-old woman is noted to have a 1.2-cm right thyroid nodule during the ninth week of pregnancy. She has no relevant medical history, and her family history is negative for thyroid cancer. Ultrasonography reveals a solid hypoechoic nodule with no other suspicious features, and FNA biopsy is deferred. At a follow-up visit, the obstetrician notices that the nodule has grown on physical examination and that the patient has some swollen lymph nodes. On repeat thyroid ultrasonography at 18 weeks' gestation, the nodule is noted to have a maximal diameter of 2.4 cm, and a 2-cm ipsilateral central compartment lymph node is noted. FNA biopsy confirms papillary thyroid cancer in both the nodule and lymph node. Her serum TSH concentration is 0.9 mIU/L (0.5-5.0 mIU/L).

Which of the following is the best next step in this patient's management?

A. Defer surgery until the third trimester
B. Perform ethanol ablation of the lymph node now; defer thyroidectomy until after delivery
C. Recommend no intervention until after delivery
D. Refer for immediate total thyroidectomy with neck dissection
E. Start levothyroxine suppressive therapy

30 A 36-year-old man presents for follow-up of a thyroid nodule that was first noted 12 months ago when it was palpated during a routine physical examination. On initial ultrasonography, the nodule was 2.3 cm, solid and hypoechoic, and had irregular margins. There were no microcalcifications and no cervical lymphadenopathy. The right lobe had a normal echotexture, with no discrete nodules. The nodule was initially biopsied 6 months ago and the interpretation was Bethesda I, nondiagnostic. FNA biopsy was repeated with an on-site cytopathologic evaluation. The results of the second biopsy were nondiagnostic.

On ultrasonography today, the nodule is now 3.1 cm, hypoechoic, and has irregular margins. A third FNA biopsy shows no follicular cells on aspirate and is interpreted as Bethesda I.

He has no compressive or obstructive symptoms.

Laboratory test result:
Serum TSH = 1.74 mIU/L (0.5-5.0 mIU/L)

Which of the following is the best next step in this patient's management?

A. Measure serum calcitonin
B. Perform ^{18}FDG PET-CT imaging
C. Perform thyroid lobectomy
D. Repeat ultrasonography in 6 to 12 months
E. Repeat ultrasound-guided FNA biopsy with molecular markers

31 A 21-year-old asymptomatic woman is referred to endocrinology after a right thyroid nodule is found on routine physical examination. The thyroid nodule is mobile and firm with no palpable cervical adenopathy. Her serum TSH concentration is 2.1 mIU/L. Thyroid ultrasonography shows a 2.5-cm nodule with moderately suspicious features (hypoechoic and solid; TI-RADS 4), with no abnormalities noted in the left thyroid lobe. FNA biopsy is interpreted to be Bethesda III (atypia of unknown significance). The biopsy specimen is sent for testing with a pathogenic variant panel and a microRNA classifier. Genetic testing does not detect any pathogenic variants, and the microRNA panel result is designated as level 1 (negative). The patient subsequently consults with a surgeon and expresses a desire to avoid surgery if her cancer risk is low.

Which of the following is the best approach to this patient's management?

A. Follow-up thyroid ultrasonography in approximately 1 year
B. Levothyroxine suppression to decrease nodule size
C. No further follow-up
D. Right lobectomy
E. Total thyroidectomy

32 A 34-year-old woman is incidentally found to have a 2.6-cm thyroid nodule after going to the emergency department for treatment of injuries sustained in a motor vehicle accident. The patient has no compressive symptoms, is clinically and biochemically euthyroid, has no family history of thyroid disorders, and no personal history of radiation exposure to the neck. Thyroid ultrasonography shows that the nodule is isoechoic with regular margins and without calcifications (*see images, arrows, following page*). No abnormal lymph nodes are seen in the lateral neck.

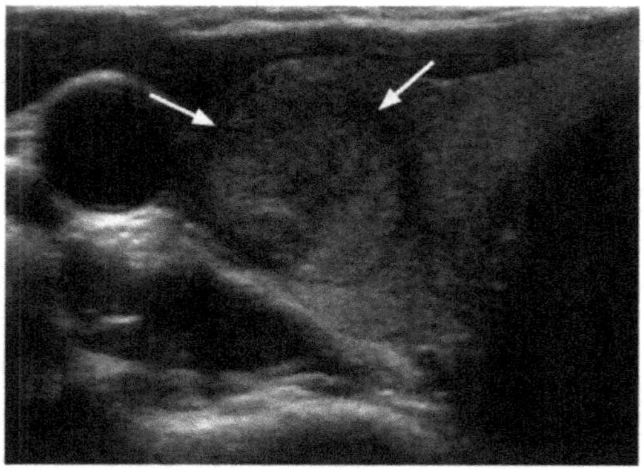

A

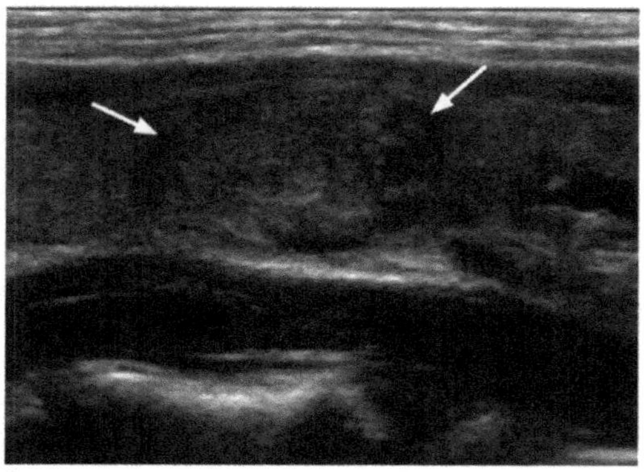

B

Panel A = transverse view; panel B = longitudinal view. Reprinted from Shin J H. *Ultrasonography*, 2017; 36(2):103-110. © The Korean Society of Ultrasound in Medicine.

The patient elects to observe the nodule, but follow-up ultrasonography performed 18 months later shows that the nodule has grown to 3.4 cm. A nodule biopsy is performed, and cytology is reported as Bethesda III (follicular lesion of undetermined significance). The cytologic material is sent for molecular testing, and an *NRAS* variant is identified as the sole pathogenic variant.

Which of the following is most likely to be found if the patient undergoes surgery?

A. Benign follicular adenoma
B. Columnar variant of papillary thyroid cancer
C. Diffuse sclerosing variant of papillary thyroid cancer
D. Hobnail variant of papillary thyroid cancer
E. Tall cell variant of papillary thyroid cancer

33

An 18-year-old man has a palpable 2-cm neck mass (*see CT images 1 and 2, arrows*). He reports previously being treated with antibiotics after he developed pain and redness in this area. Results from thyroid function tests are normal. Ultrasonography (*image 3*) confirms a cystic mass juxtaposed to the hyoid bone.

Image 1, sagittal view

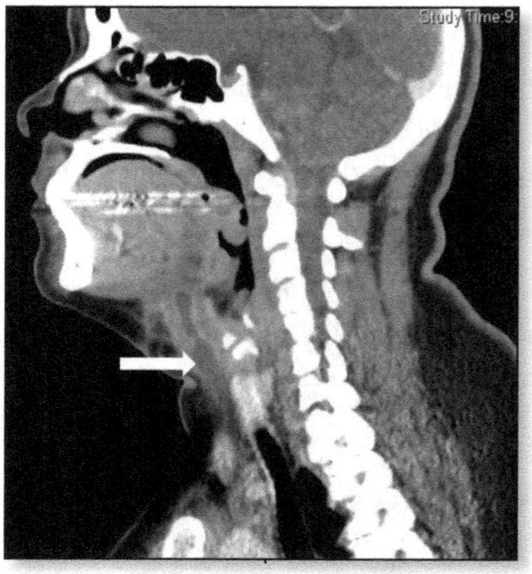

Image 2, coronal view

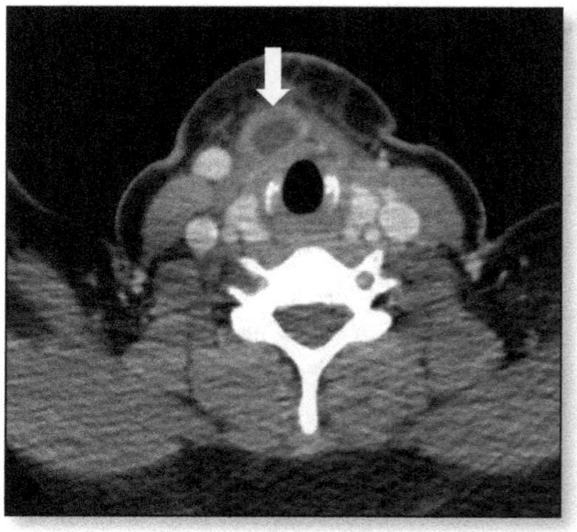

Image 3

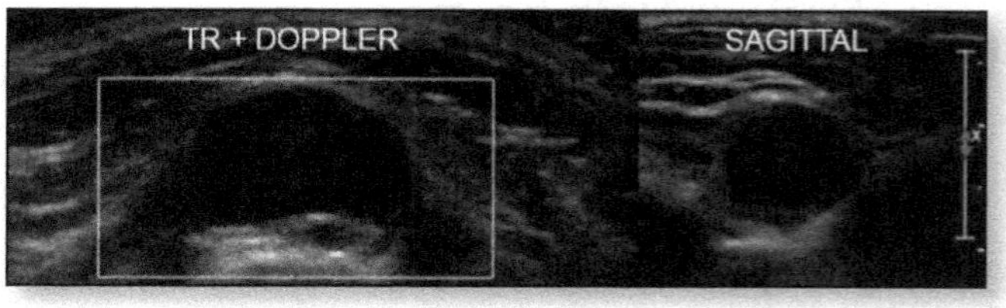

Which of the following is the best management approach for this patient?

A. Initiation of levothyroxine therapy to achieve TSH suppression
B. No treatment now; antibiotics if there is recurrence of infection
C. Radioactive iodine therapy
D. Surgical resection of the cystic mass
E. Surgical resection of the cystic mass with total thyroidectomy

34 A 32-year-old man with widely invasive follicular thyroid cancer undergoes total thyroidectomy followed by radioiodine remnant ablation with 150 mCi ^{131}I. He subsequently develops lung metastases and is treated with an additional 200 mCi, with an objective decrease in the size of the lung metastases and reduction in serum thyroglobulin levels.

Which of the following is the most likely adverse effect from this patient's radioiodine therapy?

A. Azoospermia
B. Excessive dental caries
C. Leukemia
D. Nasolacrimal duct obstruction
E. Permanent loss of taste

ENDOCRINE BOARD REVIEW

ANSWERS

Adrenal Board Review

Tobias Else, MD

1 ANSWER: C) Reassure her of the benign character of the adrenal mass

This vignette describes an incidentally discovered adrenal mass in a 10-year cancer survivor. The key characteristics are the relatively low attenuation and the minimal change in Hounsfield units following contrast administration, which indicate this mass is an adrenal cyst (no contrast uptake). It most likely arose from a hematoma, considering that the patient had received anticoagulation. The small calcifications observed in the lesion's wall are common in pseudocysts that develop from a hematoma. Further follow-up of this lesion in a patient with a history of anticoagulation is not necessary, and she should be reassured of the benign nature of the mass (Answer C). Recognizing these benign lesions is important, and they are usually not addressed in the general guidelines regarding incidentally discovered adrenal masses.

While cancer can certainly recur 10 years after initial diagnosis, metastasis would take up contrast and show delayed washout.

Surgery for adrenal cysts (Answer E) can be considered if a patient is symptomatic, which is not the case in this vignette.

Because the adrenal lesion in this patient does not consist of any reasonable "living" tissue, ^{18}FDG-PET (Answer A), biopsy (Answer D), or biochemical workup (Answer B) is unnecessary. Moreover, she does not have symptoms or signs of hypercortisolism or adrenal insufficiency (Answer B). Occasionally pheochromocytomas are cystic, but this patient's biochemical workup was negative.

EDUCATIONAL OBJECTIVE

Identify adrenal cysts or adrenal hematoma as adrenal masses that generally do not require further workup.

REFERENCE(S)

Fassnacht M, Tsagarakis S, Terzolo M, et al. European Society of Endocrinology clinical practice guidelines on the management of adrenal incidentalomas, in collaboration with the European Network for the Study of Adrenal Tumors. *Eur J Endocrinol.* 2023;189(1):G1-G42. PMID: 37318239

Wang MX, Mahmoud HS, Klimkowski S, et al. Cystic adrenal masses: spectrum of multimodality imaging features and pathological correlation. *Clin Radiol.* 2022;77(7):479-488. PMID: 35428471

2 ANSWER: A) Educate about symptoms and signs of adrenal insufficiency; ask her to call if she has any symptoms after stopping prednisone

This patient has been on short-term supraphysiologic glucocorticoid therapy for treatment of an urticarial rash. She was treated for 3 weeks, followed by 1 week of physiologic daily dose equivalent (prednisone 4-6 mg or hydrocortisone 15 to 25 mg). Short-term therapy (<4 weeks) very rarely leads to hypothalamic-pituitary-adrenal axis suppression that would last beyond cessation of therapy and would be clinically important. Therefore, in general, following short-term treatment, glucocorticoids can simply be stopped. It is good practice to inform the patient of potential signs and symptoms of adrenal insufficiency (Answer A).

If the patient had been on long-term therapy (>4 weeks), switching to hydrocortisone

(Answer E) as a shorter-acting glucocorticoid that can be more easily tapered would be a good idea.

Long-term glucocorticoid therapy can usually be tapered while simply watching for symptoms, but biochemical testing could be performed if necessary or considered if the patient or physician desires it. In that scenario, an 8 AM cortisol measurement (Answer B) would be a good choice, but ACTH measurement (Answer C) or cosyntropin-stimulation testing (Answer D) would rarely be necessary.

EDUCATIONAL OBJECTIVE

Evaluate, diagnose, and treat patients who are tapering exogenous glucocorticoid therapy.

REFERENCE(S)

Broersen LH, Pereira AM, Jørgensen JO, Dekkers OM. Adrenal insufficiency in corticosteroids use: systematic review and meta-analysis. *J Clin Endocrinol Metab.* 2015;100(6):2171-2180. PMID: 25844620

Prete A, Bancos I. Glucocorticoid induced adrenal insufficiency. *BMJ.* 2021;374:n1380. PMID: 34253540

3 ANSWER: E) Reassure the patient she has a very low tumor risk and that surveillance recommendations are not mandatory

When considering all genetic predisposition syndromes for pheochromocytoma or paraganglioma, *SDHx*-related hereditary paraganglioma syndromes due to pathogenic variants in *SDHx* are by far the most common syndromes (more common than von Hippel-Lindau disease or multiple endocrine neoplasia type 2). With increasing use of large next-generation sequencing panels in patients with cancer or a family history of cancer, incidental findings are increasingly common. Therefore, it is important to be familiar with some of the recommendations. The general recommendation for patients with pathogenic variants in *SDHB, SDHC,* and *SDHD* is regular screening for tumors (eg, whole-body MRI every 2 years plus annual metanephrine measurement). *SDHA* pathogenic variants, however, have the highest incidence and lowest penetrance, and recent expert consensus suggests a different approach for these patients. The risk of developing a pheochromocytoma or paraganglioma with a pathogenic *SDHA* variant is very low, definitely less than 5% and most likely less than 1% to 2%. Furthermore, the *SDHA* variant diagnosed in this patient is present in up to 1 in 1500 people, clearly exceeding the prevalence of *SDHA*-related hereditary paraganglioma syndrome. The current consensus regarding recommendations for incidentally identified carriers of *SDHA* pathogenic variants without a personal or family history of associated tumors is to NOT recommend surveillance or screening for any tumors (Answer E).

For patients with an *SDHA* pathogenic variant AND a personal or family history of pheochromocytoma or paraganglioma and for all patients with an *SDHB, SDHC,* or *SDHD* pathogenic variant, initial and regular metanephrine evaluation (plasma or urine) and whole-body MRI are recommended (Answer D).

Annual plasma metanephrine measurement by itself (Answer C) or annual Ga-DOTATATE PET and plasma metanephrine measurement (Answer B) would be insufficient for surveillance.

Repeat genetic testing (Answer A) is not necessary, as germline genetic findings do not change over a patient's lifetime.

EDUCATIONAL OBJECTIVE

Explain the differences in surveillance recommendations for patients with hereditary cancer syndromes.

REFERENCE(S)

Else T, Greenberg S, Fishbein L. Hereditary paraganglioma-pheochromocytoma syndromes. In: Adam MP, Feldman J, Mirzaa GM, Pagon RA, Wallace SE, Bean LJH, Gripp KW, Amemiya A, eds. GeneReviews® [Internet]. Seattle (WA): University of Washington, Seattle; 1993-2024. PMID: 20301715

Amar L, Pacak K, Steichen O, Akker SA, et al. International consensus on initial screening and follow-up of asymptomatic SDHx mutation carriers. *Nat Rev Endocrinol.* 2021;17(7):435-444. PMID: 34021277

Hanson H, Durkie M, Lalloo F, et al; UK Cancer Genetics Centres. UK recommendations for SDHA germline genetic testing and surveillance in clinical practice. *J Med Genet.* 2023;60(2):107-111. PMID: 35260474

4 ANSWER: A) Measure 8 AM ACTH, cortisol, deoxycorticosterone, and 11-deoxycortisol

This patient has a typical, albeit late, presentation of 17-hydroxylase deficiency with hypertension and hypokalemia (due to shunting and increased production of adrenal mineralocorticoids, particularly deoxycorticosterone) and lack of significant pubertal development (due to absence of sex steroids). This patient's aldosterone was measured by immunoassay. If using mass spectrometry, most patients have very low aldosterone levels, but immunoassays cross-react with several other metabolites. The patient in this vignette could be either genetic male or genetic female—examination of internal sex organs, specifically the uterus, or karyotyping would determine her genetic sex. Although she could have primary aldosteronism, primary amenorrhea and lack of pubertal development suggest a different etiology. Thus, measuring aldosterone in a 24-hour urine collection (Answer B) is incorrect.

Abdominal CT (Answer C) would reveal enlarged adrenal glands, but not the molecular diagnosis. The same is true for pelvic ultrasonography, which would suggest the patient's genetic sex by determining the presence or absence of a uterus, but not the underlying diagnosis.

While 21-hydroxylase deficiency is best diagnosed with cosyntropin-stimulated 17-hydroxyprogesterone measurement (elevated) (Answer E), the block in 17-hydroxylase deficiency is before this step and therefore, 17-hydroxyprogesterone is low, deoxycorticosterone is elevated, cortisol is low, and ACTH is often elevated. Thus, measuring these analytes (Answer A) is the best next step. Patients with 17-hydroxylase deficiency usually do not have any overt symptoms or signs of glucocorticoid deficiency, as it is masked, in part, by the increased mineralocorticoids and the presence of corticosterone as a glucocorticoid.

A progesterone challenge (Answer D) is not indicated and would be unsuccessful because the patient either has no uterus if the karyotype is XY or has an underdeveloped uterus if XX.

EDUCATIONAL OBJECTIVE

Identify 17-hydroxylase deficiency as a cause of congenital adrenal hyperplasia.

REFERENCE(S)

Neres MS, Auchus RJ, Shackleton CH, Kater CE. Distinctive profile of the 17-hydroxylase and 17,20-lyase activities revealed by urinary steroid metabolomes of patients with CYP17 deficiency. *Arq Bras Endocrinol Metabol.* 2010;54(9):826-832. PMID: 21340176

Maheshwari M, Arya S, Ranjan Lila A, et al. 117α-hydroxylase/17,20-lyase deficiency in 46,XY: our experience and review of literature. *J Endocr Soc.* 2022;6(3):bvac001. PMID: 35178494

5 ANSWER: D) Perform a 1-mg dexamethasone test with measurement of cortisol only

This patient has an incidentally discovered adrenal mass and no overt hypercortisolism. However, testing for mild autonomous cortisol excess with a 1-mg dexamethasone-suppression test is indicated (Answer D). Although commonly pursued, measurement of dexamethasone (Answer C) is generally not indicated (>95% of patients will achieve sufficient dexamethasone levels), and there is no suggestion that this patient would have increased metabolism (no CYP3A4-inducing medication present). Cost-effectiveness is important, and in the event of an unexpectedly high cortisol value after administering 1 mg dexamethasone, one could either repeat the 1-mg dexamethasone-suppression test with dexamethasone measurement or simply use a higher dexamethasone dose (eg, 2 mg).

Measurement of random morning cortisol and ACTH (Answer B) is not helpful in the workup of hypercortisolism.

In the absence of hypertension or hypokalemia, screening for primary aldosteronism is unnecessary, and no screening for pheochromocytoma (Answer A) is indicated in a patient with an adrenal lesion that has definitive characteristics of a lipid-rich adenoma.

There is also no concern that the lesion is malignant, so an ^{18}FDG-PET (Answer E) is unnecessary.

EDUCATIONAL OBJECTIVE

Guide the most cost-effective workup for hypercortisolism.

REFERENCE(S)

Genere N, Kaur RJ, Athimulam S, et al. Interpretation of abnormal dexamethasone suppression test is enhanced with use of synchronous free cortisol assessment. *J Clin Endocrinol Metab.* 2022;107(3):e1221-e1230. PMID: 34648626

Fassnacht M, Tsagarakis S, Terzolo M, et al. European Society of Endocrinology clinical practice guidelines on the management of adrenal incidentalomas, in collaboration with the European Network for the Study of Adrenal Tumors. *Eur J Endocrinol.* 2023;189(1):G1-G42. PMID: 37318239

6 ANSWER: B) Li-Fraumeni syndrome

This patient has a history of an androgen-producing adrenal mas, likely an adrenocortical carcinoma, diagnosed in childhood. In addition, she has a family history of bilateral breast cancer at young age and osteosarcoma. All 3 tumors are typical of Li-Fraumeni syndrome (Answer B), and the patient most likely has a pathogenic variant in the *TP53* gene.

Pathogenic variants in *BRCA1* or *BRCA2* (Answer A) are not associated with adrenal tumors.

While patients with McCune-Albright syndrome (Answer D) can have hypercortisolism, this condition is never inherited, and the patient lacks any other features of this syndrome.

Lynch syndrome (Answer C) is observed in up to 4% of patients with adrenal cancer, but one would expect colon and uterine cancer in the family history.

While patients with multiple endocrine neoplasia type 1 (Answer E) can develop benign and malignant adrenal lesions, there are no other associated findings such as early-onset hyperparathyroidism reported in the family.

EDUCATIONAL OBJECTIVE

Identify hereditary syndromes with increased risk for adrenal malignancies.

REFERENCE(S)

Petr EJ, Else T. Adrenocortical carcinoma (ACC): when and why should we consider germline testing? *Presse Med.* 2018;47(7-8 Pt 2):e119-e125. PMID: 30104051

Fassnacht M, Dekkers OM, Else T, et al. European Society of Endocrinology Clinical Practice Guidelines on the management of adrenocortical carcinoma in adults, in collaboration with the European Network for the Study of Adrenal Tumors. *Eur J Endocrinol.* 2018;179(4):G1-G46. PMID: 30299884

7 ANSWER: E) Repeat the 1-mg dexamethasone-suppression test

This patient's clinical findings and symptoms are very suggestive of hypercortisolism, and there is a high pretest probability. Therefore, further evaluation should be pursued. Although the 1-mg dexamethasone-suppression test is a good test for hypercortisolism, the patient had just recently finished a course of antiviral medications, including ritonavir, which is a very potent CYP3A4 inhibitor that likely dramatically increased dexamethasone during the suppression test. Ritonavir can produce false-negative results, and current postdexamethasone cortisol value is unreliable. Thus, 1-mg dexamethasone-suppression testing, 24-hour urinary collection for cortisol, or salivary cortisol measurements should be repeated (thus, Answer E is correct and Answer D is incorrect).

Although the possibility that the patient is using synthetic steroids should be considered

(Answer B), endogenous production should be excluded first. Although ACTH can help distinguish between ACTH-dependent vs ACTH-independent hypercortisolism in patients with established hypercortisolism, random measurement before establishment of hypercortisolism is not helpful, and neither is a random 8 AM cortisol measurement (Answer A).

If the patient is documented to have hypercortisolism, a pituitary tumor is a likely cause. However, the biochemical diagnosis must be established before performing pituitary-directed MRI (Answer C).

EDUCATIONAL OBJECTIVE

Identify medications that affect dexamethasone and glucocorticoid metabolism.

REFERENCE(S)

M E Hillebrand-Haverkort, M F Prummel, J H ten Veen. Ritonavir-induced Cushing's syndrome in a patient treated with nasal fluticasone. *AIDS.* 1999;13(13):1803. PMID: 10509596

Valin N, De Castro N, Garrait V, Bergeron A, Bouche C, Molina JM. Iatrogenic Cushing's syndrome in HIV-infected patients receiving ritonavir and inhaled fluticasone: description of 4 new cases and review of the literature. *J Int Assoc Physicians AIDS Care (Chic).* 2009;8(2):113-121. PMID: 19270151

8 ANSWER: E) Start therapy with mitotane and continue for at least 2 years

This patient has a new diagnosis of adrenocortical carcinoma, stage 2, likely with no presurgical hormone excess. In general, care for patients with adrenal cancer should occur at sites that have multidisciplinary teams dedicated to the care of adrenal neoplasia, but she would like to continue therapy locally. The mainstay of adjuvant therapy for patients with adrenal cancer with any high-risk features (eg, stage 3 or 4, Ki67 index >10%) is mitotane therapy only (Answer E). Recommending no therapy (Answer A) would be inappropriate as there is strong evidence that adjuvant mitotane therapy prevents, or at least delays recurrences.

Radiation therapy (Answer B) is mainly used for patients with non-R0 resections and at some centers for patients with high-grade stage 3 cancers, but not for R0 stage 2 cancers.

Both adjuvant cytotoxic chemotherapy and adjuvant immunotherapy (Answers C and D) are being investigated in clinical trials, but these treatments should otherwise be reserved for patients with multiple high-risk features.

EDUCATIONAL OBJECTIVE

Discuss guideline-based recommendations for adjuvant adrenal cancer therapy.

REFERENCE(S)

Fassnacht M, Dekkers OM, Else T, et al. European Society of Endocrinology Clinical Practice Guidelines on the management of adrenocortical carcinoma in adults, in collaboration with the European Network for the Study of Adrenal Tumors. *Eur J Endocrinol.* 2018;179(4):G1-G46. PMID: 30299884

9 ANSWER: B) Cosyntropin-stimulation test measuring 17-hydroxyprogesterone and cortisol

The evaluation of chronic, nonprogressive androgen excess without virilization in a young woman is primarily to distinguish polycystic ovary syndrome (PCOS) from other causes of hyperandrogenism: Cushing syndrome, hyperprolactinemia, and nonclassic congenital adrenal hyperplasia. This patient has no clinical features of Cushing syndrome (and no directed tests are necessary or given as options) and a normal serum prolactin concentration. Her history and physical examination findings are atypical for PCOS in that she had onset of androgen excess in childhood before menses, she does not have obesity, and she has a normal glucose concentration without evidence of insulin resistance. Thus, nonclassic 21-hydroxylase deficiency should be considered. A morning follicular-phase 17-hydroxyprogesterone concentration less than 200 ng/dL (<6.1 nmol/L) excludes nonclassic 21-hydroxylase deficiency, and a value greater than 1000 ng/dL (>30.3 nmol/L) establishes the diagnosis. Serum 17-hydroxyprogesterone varies with the time of day and across the menstrual cycle.

Given this patient's suspicious history and an equivocal random value of 300 ng/dL (9.1 nmol/L), a formal cosyntropin-stimulation test for 17-hydroxyprogesterone (Answer B) is warranted.

Adrenal-directed CT (Answer A) is recommended if the testosterone concentration is markedly elevated (>150 ng/dL [>5.2 nmol/L]).

Nonclassic 3β-hydroxysteroid dehydrogenase/isomerase type 2 (3β-HSD2) deficiency is exceedingly rare and is only considered in unusual cases after nonclassic 21-hydroxylase deficiency has been excluded. Furthermore, 17-hydroxyprogesterone is also elevated in 3β-HSD2 deficiency because of the type 1 enzyme, and the most discriminatory parameter for this condition is the 17-hydroxypregnenolone-to-cortisol ratio. Thus, 11-deoxycortisol measurement (Answer E) is incorrect.

Plasma ACTH measurement (Answer D) would not aid in this patient's diagnosis.

In a patient with childhood-onset androgen excess sufficient to advance bone age, a diagnosis should be pursued. Thus, no further testing (Answer C) is incorrect.

EDUCATIONAL OBJECTIVE

Guide the biochemical evaluation of adrenal androgen excess.

REFERENCE(S)

Auchus RJ. The classic and nonclassic congenital adrenal hyperplasias. *Endocr Pract.* 2015;21(4):383-389. PMID: 25536973

Witchel SF. Nonclassic congenital adrenal hyperplasia. *Curr Opin Endocrinol Diabetes Obes.* 2012;19(3):151-158. PMID: 22499220

Carbunaru G, Prasad P, Scoccia B, et al. The hormonal phenotype of nonclassic 3β-hydroxysteroid dehydrogenase (HSD3B) deficiency in hyperandrogenic females is associated with insulin-resistant polycystic ovary syndrome and is not a variant of inherited HSD3B2 deficiency. *J Clin Endocrinol Metab.* 2004;89(2):783-794. PMID: 14764797

Speiser PW, Arlt W, Auchus RJ, et al. Congenital adrenal hyperplasia due to steroid 21-hydroxylase deficiency: an Endocrine Society clinical practice guideline. *J Clin Endocrinol Metab.* 2018;103(11):4043-4088. PMID: 30272171

10 ANSWER: B) Her risk of having a child with *classic* 21-OHD is >0.5%

The prevalence of classic and nonclassic 21-OHD in the general population is 1 in 16,000 and 1 in 1000, respectively. To have classic 21-OHD, an individual must either have no functional *CYP21A2* alleles or have less than 2% residual enzyme activity. Nearly all patients with classic 21-OHD are identified in infancy because of atypical genitalia, adrenal insufficiency, and/or abnormal newborn screening results (now available in many countries, including the United States). Most cases of nonclassic 21-OHD are never diagnosed, particularly when the affected individual is male. To have nonclassic 21-OHD, an individual must have at least 1 partially functional allele with 10% to 20% of residual enzyme activity and no wild-type allele. The other allele can be a classic 21-OHD variant or deletion (0%-2% activity) or a second nonclassic 21-OHD allele. Studies have shown that about 70% of patients who are diagnosed with nonclassic 21-OHD are compound heterozygotes for a nonclassic allele and a classic allele. Furthermore, 4% of parents with children affected by classic 21-OHD actually have occult nonclassic 21-OHD, and they themselves are compound heterozygotes for classic and nonclassic 21-OHD alleles. Consequently, even without knowing this patient's genotype, we know she is at higher-than-average risk for having a child with classic 21-OHD.

To understand the calculations, one needs to know the carrier frequency of classic 21-OHD, which is ~2%. Therefore, there is a 1 in 50 chance that the patient's partner carries a classic 21-OHD allele and 25% of their offspring will be homozygous for the classic allele: 1 in 200 (0.5%). The largest 2 studies of such patients documented the risk to be even a little higher than the theoretical risk, in the range of 1.5% to 2.5% (thus, Answer B is correct).

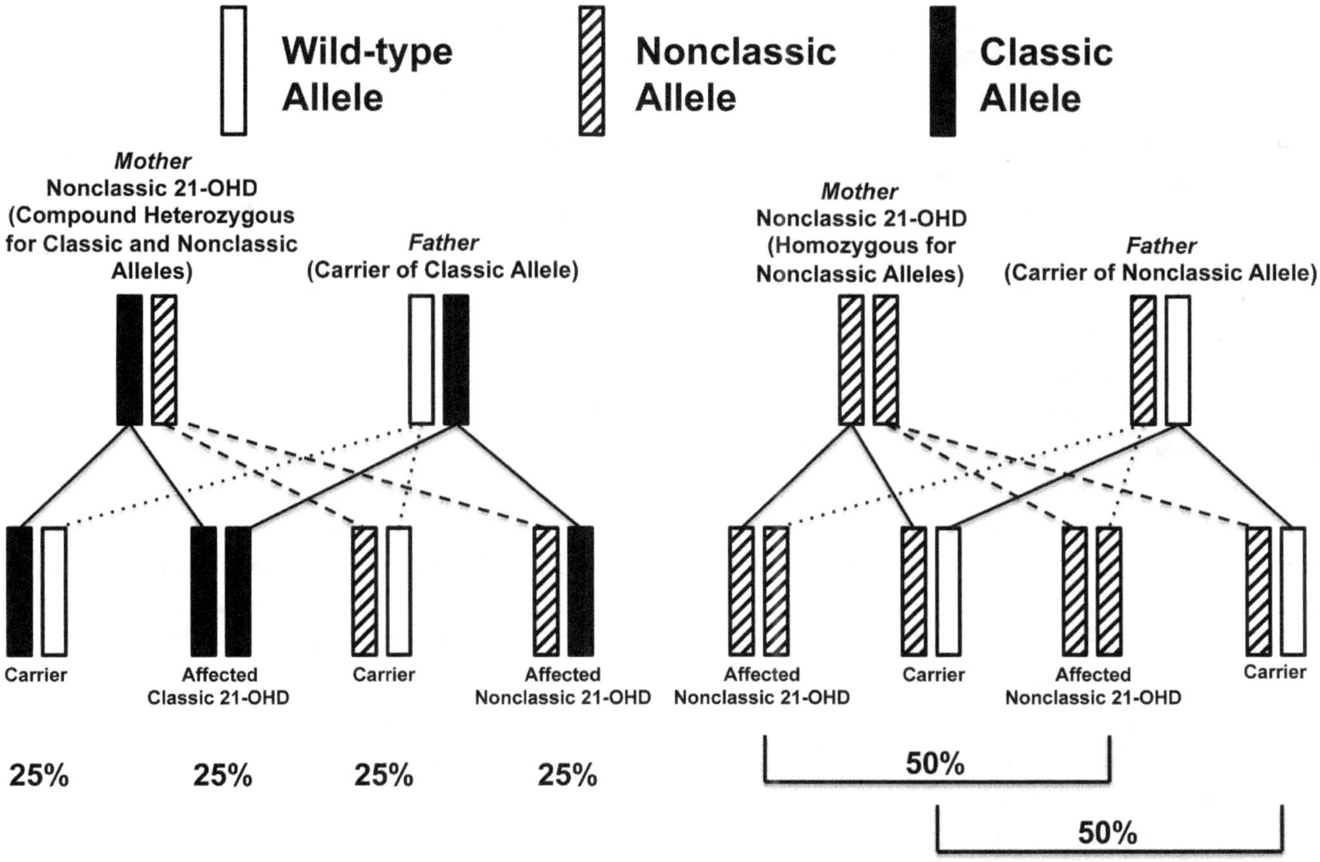

The patient could be a compound heterozygote with 1 classic 21-OHD allele and 1 nonclassic allele, and if her partner is also a carrier of a classic allele, she could have children with classic 21-OHD (thus, Answer C is incorrect).

The risk of 0.01% translates to the general population risk (1/16,000) (thus, Answer A is incorrect).

If both the patient and her partner were to have a clinical diagnosis of nonclassic 21-OHD, it would be possible that both are homozygous for nonclassic 21-OHD alleles (and hence not at risk for having a child with classic 21-OHD). As discussed above, this couple is at risk of having a child with classic 21-OHD if the patient has a classic allele and her partner is simply a carrier of a classic allele (not affected with 21-OHD) (thus, Answer D is incorrect). If she and her partner are both carriers of a classic allele, then the probability of having a child affected with classic 21-OHD is 25% with each pregnancy. The diagram illustrates 2 of several possibilities.

EDUCATIONAL OBJECTIVE

Counsel a patient on the genetics of 21-hydroxylase deficiency and the frequencies of classic and nonclassic alleles.

REFERENCE(S)

Finkielstain GP, Chen W, Mehta SP, et al. Comprehensive genetic analysis of 182 unrelated families with congenital adrenal hyperplasia due to 21-hydroxylase deficiency. *J Clin Endocrinol Metab.* 2011;96(1):E161-E172. PMID: 20926536

Nandagopal R, Sinaii N, Avila NA, et al. Phenotypic profiling of parents with cryptic nonclassic congenital adrenal hyperplasia: findings in 145 unrelated families. *Eur J Endocrinol.* 2011;164(6):977-984. PMID: 21444649

Moran C, Azziz R, Weintrob N, et al. Reproductive outcome of women with 21-hydroxylase-deficient nonclassic adrenal hyperplasia. *J Clin Endocrinol Metab.* 2006;91(9):3451-3456. PMID: 16822826

11 ANSWER: C) Normal testosterone, high androstenedione, low LH

This patient has a history of adrenal insufficiency with bilateral testicular masses and medication nonadherence. This is an unfortunately common situation for young men with classic 21-hydroxylase deficiency who develop testicular adrenal rest tumors (TARTs). These are ACTH-responsive masses that are either ectopic adrenal tissue or reprogrammed steroidogenic stem cells in the testes that grow and produce a pattern of steroids similar to that of the adrenal cortex of these patients. The major clue is the bilateral nature of the tumors and their firm, irregular texture. In 21-hydroxylase deficiency, the adrenal produces abundant androstenedione and inefficiently converts this precursor to testosterone, so the major laboratory feature is elevated androstenedione, disproportionate to testosterone, which is typically "normal" but not derived from the normal testicular Leydig cells. The high adrenal androgen production suppresses LH. Initially, FSH is also low, but with time the masses compromise blood flow to the normal testis and cause irreversible damage to the Sertoli and germ cells, and FSH rises. Both the testicular mass and the suppressed gonadotropins cause infertility. TARTs and high FSH are poor prognostic factors for fertility in men with classic 21-hydroxylase deficiency. Intensification of glucocorticoid therapy can allow regression of the rests and restoration of fertility, but this can take many months. Surgical removal of TARTs often provides long-term control of the tumors, but it does not restore testicular function. The pattern of laboratory results expected in this patient is normal testosterone, high androstenedione, and low LH (Answer C).

The pattern in Answer A implies LH-dependent androstenedione and testosterone production, which is incorrect.

The pattern in Answer B is typical of a Leydig-cell tumor producing estradiol, but this presents as a solitary, often small and round mass in one testis.

The pattern in Answer D is typical of primary testicular failure and ignores the adrenal-derived androgens.

The pattern in Answer E is typical of a nonfunctional testicular tumor such as a seminoma early in the disease course, and these cancers are also unilateral.

EDUCATIONAL OBJECTIVE

Diagnose testicular adrenal rest tumors in a man with 21-hydroxylase deficiency and predict patterns of laboratory test results.

REFERENCE(S)

Arlt W, Willis DS, Wild SH, et al; United Kingdom Congenital Adrenal Hyperplasia Adult Study Executive (CaHASE). Health status of adults with congenital adrenal hyperplasia: a cohort study of 203 patients. *J Clin Endocrinol Metab.* 2010;95(10):5110-5121. PMID: 20719839

Auchus RJ, Arlt W. Approach to the patient: the adult with congenital adrenal hyperplasia. *J Clin Endocrinol Metab.* 2013;98(7):2645-2655. PMID: 23837188

Reisch N, Rottenkolber M, Greifenstein A, et al. Testicular adrenal rest tumors develop independently of long-term disease control: a longitudinal analysis of 50 adult men with congenital adrenal hyperplasia due to classic 21-hydroxylase deficiency. *J Clin Endocrinol Metab.* 2013;98(11):E1820-E1826. PMID: 23969190

Claahsen-van der Grinten HL, Otten BJ, Takahashi S, et al. Testicular adrenal rest tumors in adult males with congenital adrenal hyperplasia: evaluation of pituitary-gonadal function before and after successful testis-sparing surgery in eight patients. *J Clin Endocrinol Metab.* 2007;92(2):612- 615. PMID: 17090637

King TF, Lee MC, Williamson EE, Conway GS. Experience in optimizing fertility outcomes in men with congenital adrenal hyperplasia due to 21 hydroxylase deficiency. *Clin Endocrinol (Oxf).* 2016;84(6):830-836. PMID: 26666213

12 ANSWER: B) Measurement of plasma free fractionated metanephrines

The finding of an incidental adrenal nodule in a patient with a known malignancy always raises the possibility of metastatic disease. The primary malignancies most commonly associated with adrenal metastasis include lung cancer, breast cancer, gastrointestinal cancers, and melanoma. The history of breast cancer, the large right adrenal nodule with a high attenuation value, and the positive PET scan should raise the possibility of metastatic disease in this patient. A percutaneous CT-guided aspiration biopsy (Answer D) is certainly warranted in patients in whom metastatic disease may change the prognosis or therapeutic plan. However, biochemical evaluation of an adrenal nodule (Answer B) is *always* required before any attempts to perform a CT-guided biopsy or to remove the nodule surgically (Answer E).

Pheochromocytoma must always be excluded in patients with incidental adrenal nodules that have an attenuation value greater than 15 Hounsfield units. An aspiration biopsy may result in a catastrophic outcome in a patient with an unsuspected pheochromocytoma. FDG-PET yields positive uptake in 70% to 80% of patients with both benign and malignant pheochromocytomas. Therefore, plasma free fractionated metanephrines (Answer B) or 24-hour urinary catecholamines and metanephrines should be measured before any further intervention in this patient. This woman had marked elevation of plasma free metanephrines and eventually had successful laparoscopic right adrenalectomy for removal of her pheochromocytoma.

In this vignette, the overnight low-dose (1-mg) dexamethasone-suppression test yielded an abnormal cortisol concentration of 2.2 μg/dL (60.7 nmol/L) (normal, <1.8 μg/dL [<49.7 nmol/L]). However, in this patient, the abnormal result is confounded by the use of tamoxifen. Similar to estrogen, tamoxifen raises the level of the binding protein for cortisol—corticosteroid-binding globulin—and makes it impossible to interpret the result of a dexamethasone-suppression test. Thus, performing a high-dose dexamethasone-suppression test (Answer A) is incorrect. If there is concern for an aldosterone-producing adenoma (hypertension, hypokalemia), renin and aldosterone should be measured (Answer C) to screen for primary aldosteronism. Adrenal venous sampling is only indicated to distinguish a steroid-secreting neoplasm (usually aldosterone-secreting) from bilateral adrenal hyperplasia.

EDUCATIONAL OBJECTIVE

Order appropriate biochemical tests to exclude pheochromocytoma in patients with adrenal nodules and an indeterminate attenuation value.

REFERENCE(S)

Vikram R, Yeung HDW, Macapinlac HA, Iyer RB. Utility of PET/CT in differentiating benign from malignant adrenal nodules in patients with cancer. *Am J Roentgenol.* 2008;191(5):1545-1551. PMID: 18941099

Shulkin BL, Thompson NW, Shapiro B, Francis IR, Sisson JC. Pheochromocytomas: imaging with 2-[fluorine- 18]fluoro-2-deoxyglucose-D-glucose PET. *Radiology.* 1999;212(1):35-41. PMID: 10405717

Yu R, Nissen NN, Dhall D, Wei M. Pheochromocytoma in patients suspected of harboring adrenal metastasis: management and clinical predictors. *Endocr Pract.* 2008;14(8):967-972. PMID: 19095594

13 ANSWER: B) No further testing

During critical illness, cortisol rises and remains elevated without circadian rhythm for days to weeks until recovery occurs. Furthermore, cortisol production is resistant to suppression from exogenous glucocorticoids such as dexamethasone. The more gravely ill the patient, the greater the stimulus for cortisol production and the less the cortisol rises with cosyntropin. Viewed this way, cortisol and its attenuated rise with cosyntropin are prognostic factors in critical illness. In addition, many critically ill patients are hypoproteinemic, with low albumin and low plasma cortisol-binding capacity as in this patient, such that the total serum cortisol underestimates the concentration of free and biologically active cortisol. For patients with serum albumin concentrations less than 2.5 g/dL (<25 g/L), the serum free cortisol is uniformly normal, even when the serum total stimulated cortisol concentration is 12 to 18 μg/dL (331.1-496.6 nmol/L), which is below the conventional cutoff for a normal response. In addition, newer cortisol immunoassays and mass spectrometry assays yield values about 30% lower than older immunoassays. For these reasons, this patient does not have adrenal insufficiency and requires no further testing or therapy (Answer B).

Serum DHEA-S (Answer D) is a useful measure of adrenal function in combination with cortisol, as DHEA-S production is also ACTH-dependent. However, in critical illness, DHEA-S falls and DHEA rises. Thus, serum DHEA-S cannot be used to adjudicate adrenal function in critical illness.

Plasma ACTH (Answer C) will not influence the interpretation of the cosyntropin-stimulation test, and it can be low or low-normal after several days of critical illness.

Critical illness is a contraindication to an insulin tolerance test, and cortisol values from a low-dose cosyntropin-stimulation test (Answer A) would have to be corrected for hypoproteinemia as well.

The patient does not have adrenal insufficiency and therefore measurement of synthetic glucocorticoids (Answer E) as a possible cause of adrenal insufficiency is unnecessary.

EDUCATIONAL OBJECTIVE

Interpret cortisol dynamics in critical illness.

REFERENCE(S)

Sprung CL, Annane D, Keh D, et al; CORTICUS Study Group. Hydrocortisone therapy for patients with septic shock. *N Engl J Med.* 2008;358(2):111-124. PMID: 18184957

Arafah BM. Hypothalamic pituitary adrenal function during critical illness: limitations of current assessment methods. *J Clin Endocrinol Metab.* 2006;91(10):3725-3745. PMID: 16882746

Sam S, Corbridge TC, Mokhlesi B, Comellas AP, Molitch ME. Cortisol levels and mortality in severe sepsis. *Clin Endocrinol (Oxf).* 2004;60(1):29-35. PMID: 14678284

Hamrahian AH, Oseni TS, Arafah BM. Measurements of serum free cortisol in critically ill patients. *N Engl J Med.* 2004;350(16):1629-1638. PMID: 15084695

Annane D, Sebille V, Troche G, Raphael JC, Gajdos P, Bellissant E. A 3-level prognostic classification in septic shock based on cortisol levels and cortisol response to corticotropin. *JAMA.* 2000;283(8):1038-1045. PMID: 10697064

14 ANSWER: C) Increase the hydrocortisone dosage to 40 mg on arising and 20 mg in the early afternoon

This woman had severe Cushing disease for a prolonged period. Her pituitary surgery was successful with histologic confirmation of adenoma resection plus undetectable cortisol and ACTH. She had a low DHEA-S concentration, which is often elevated in Cushing disease before surgery, but it significantly drops as a result of the absent ACTH stimulation of the adrenal cortex. Her hypothalamic-pituitary-adrenal axis will remain suppressed for many months, and she requires cortisol replacement therapy. Not surprisingly, she is experiencing cortisol withdrawal syndrome. Laboratory testing confirms central adrenal insufficiency, so no further testing for recurrent disease (Answers D and E) is required. Instead, her hydrocortisone dosage should be increased (Answer C). While the current dosage might seem supraphysiologic, it is still very low relative to her cortisol exposure when she had Cushing disease. Patients even experience cortisol withdrawal syndrome when their Cushing disease is not cured but ACTH and cortisol production is significantly lowered.

Because her cortisol deficiency is central, her renin-angiotensin-aldosterone axis is functional, and both standing blood pressure and serum potassium are normal. Fludrocortisone (Answer B) is therefore unnecessary.

DHEA-S decreases following cure of Cushing disease and can remain low for years despite recovery of cortisol production. Some literature suggests that DHEA replacement (Answer A) is beneficial for women with permanent adrenal insufficiency in the chronic setting, but the benefits are mostly for sexuality and do not address cortisol withdrawal. In several months, it might be appropriate to consider DHEA supplementation.

Ancillary medications to aid symptoms include selective serotonin reuptake inhibitors for mood problems and nonsteroidal anti-inflammatory drugs for myalgias. The hydrocortisone dosage is gradually tapered as symptoms abate to allow axis recovery. For those with severe glucocorticoid-induced myopathy, physical therapy is very important from the midpoint of the recovery phase.

EDUCATIONAL OBJECTIVE

Manage cortisol withdrawal syndrome following cure of Cushing disease.

REFERENCE(S)

Bhattacharyya A, Kaushal K, Tymms DJ, Davis JR. Steroid withdrawal syndrome after successful treatment of Cushing's syndrome: a reminder. *Eur J Endocrinol.* 2005;153(2):207-210. PMID: 16061825

Kleiber H, Rey F, Temler E, Gomez F. Dissociated recovery of cortisol and dehydroepiandrosterone sulphate after treatment for Cushing's syndrome. *J Endocrinol Invest.* 1991;14(6):489-492. PMID: 1663528

El Asmar N, Rajpal A, Selman WR, Arafah BM. The value of perioperative levels of ACTH, DHEA, and DHEA-S and tumor size in predicting recurrence of Cushing disease. *J Clin Endocrinol Metab.* 2018;103(2):477-445. PMID: 29244084

Nieman LK, Biller BM, Findling JW, et al; Endocrine Society. Treatment of Cushing's syndrome: an Endocrine Society Clinical Practice Guideline. *J Clin Endocrinol Metab.* 2015;100(8):2807-2831. PMID: 26222757

Zhang CD, Li D, Singh S, et al. Glucocorticoid withdrawal syndrome following surgical remission of endogenous hypercortisolism: a longitudinal observational study. *Eur J Endocrinol.* 2023;188(7):592-602. PMID: 37395115

15 ANSWER: B) Medication given as prophylaxis for postoperative nausea

This patient with obesity, diabetes, and hypertension has had an episode of mild postsurgical hypotension and tachycardia, responsive to fluid resuscitation. She has hyperglycemia and mild hyponatremia. Clinically, the rapid resolution of symptoms with intravenous fluids, as well as the presence of hyperglycemia are not consistent with adrenal insufficiency. Hyperglycemia and low cortisol are most likely due to the presurgical administration of dexamethasone (Answer B). Dexamethasone, 4 to 8 mg, is routinely given to patients with risk factors for postoperative nausea and vomiting (female sex, nonsmoker, emetogenic surgery).

Inhaled anesthetics (Answer A) are not associated with adrenal insufficiency. Etomidate, sometimes used in anesthetic protocols, can induce a transient adrenally insufficient state due to 11-hydroxylase inhibition.

While opioids in the acute and chronic setting can alter the hypothalamic-pituitary-adrenal axis, nonopioid drugs or low-dosage tramadol (Answer D) do not pose this risk.

Metastasis from solid tumors (Answer C) almost never causes adrenal insufficiency. Indeed, the adrenal cortex gets pushed to the periphery, but remains present and functional with even large metastasis. Moreover, adrenal metastasis from colon cancer is rare. Adrenal metastases are more typical of lung cancer, breast cancer, kidney cancer, or melanoma.

This patient has no other risk factors, symptoms, or signs consistent with preexisting adrenal insufficiency (Answer E). When considering adrenal insufficiency in the acute postsurgical setting, it is important to evaluate for anticoagulation or bleeding disorders, which predispose to adrenal hemorrhage. However, the clinical scenario would be much more serious.

If the patient did not receive any glucocorticoids for postoperative nausea and vomiting, it would be worthwhile to explore previous use of glucocorticoids in inhalers, nasal spray, musculoskeletal injections, or topical application, all of which can suppress the hypothalamic-pituitary-adrenal axis.

EDUCATIONAL OBJECTIVE

List the various conditions treated with glucocorticoids and explain their effect on adrenal function.

REFERENCE(S)

Gan TJ, Diemunsch P, Habib AS, et al; Society for Ambulatory Anesthesia. Consensus guidelines for the management of postoperative nausea and vomiting [published corrections appear in *Anesth Analg.* 2014;118(3):689 and *Anesth Analg.* 2015;120(2):494]. *Anesth Analg.* 2014;118(1):85-113. PMID: 24356162

Bornstein SR, Allolio B, Arlt W, et al. Diagnosis and treatment of primary adrenal insufficiency: an Endocrine Society clinical practice guideline. *J Clin Endocrinol Metab.* 2016;101(2):364-389. PMID: 26760044

16 ANSWER: D) Low plasma renin activity and low serum aldosterone

For many years, licorice consumption has been appreciated as a cause of hypertension and hypokalemic metabolic alkalosis. The state of mineralocorticoid excess is clinically similar to that in patients with primary hyperaldosteronism; however, patients with primary aldosteronism could be expected to have an elevated aldosterone concentration and low plasma renin activity (Answer B). In licorice-induced hypertension and hypokalemia, normal amounts of cortisol act as a mineralocorticoid. Licorice contains glycyrrhizic acid, which is hydrolyzed to glycyrrhetinic acid after ingestion. Glycyrrhetinic acid inhibits 11β-hydroxysteroid dehydrogenase type 2, an enzyme that reversibly catalyzes the conversion of cortisol to cortisone in the distal renal tubule. This conversion of cortisol to its inactive metabolite cortisone protects the mineralocorticoid receptor from cortisol. The inhibition of this enzyme by glycyrrhetinic acid raises intrarenal cortisol levels, providing free access to the mineralocorticoid receptor and causing potassium wasting, sodium retention, hypertension, and suppression of the renin-angiotensin-aldosterone system (thus, Answer D is correct).

Not unexpectedly, urinary cortisol measurements may also be increased in patients consuming licorice. It is a common misconception that licorice products (confections, dietary supplements, chewing tobacco) sold in the United States do not contain glycyrrhizic acid; on the contrary, many products contain variable amounts of the active ingredients of licorice.

Renovascular hypertension with secondary hyperaldosteronism may present in this fashion but would be associated with elevations of both aldosterone and plasma renin activity (thus, Answer A is incorrect). The use of an ACE inhibitor or an angiotensin-receptor blocker would induce an elevation in plasma renin activity and a decrease in serum aldosterone (Answer C).

Of course, normal levels of plasma renin activity and aldosterone (Answer E) would not provide any insight into the cause of the hypertension and hypokalemia in this patient.

EDUCATIONAL OBJECTIVE

Explain the biochemical mechanism of licorice-induced hypertension and hypokalemia.

REFERENCE(S)

Walker BR, Edwards CR. Licorice-induced hypertension and syndromes of apparent mineralocorticoid excess. *Endocrinol Metab Clin North Am.* 1994;23(2):359-377. PMID: 8070427

Epstein MT, Espiner EA, Donald RA, Hughes H, Cowles RJ, Lun S. Licorice raises urinary cortisol in man. *J Clin Endocrinol Metab.* 1978;47(2):397-400. PMID: 233669

Lalande BM, Findling JW. Amelioration of licorice-induced hypokalemic rhabdomyolysis with dexamethasone: a case report and review of the literature. *Endocrinologist.* 1998;8:359-363.

17 ANSWER: E) No further diagnostic studies

Approximately 15% to 20% of aldosterone-producing adenomas larger than 1.5 cm co-secrete cortisol. The autonomous cortisol secretion is usually mild, and affected patients often lack any overt evidence of hypercortisolism. Aldosterone-producing adenomas rarely consist of only zona glomerulosa–derived cells. As an aldosterone-producing adenoma grows, glucocorticoid oversecretion by the tumor may become apparent or detectable by biochemical testing. After adrenalectomy, the patient may have suppression of the endogenous hypothalamic-pituitary-adrenal axis with hypocortisolism and, as expected, suppression of the renin-angiotensin system with hypoaldosteronism. Accordingly, patients may experience signs and symptoms of adrenal insufficiency and glucocorticoid withdrawal, as well as hyperkalemia. There have been reports of adrenal insufficiency after unilateral adrenalectomy for a "nonsecretory" adrenal nodule. Patients with both primary aldosteronism and autonomous cortisol secretion have a high incidence of cardiovascular events, which mandates an aggressive diagnostic and therapeutic strategy.

Because the degree of ACTH-independent hypercortisolism is mild and subclinical, the hypothalamic-pituitary-adrenal axis often recovers promptly, and the patient may do well and not need any diagnostic testing or therapeutic intervention. The recovery of the hypothalamic-pituitary-adrenal axis after suppression by either endogenous or exogenous corticosteroid excess follows a typical pattern. Initially, the hypothalamus and pituitary recover until ACTH levels actually exceed the normal range to provoke growth and increased steroidogenesis from the atrophic adrenal cortex. Thus, the elevated ACTH and low cortisol mimic the biochemical findings of primary adrenal insufficiency, but, in fact, provide reassurance that hypothalamic-pituitary-adrenal function is recovering nicely. Basal physiologic hydrocortisone therapy and stress-dose management are usually required until adrenal function has fully recovered. No further diagnostic studies are needed in this patient (Answer E). The hypoaldosteronism can usually be managed conservatively by encouraging liberal salt intake (increasing distal renal sodium delivery) and a low-potassium diet. Occasionally, patients need mineralocorticoid replacement with fludrocortisone.

This patient's biochemical findings clearly show postoperative hypocortisolism. Because oral contraceptives increase the major binding protein for cortisol (corticosteroid-binding globulin), the low cortisol concentration is enough to establish a diagnosis of cortisol deficiency.

21-Hydroxylase antibodies (Answer C) are a hallmark of classic autoimmune adrenalitis, which is unlikely in this patient. Her elevated ACTH and low serum cortisol provide enough evidence for adrenal insufficiency.

Since adrenal androgen production is decreased in both primary and secondary adrenal insufficiency, measuring DHEA-S (Answer B) may be a sensitive indicator of impaired adrenal function; however, hypoadrenalism is already apparent in this patient.

Pituitary imaging (Answer D) would not provide any insight into the recovery of adrenocortical function.

The patient is recovering from surgery to remove a cortisol-producing lesion. Although there are occasional diagnoses of primary adrenal insufficiency that can be supported by imaging findings (eg, lymphoma, tuberculosis, hemorrhage), this is not expected in this patient. Thus, an adrenal protocol CT (Answer A) is not indicated.

EDUCATIONAL OBJECTIVE

Diagnose adrenal insufficiency after unilateral adrenalectomy for an aldosterone-producing adenoma and recognize the frequency of concomitant and covert autonomous cortisol secretion from some aldosterone-producing adenomas.

REFERENCE(S)

Spath M, Korovkin S, Antke C, Anlauf M, Willenberg HS. Aldosterone- and cortisol-co-secreting adrenal tumors: the lost subtype of primary aldosteronism. *Eur J Endocrinol.* 2011;164(4):447-455. PMID: 21270113

Fisher E, Hanslik G, Pallauf A, et al. Prolonged zona glomerulosa insufficiency causing hyperkalemia in primary aldosteronism after adrenalectomy. *J Clin Endocrinol Metab.* 2012;97(11):3965-3973. PMID: 22893716

Graber AL, Ney RL, Nicholson WE, Island DP, Liddle GW. Natural history of pituitary-adrenal recovery following long-term suppression with corticosteroids. *J Clin Endocrinol Metab.* 1965;25:11-16. PMID: 14252277

Reincke M, Nieke J, Krestin GP, Saeger W, Allolio B, Winkelmann W. Preclinical Cushing's syndrome in adrenal "incidentalomas": comparison with adrenal Cushing's syndrome. *J Clin Endocrinol Metab.* 1992;75(3):826-832. PMID: 1517373

Nakajima Y, Yamada M, Taguchi R, et al. Cardiovascular complications of patients with aldosteronism associated with autonomous cortisol secretion. *J Clin Endocrinol Metab.* 2011;96(8):2512-2518. PMID: 21593113

18 ANSWER: D) Homocysteine and methylmalonic acid measurement

Autoimmune polyendocrine syndromes (APS) can be grouped into APS type 1 and APS type 2. APS type 1 is an autosomal recessive disorder caused by pathogenic variants in the *AIRE* gene. The main manifestations are primary adrenal insufficiency, hypoparathyroidism, and mucocutaneous candidiasis, but other autoimmune endocrinopathies can also occur (eg, hypothyroidism [20%], pernicious anemia [15%]). This patient lacks the core manifestations of hypoparathyroidism and mucocutaneous candidiasis, but she most likely has 2 manifestations of APS type 2. The main manifestations of APS type 2 in patients with adrenal insufficiency are hypothyroidism (40%), type 1 diabetes (10%), vitamin B_{12} deficiency (10%), and vitiligo (10%).

Further evaluation for atrophic gastritis and vitamin B_{12} deficiency usually identifies this reversible cause of the patient's neurologic symptoms. While vitamin B_{12} values well below the lower limit of normal are often diagnostic of deficiency, borderline levels (200-300 pg/mL) are best followed up by homocysteine and methylmalonic acid level measurement (Answer D). Methylmalonic acid is the most specific and sensitive marker for vitamin B_{12} deficiency. Treatment consists of vitamin B_{12} supplementation, either with intramuscular B_{12} or high oral doses. Atrophic gastritis and vitamin B_{12} deficiency can present with neurologic symptoms without any hematologic or gastrointestinal symptoms or signs.

Celiac disease is best diagnosed with esophagogastroduodenoscopy and deep duodenal biopsies (Answer A). Celiac disease coexists in about 5% of patients with APS type 2. Celiac disease is associated with a broad spectrum of neurologic manifestations, but other symptoms or signs are commonly present. Assessing for tissue transglutaminase-IgA antibodies is the screening of choice for celiac disease. IgA deficiency can lead to false-negative screening, but in this case tissue transglutaminase-IgG was also negative, and measurement of total IgA (Answer E) is not necessary.

Diminished ankle reflexes, particularly with a delayed relaxation phase, are associated with hypothyroidism. However, there is no concern in this patient that the slightly increased/upper-limit TSH reflects current severe underreplaced hypothyroidism and no other hypothyroid symptoms are present. Thus, free T_4 measurement (Answer B) is not necessary.

Adrenoleukodystrophy (Answer C) is an X-linked recessive disorder that can initially present with adrenal insufficiency and later with myelopathy with the neurologic manifestations of sensory ataxia and neurogenic bladder dysfunction. Although female carriers can develop myelopathy, adrenal insufficiency in female carriers is exceedingly rare.

EDUCATIONAL OBJECTIVE

Identify atrophic gastritis as an autoimmune disorder that occurs with adrenal insufficiency.

REFERENCE(S)

Erichsen MM, Løvås K, Skinningsrud B, et al. Clinical, immunological, and genetic features of autoimmune primary adrenal insufficiency: observations from a Norwegian registry. *J Clin Endocrinol Metab.* 2009;94(12):4882-4890. PMID: 19858318

Bruserud O, Oftedal BE, Landegren N, et al. A longitudinal follow-up of autoimmune polyendocrine syndrome type 1. J Clin Endocrinol Metab. 2016;101(8):2975-2983. PMID: 27253668

Green R, Allen LH, Bjørke-Monsen A-L, et al. Vitamin B_{12} deficiency. *Nat Rev Dis Primers.* 2017;3:17040. PMID: 28660890

Kemp S, Huffnagel IC, Linthorst GE, Wanders RJ, Engelen M. Adrenoleukodystrophy - neuroendocrine pathogenesis and redefinition of natural history. *Nat Rev Endocrinol.* 2016;12(10):606-615. PMID: 27312864

19 ANSWER: E) Unable to localize

For adrenal venous sampling, the cortisol concentrations in the adrenal vein samples are used to determine whether the adrenal veins were accessed and to correct for the fractional dilution of the adrenal vein blood with mixed venous blood. This ratio of cortisol in the adrenal vein blood to the cortisol in the mixed venous blood is often called the selectivity index. The selectivity index on both sides should be greater than 2 if adrenal venous sampling is performed without cosyntropin and greater than 3 if performed with cosyntropin infusion. Otherwise, the sample does not contain sufficient adrenal vein blood to interpret the results, and the study should not be interpreted unless both selectivity indices are greater than these minimum values. Usually, the right side, which is more difficult to access, fails the selectivity index test. If the aldosterone-to-cortisol ratio in the left adrenal vein is much lower than in the mixed venous blood, also called "contralateral suppression," aldosterone production can sometimes be confidently localized to the right adrenal, but conclusive cut-off values are not known. Note that contralateral suppression is not always observed in studies with convincing lateralization, so lack of contralateral suppression does not equate to bilateral aldosterone production.

Because the selectivity index on the right side is only 1.1 times higher than that of the mixed venous blood, the study was not successful (thus, Answer E is correct and Answer B is incorrect). Although it is possible that both adrenal glands are the source (Answer A), this conclusion cannot be drawn because of the low selectivity index on the right side. For the reasons stated above, the adrenal venous sampling study did not yield enough information to localize the aldosterone production (thus, Answers C and D are incorrect), even though all the information required for interpretation (aldosterone and cortisol from the adrenal veins and mixed venous blood) was available. Plasma metanephrines can also be used to confirm successful access of the adrenal veins, but the values cannot be used mathematically to correct for dilution with mixed venous blood.

EDUCATIONAL OBJECTIVE

Interpret results of adrenal venous sampling.

REFERENCE(S)

Rossi GP, Auchus RJ, Brown M, et al. An expert consensus statement on the use of adrenal vein sampling for the subtyping of primary aldosteronism. *Hypertension.* 2014;63(1):151-160. PMID: 24218436

Dekkers T, Deinum J, Schultzekool LJ, et al. Plasma metanephrine for assessing the selectivity of adrenal venous sampling. *Hypertension.* 2013;62(6):1152-1157. PMID: 24082051

Funder JW, Carey RM, Mantero F, et al. The management of primary aldosteronism: case detection, diagnosis, and treatment: an Endocrine Society Clinical Practice Guideline. *J Clin Endocrinol Metab.* 2016;101(5):1889-1916. PMID: 26934393

20 ANSWER: B) CT of the adrenal glands

Determining the cause of endogenous Cushing syndrome is essential to recommending appropriate therapy. The differential diagnostic challenge in this woman is deciding whether she has ACTH-dependent or ACTH-independent hypercortisolism. Reliable ACTH assays are necessary to distinguish between elevated and, more importantly, subnormal ACTH levels. Plasma ACTH assays have certainly improved since the first radioimmunoassays; however, a recent critical evaluation of plasma ACTH assays demonstrates a high degree of variability. Most ACTH assays cannot correctly identify patients with suppressed ACTH concentrations. This patient poses a particular diagnostic difficulty because her plasma ACTH concentration is 14.0 pg/mL (3.1 pmol/L). This plasma ACTH value does not establish the diagnosis of ACTH-dependent Cushing syndrome. A repeated ACTH measurement (possibly in a different reference laboratory) should be obtained to see if a more definitive value is secured. Another reasonable approach is to perform an ovine corticotropin-releasing hormone–stimulation test (1 mcg/kg intravenously with ACTH and cortisol measurements at 15-minute intervals for 1 hour). Patients with ACTH-independent (adrenal-dependent) Cushing syndrome would be expected to have a blunted ACTH response, and those with pituitary ACTH-dependent hypercortisolism would be expected to exhibit a robust ACTH response.

The major clue in this woman is the very low DHEA-S. DHEA-S is usually low in patients with benign causes of adrenal-dependent (ACTH-independent) Cushing syndrome, while it is usually normal (sometimes elevated) in patients with ACTH-dependent hypercortisolism. In addition, most patients with mild-to-moderate hypercortisolism due to Cushing disease demonstrate some reduction in basal cortisol after even a 1-mg overnight dexamethasone-suppression test, and one would expect some suppression of cortisol after a high dose of dexamethasone in a young woman with mild pituitary Cushing syndrome. This patient is more likely to have adrenal-dependent hypercortisolism and, therefore, CT of the adrenal glands (Answer B) should be performed.

Because most plasma ACTH assays cannot reliably detect subnormal or suppressed levels, experts suggest proceeding with adrenal imaging in patients with endogenous hypercortisolism who have ACTH concentrations less than 25 pg/mL (<5.5 pmol/L).

The finding of a 2-mm pituitary lesion should be viewed with great caution. Endocrinologists should carefully review all pituitary imaging in patients with Cushing syndrome. In this case, no evidence of a pituitary tumor was seen by an experienced endocrinologist. Thus, under no circumstances should this woman undergo pituitary surgery (Answer E) without further evaluation.

Inferior petrosal sinus sampling for ACTH (Answer A) is recommended for patients with ACTH-dependent hypercortisolism in whom there are normal or equivocal findings on pituitary imaging. However, the diagnosis of ACTH-dependent Cushing syndrome has not yet been confirmed in this young woman.

Although the patient had relatively rapid onset of Cushing syndrome, ectopic ACTH syndrome seems very unlikely. Most patients with ectopic ACTH secretion have elevated (or at least high-normal) plasma ACTH levels. Furthermore, chest CT (Answer C) and DOTATATE PET-CT (Answer D) should only be performed if inferior petrosal sinus sampling demonstrates the lack of a pituitary ACTH gradient. Without establishing a clear differential diagnosis, extensive imaging in patients with Cushing syndrome can lead to surgical misadventures.

Another measurement of this patient's basal ACTH concentration (performed at a more reliable laboratory) was less than 1.0 pg/mL (<0.22 pmol/L), and it did not stimulate after administration of ovine corticotropin-releasing hormone. CT of the adrenal glands showed a 3-cm right adrenal nodule with low attenuation values. Removal of the cortisol-secreting adrenal adenoma resulted in secondary adrenal insufficiency. She had complete resolution of Cushing syndrome.

EDUCATIONAL OBJECTIVE

Identify the hormonal profiles of the different subtypes of Cushing syndrome and the key issues in interpreting plasma ACTH and DHEA-S measurements.

REFERENCE(S)

Pecori Giraldi F, Saccani A, Cavagnini F; Study Group on the Hypothalamo-Pituitary-Adrenal Axis of the Italian Society of Endocrinology. Assessment of ACTH assay variability: a multi-center study. *Eur J Endocrinol.* 2011;164:505-515. PMID: 21252174

Javorsky BR, Carroll TB, Findling JW. Differential diagnosis of Cushing syndrome. In: Swearingen B, Biller BMK, eds. *Cushing's Disease.* New York, NY: Springer; 2011:85-106.

Flecchia D, Mazza E, Carlini M, et al. Reduced serum levels of dehydroepiandrosterone sulfate in adrenal incidentalomas: a marker of adrenocortical tumour. *Clin Endocrinol (Oxf).* 1995;42(2):129-134. PMID: 7704956

21 ANSWER: A) Counsel to seek alternatives to facet injections

This scenario is a common reason for referral to an adrenal clinic. The patient has received exogenous steroids over the course of years (facet joint injections), has symptoms and signs of hypercortisolism (weight gain, hypertension, and worsening diabetes), suppressed cortisol, and an incidental adrenal nodule. The correct recommendation is to reduce exogenous steroids and seek alternative strategies for back pain management (Answer A). Exogenous steroids received by injection are often highly potent and can suppress the adrenal axis 4 weeks or longer.

This patient's adrenal nodule is small and has a benign appearance. Any clinically significant cortisol production by the small nodule (cortisol-producing adenomas tend to be 2-4 cm) is unlikely and would result in normal or high cortisol levels. Further evaluation for hypercortisolism is not needed.

The patient has hypertension and an adrenal nodule and is on 2 antihypertensive medications. This warrants screening for primary aldosteronism with aldosterone and renin, but not a confirmatory study with 24-hour urine collection following salt loading (Answer C).

Although opioids can lead to adrenal insufficiency, this would not occur in the absence of symptoms. Thus, opioids do not need to be stopped (Answer B).

He has a low morning cortisol level, which is explained by suppression of the adrenal axis by exogenous steroids. He does not have any symptoms or signs of adrenal insufficiency and therefore no further workup or therapy is needed (Answers D and E). The adrenal nodule does not need further imaging, as it has benign imaging features. One could consider continued sporadic tests for hypercortisolism after avoiding exogenous glucocorticoids.

EDUCATIONAL OBJECTIVE

Identify causes of exogenous Cushing syndrome.

REFERENCE(S)

Stout A, Friedly J, Standaert CJ. Systemic absorption and side effects of locally injected glucocorticoids. *PM R*. 2019;11(4):409-419. PMID: 30925034

22 ANSWER: B) CT-guided percutaneous adrenal biopsy

The diagnosis of primary adrenal insufficiency may be suspected on the basis of many nonspecific signs and symptoms, volume depletion, hyponatremia, hyperkalemia, and, less commonly, incidentally discovered bilateral adrenal imaging abnormalities. This patient has many clinical features of adrenal insufficiency. Confirmation of primary adrenal insufficiency was secured with just basal biochemical studies. When ACTH concentrations exceed 80 to 100 pg/mL (17.6-22.0 pmol/L), maximum adrenocortical stimulation is achieved and cortisol values greater than 18 µg/dL (>497 nmol/L) would be expected. This patient's markedly elevated ACTH level and his suboptimal cortisol response confirm the presence of primary adrenal insufficiency. Assessment of the renin-angiotensin-aldosterone system provides further confirmation, with markedly elevated plasma renin activity and low serum aldosterone. The differential diagnosis in this setting includes infiltrative and inflammatory processes, metastatic disease, bilateral adrenal hemorrhage, and primary adrenal lymphoma. The best option to establish the correct diagnosis in this patient is CT-guided percutaneous adrenal biopsy (Answer B). Pheochromocytoma should always be excluded before this procedure, but the trivial elevation of normetanephrine is inconsistent with functional tumors of that size and is due to volume depletion. Causes of false-positive elevations in plasma and urinary metanephrines include tricyclic antidepressants, serotonin norepinephrine reuptake inhibitors, clonidine withdrawal, and sleep apnea. In this patient, CT-guided percutaneous adrenal biopsy demonstrated findings consistent with histoplasmosis. He is from an area near the confluence of the Ohio and Mississippi Rivers, where histoplasmosis is endemic. Part of the biopsy sample should also be used for acid fast bacilli culture. An interferon-gamma release assay should be used to test for tuberculosis, as this can present with the same clinical picture with adrenal insufficiency and increased adrenal gland size.

Patients with autoimmune adrenalitis have small rather than large adrenal glands, so 21-hydroxylase antibodies (Answer D), even if paradoxically positive, would not aid in the diagnosis.

Urinary free cortisol (Answer E) is not used to diagnose cortisol deficiency.

Because this patient clearly has primary adrenal insufficiency, pituitary imaging (Answer C) is unnecessary.

Adrenal venous sampling (Answer A) is of no use in the evaluation of adrenal insufficiency.

Assessing for the presence of histoplasmosis antigen in the urine would be a reasonable alternative approach, but this was not listed as an answer option in this vignette.

EDUCATIONAL OBJECTIVE

Select the appropriate diagnostic test for the evaluation of adrenal insufficiency with bilateral adrenal gland enlargement.

REFERENCE(S)

Bornstein SR, Allolio B, Arlt W, et al. Diagnosis and treatment of primary adrenal insufficiency: an Endocrine Society Clinical Practice Guideline. *J Clin Endocrinol Metab.* 2016;101(2):364-389. PMID: 26760044

Kumar N, Singh S, Govil S. Adrenal histoplasmosis: clinical presentation and imaging features in nine cases. *Abdom Imaging.* 2003;28(5):703-708. PMID: 14628881

Zhou L, Peng W, Wang C, Liu X, Shen Y, Zhou K. Primary adrenal lymphoma: radiological; pathological, clinical correlation. *Eur J Radiol.* 2012;81(3):401-405. PMID: 21146945

Zieger MA, Siegelman SS, Hamrahian AH. Medical and surgical evaluation and treatment of adrenal incidentalomas. *J Clin Endocrinol Metab.* 2011;96(7):2004-2015. PMID: 21632813

Bone Board Review

Natalie E. Cusano, MD, MS

1 ANSWER: C) Milk-alkali syndrome

This is a classic case of milk-alkali syndrome (Answer C) leading to a hypercalcemic crisis. The classic triad of milk-alkali syndrome is hypercalcemia, kidney failure, and metabolic alkalosis. Milk-alkali syndrome was originally described in the 1930s during therapy for peptic ulcer disease with sodium bicarbonate and milk. Beall et al described a "modern version" of the syndrome in 2006 in the setting of ingesting large quantities of calcium carbonate. Milk-alkali syndrome is the third most common cause of hospitalization due to hypercalcemia, behind malignancy and primary hyperparathyroidism.

After intravenous hydration, the patient's mental state improved and she was able to provide additional history of taking a calcium carbonate antacid (9 to 15 g of elemental calcium) in addition to her usual calcium supplementation. As an outpatient, after resolution of her acute on chronic kidney failure, alendronate was discontinued and she received zoledronic acid, 5 mg intravenously over 30 minutes with additional intravenous fluids. Symptoms of gastroesophageal reflux disease improved.

In the setting of excess calcium/alkali ingestion, hypercalcemia causes kidney vasoconstriction, decreases the glomerular filtration rate, and increases bicarbonate reabsorption. Metabolic alkalosis further increases renal tubular reabsorption of calcium, and hypovolemia from nausea/vomiting reduces the glomerular filtration rate. A vicious cycle can occur with rapid clinical deterioration and death. Hyperphosphatemia may also be seen with excessive ingestion of milk as the calcium source.

None of the other answers best address the patient's alkalosis. Dehydration (Answer A) was certainly present, but this was not the underlying etiology of the patient's presentation.

She was noted to have a low TSH concentration due to nonthyroidal illness, with subsequent normalization of her value after hospital discharge. Thus, thyrotoxicosis (Answer D) is not the most likely etiology.

Humeral hypercalcemia of malignancy (Answer B) would be rare in a patient with a history of stage 1 breast cancer and would be associated with an elevated PTHrP value.

Vitamin D intoxication (Answer E) should not cause alkalosis, and vitamin D toxicity does not generally present unless the 25-hydroxyvitamin D concentration exceeds 150 ng/mL (>374.4 nmol/L).

In patients with milk-alkali syndrome, simply stopping the exogenous calcium and alkali and providing vigorous saline hydration to increase the glomerular filtration rate and help clear the calcium and bicarbonate can rapidly reverse the metabolic disarray. Treatment of acute milk-alkali syndrome can lead to an acute drop in serum calcium to hypocalcemic levels (with rebound increase in PTH). More chronic cases with nephrocalcinosis take much longer to resolve.

Acute management of a hypercalcemic crisis generally involves saline hydration, subcutaneous calcitonin for 24 to 48 hours, intravenous bisphosphonate (or subcutaneous denosumab in selected patients), and treatment of the underlying disease. Furosemide should be added only when there is clinical evidence of volume overload or congestive heart failure. In cases of vitamin D–mediated hypercalcemia, prednisone, 40 to 60 mg daily, or another glucocorticoid equivalent may be useful, but it should not be given without biochemical evidence of inappropriate vitamin D levels. Finally, in patients with hypercalcemic crisis due to primary hyperparathyroidism, cinacalcet can be a "bridge" to parathyroidectomy.

EDUCATIONAL OBJECTIVE

Diagnose milk-alkali syndrome.

REFERENCE(S)

Beall DP, Henslee HB, Webb HR, Scofield RH. Milk-alkali syndrome: a historical review and description of the modern version of the syndrome. *Am J Med Sci.* 2006;331(5):233-242. PMID: 16702792

Bondje S, Barnes C, Kaplan F. Another case of milk–alkali syndrome or a learning opportunity? *Endocrinol Diabetes Metab Case Rep.* 2022;2022:21-0151.

2 ANSWER: B) Review her bone density images

This patient has a history of lumbar spinal fusion, yet L1-L4 were included in the bone density report. Her bone density at L4 was falsely elevated due to hardware and was 2 standard deviations above her value at L3. L4 was incorrectly included in the calculation of her T-score (*figure and table*). When L4 was excluded, her T-score at the lumbar spine L1-L3 was −2.8, indicating osteoporosis treatment is warranted. Thus, the best next step is to review this patient's bone density images (Answer B).

Increasing her calcium and vitamin D intake (Answer D) is not correct because her calcium intake is sufficient by history and her 25-hydroxyvitamin D value is within the sufficient range.

Hormone therapy (Answer E) can be considered for symptomatic relief of moderate to severe vasomotor symptoms in some women, but it is not indicated as specific therapy for osteoporosis unless a bisphosphonate or denosumab is not appropriate.

Starting ibandronate (Answer C) before reviewing her bone density values is premature. Of note, ibandronate is not a preferred agent in many guideline statements because it lacks nonvertebral fracture efficacy.

Waiting to repeat DXA in 2 years (Answer A) would be incorrect without first reviewing her bone density images to determine whether therapy is needed.

Figure. Lumbar Spine DXA Images

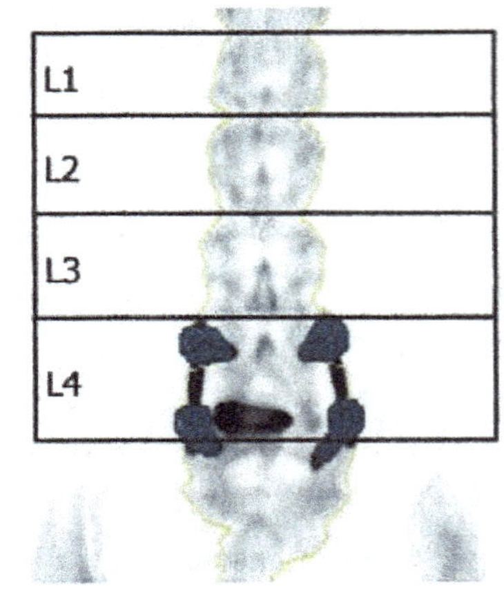

Region	BMD (g/cm²)	Young-Adult T-Score	Age-Matched Z-Score
L1	0.801	-2.8	-1.2
L2	0.820	-3.2	-1.7
L3	0.883	-2.7	-1.1
L4	1.443	1.7	3.3
L1-L4	1.039	-1.3	0.3

EDUCATIONAL OBJECTIVE

Carefully review DXA images and identify common technical errors.

REFERENCE(S)

Watts NB. Fundamentals and pitfalls of bone densitometry using dual-energy X-ray absorptiometry (DXA). *Osteoporos Int.* 2004;15(11):847-854. PMID: 15322740

Schousboe JT, Shepherd JA, Bilezikian JP, Baim S. Executive summary of the 2013 international society for clinical densitometry position development conference on bone densitometry. *J Clin Densitom.* 2013;16(4):455-466. PMID: 24183638

3 ANSWER: C) PTH = 15 pg/mL (SI: 1.59 pmol/L); phosphate = 4.7 mg/dL (SI: 1.52 mmol/L); 1,25-dihydroxyvitamin D = 80 pg/mL (SI: 208 mmol/L)

The pattern of laboratory values in Answer C is typical of hypercalcemia due to granulomatous disease, such as sarcoidosis, tuberculosis, or silicone-induced granulomas. In granulomatous diseases or lymphoma, 1,25-dihydroxyvitamin D levels are elevated due to extrarenal production of the hormone. In the setting of hypercalcemia and low PTH, 1,25-dihydroxyvitamin D is typically suppressed, not elevated. Patients with granulomatous diseases may have an elevated phosphate concentration since 1,25-dihydroxyvitamin D increases absorption of phosphate from the intestines and increases urinary phosphate absorption. Non–PTH-mediated hypercalcemia suppresses PTH below 20 to 25 pg/mL (<2.12-2.65 pmol/L) and in some cases to undetectable levels.

Hypercalcemia due to excessive secretion of PTHrP is the most common cause of hypercalcemia of malignancy and is the most common cause of hypercalcemia in the inpatient setting. Affected patients can have low PTH, low phosphate, and normal 1,25-dihydroxyvitamin D levels, similar to the pattern in Answer A. Hypercalcemia can be considered PTH-mediated if PTH concentrations are 25 pg/mL or greater (≥2.65 pmol/L). PTH-dependent causes of hypercalcemia include primary hyperparathyroidism, tertiary hyperparathyroidism, familial hypocalciuric hypercalcemia, and neonatal hyperparathyroidism. Individuals with hypercalcemia due to primary hyperparathyroidism have high or inappropriately normal PTH values and normal or low phosphate (Answer E). 1,25-Dihydroxyvitamin D levels can be normal or elevated due to PTH's stimulation of 25-hydroxyvitamin D_3 1α-hydroxylase. Individuals with primary hyperparathyroidism do not have low PTH levels unless biotin is interfering with the specific assay (not common with most laboratory assays).

The values listed in Answers B and D are not typical of any disease process.

EDUCATIONAL OBJECTIVE

Diagnose 1,25-dihydroxyvitamin D–mediated hypercalcemia.

REFERENCE(S)

Tebben PJ, Singh RJ, Kumar R. Vitamin D-mediated hypercalcemia: mechanisms, diagnosis, and treatment. *Endocr Rev.* 2016;37(5):521-547. PMID: 27588937

4 ANSWER: D) Omeprazole

Hypomagnesemia due to proton-pump inhibitor use (Answer D) impairs PTH release in response to low calcium and causes skeletal resistance to PTH. PTH resistance can occur with magnesium levels below 0.8 mg/dL (<0.33 mmol/L), with a decrease in PTH secretion occurring with more profound hypomagnesemia. Hypomagnesemia is most commonly due to malabsorption; chronic alcoholism; and medications such as proton-pump inhibitors, diuretics, and cisplatin. Magnesium disorders are the only reversible cause of hypoparathyroidism, and parenteral magnesium repletion resulted in a significant rise in this patient's PTH concentration. Calcium supplementation alone cannot correct hypocalcemia in the setting of magnesium deficiency.

Parenteral antiresorptive medications such as pamidronate, zoledronic acid, and denosumab can cause hypocalcemia, particularly in patients with profound vitamin D deficiency and/or chronic kidney disease. Oral bisphosphonate therapy (Answer A) is unlikely to result in hypocalcemia and would cause an elevation, not a decrease, in the PTH concentration.

Hypomagnesemia can induce hypokalemia through urinary potassium wasting. Hypokalemia (Answer B) does not cause hypomagnesemia or hypocalcemia.

While profound vitamin D deficiency (Answer E) most likely contributed to this patient's low serum calcium, hypomagnesemia is the primary etiology in this case as evidenced by the low, not elevated, PTH concentration.

Hypoparathyroidism (Answer C) is a rare disorder that most commonly occurs after parathyroid surgery or is associated with autoimmune disease. This patient has no evidence of neck surgery or other autoimmune conditions on physical examination. Hypoparathyroidism would not account for her hypomagnesemia or hypokalemia.

EDUCATIONAL OBJECTIVE

Identify proton-pump inhibitors as a cause of hypomagnesemia leading to hypocalcemia.

REFERENCE(S)

Chase LR, Slatopolsky E. Secretion and metabolic efficacy of parathyroid hormone in patients with severe hypomagnesemia. *J Clin Endocrinol Metab.* 1974;38(3):363-371. PMID: 4360918

Fatemi S, Ryzen E, Flores J, Endres DB, Rude RK. Effect of experimental human magnesium depletion on parathyroid hormone secretion and 1,25-dihydroxyvitamin D metabolism. *J Clin Endocrinol Metab.* 1991;73(5):1067-1072. PMID: 1939521

Epstein M, McGrath S, Law F. Proton-pump inhibitors and hypomagnesemic hypoparathyroidism. *N Engl J Med.* 2006;355(17):1834-1836. PMID: 17065651

5 ANSWER: A) Continue alendronate

This patient is at very high risk for future fracture based on her history of low-trauma hip fracture and continued osteoporosis at the femoral neck. Guidance from the American Society for Bone and Mineral Research identified patients at high fracture risk, including older women and patients with low hip T-score or high fracture risk score, previous major osteoporotic fracture, and fracture while on therapy. In women at high risk, treatment continuation for up to 10 years (oral bisphosphonate) or 6 years (intravenous bisphosphonate) should be considered. The American Association of Clinical Endocrinology agrees with this algorithm. US FDA guidance also states that in patients at increased fracture risk (eg, older patients with a fracture history and bone mineral density in the osteoporotic range), benefits of continued therapy after 5 years may outweigh risks. Thus, continuation of alendronate is recommended (thus, Answer A is correct and Answer E is incorrect).

Certainly, for a patient in whom there is a lack of densitometric response to alendronate, switching to alternative therapies, such as zoledronic acid, denosumab, teriparatide, or abaloparatide, should be considered, but they were not presented as options here.

Romosozumab (Answer D) is not a good choice given her recent history of cerebrovascular accident. There is a black box warning on romosozumab's FDA label for patients with a myocardial infarction or stroke within the preceding year.

Combination alendronate and teriparatide therapy (Answer B) has not been demonstrated to be beneficial and it would not be covered by insurance. Of note, if the patient is right-handed, she may need assistance with administration of teriparatide.

Ibandronate (Answer C) has not been demonstrated to reduce the risk of nonvertebral fractures, and it is not considered a first-line therapy for this reason in many guideline statements.

EDUCATIONAL OBJECTIVE

Recommend antiresportive therapy for up to 10 years in a patient at high fracture risk.

REFERENCE(S)

Food and Drug Administration. Background document for meeting of Advisory Committee for Reproductive Health Drugs and Drug Safety and Risk Management Advisory Committee. September 9, 2011 https://public4.pagefreezer.com/browse/FDA/20-04-2024T15:35/https://www.fda.gov/drugs/drug-safety-and-availability/fda-drug-safety-communication-safety-update-osteoporosis-drugs-bisphosphonates-and-atypical

Adler RA, El-Hajj Fuleihan G, Bauer DC, et al. Managing osteoporosis in patients on long-term bisphosphonate treatment: report of a Task Force of the American Society for Bone and Mineral Research. *J Bone Miner Res.* 2016;31(1):16-35. PMID: 26350171

Camacho PM, Petak SM, Binkley N, et al. American Association of Clinical Endocrinologists/American College of Endocrinology clinical practice guidelines for the diagnosis and treatment of postmenopausal osteoporosis-2020 update. *Endocr Pract.* 2020;26(5):564-570. PMID: 32427503

6 ANSWER: B) Hypophosphatasia

Hypophosphatasia (Answer B) is a rare genetic disease caused by loss-of-function pathogenic variants in the *ALPL* gene, which encodes the tissue-nonspecific isoenzyme of alkaline phosphatase (TNSALP). TNSALP is particularly abundant in the bone, liver, and kidneys but is also expressed in other tissues, including cartilage and teeth. The main physiologic substrates of TNSALP are inorganic pyrophosphate and pyridoxal-5′-phosphate (the active metabolite of vitamin B_6). Loss of function of TNSALP results in a generalized reduction in alkaline phosphatase activity and accumulation of TNSALP substrates, including inorganic pyrophosphate and vitamin B_6. The prevalence of severe hypophosphatasia is approximately 1 in 100,000 in Anglo-Saxon populations and is more prevalent among Mennonites in Manitoba, Canada, where 1 in every 25 persons is a carrier. Inheritance is autosomal recessive for the infantile forms but is either autosomal recessive or autosomal dominant for the milder adult forms, with variable penetrance. The clinical presentation and severity of hypophosphatasia are variable due to many different pathogenic variants in the *ALPL* gene.

Therapy for hypophosphatasia can include enzyme replacement therapy with asfotase alfa, which rapidly and markedly increases serum alkaline phosphatase levels (to as high as 24,000 U/L [400.8 μkat/L]) within 4 weeks of starting treatment. Alkaline phosphatase remains elevated (3000-6000 IU/L [50.1-100.2 μkat/L]) after 5 years of continuous therapy. To date, these markedly elevated alkaline phosphatase levels do not appear to have any detrimental effects. Patients on asfotase alfa therapy should be monitored with ophthalmic examination at baseline and annually or as clinically indicated to identify ectopic eye calcification. Kidney ultrasonography and urinary calcium/creatinine should be assessed at baseline and every 6 months, as clinically indicated, to monitor for nephrocalcinosis.

The other disorders listed are associated with elevated alkaline phosphatase levels, although not to such a degree (*box*; thus, Answers A, C, D, and E are incorrect). X-linked hypophosphatemic rickets is an X-linked dominant form of rickets that is relatively unresponsive to vitamin D. Hypophosphatemia arises as a consequence of a defective *PHEX* gene product (phosphate-regulating gene with homology to endopeptidases on the X chromosome) that ultimately results in elevated FGF-23 levels and impaired renal proximal tubule phosphate reabsorption. Although infrequent, elevated serum alkaline phosphatase levels can occur in adults with X-linked hypophosphatemic rickets, and this most likely indicates the presence of extensive osteomalacia.

Fibrous dysplasia is a disease where abnormal fibrous tissue replaces healthy bone.

Box. Causes of Elevated Bone-Specific Alkaline Phosphatase

Severe primary hyperparathyroidism
Hyperthyroidism
Metastatic cancer in bone
Paget disease of bone
Recent large bone fracture
Osteomalacia
Severe (<8-10 ng/mL) vitamin D deficiency
Space travel
Immobilization
Osteoanabolic therapy (teriparatide, abaloparatide, romosozumab, rhPTH[1–84])
Treatment with strontium ranelate
Treatment with asfotase alfa
High bone turnover osteoporosis
Kidney bone disease: either hyperparathyroid disease or osteomalacia

EDUCATIONAL OBJECTIVE

Identify asfotase alfa as the cause of elevated alkaline phosphatase in a patient with hypophosphatasia.

REFERENCE(S)

Bowden SA, Foster BL. Profile of asfotase alfa in the treatment of hypophosphatasia: design, development, and place in therapy. *Drug Des Devel Ther.* 2018;12:3147-3161. PMID: 30288020

Kishnani PS, Rush ET, Arundel P, et al. Monitoring guidance for patients with hypophosphatasia treated with asfotase alfa. *Mol Genet Metab.* 2017;122(1-2):4-17. PMID: 28888853

Lewiecki EM, Bilezikian JP, Bukata SV, et al. Proceedings of the 2016 Santa Fe Bone Symposium: new concepts in the management of osteoporosis and metabolic bone diseases. *J Clin Densitom.* 2017;20(2):134-152. PMID: 28185765

7 ANSWER: E) Calcium, normal; phosphate, decreased; PTH, normal or increased; 25-hydroxyvitamin D, normal; 1,25-dihydroxyvitamin D, normal or decreased

The laboratory pattern in Answer E is typical for X-linked hypophosphatemic rickets. X-linked hypophosphatemic rickets is an X-linked dominant form of rickets that is relatively unresponsive to vitamin D. Hypophosphatemia arises as a consequence of a defective *PHEX* gene product (phosphate-regulating gene with homology to endopeptidases on the X chromosome), which ultimately results in elevated FGF-23 levels and impaired renal proximal tubule phosphate reabsorption. In addition, despite severe hypophosphatemia, 1,25-dihydroxyvitamin D_3 production is not appropriately enhanced due to FGF-23–mediated suppression of 1α-hydroxylase activity. Thus, the "normal" level of 1,25-dihydroxyvitamin D_3 is inappropriate in the setting of elevated PTH and low serum phosphate. The patterns in Answers A, B, and C are typical of calcipenic rickets, which, as the name suggests, is primarily due to a lack of calcium, typically because of a lack of vitamin D effects, either from deficiency or defective functioning.

The pattern in Answer A is typical of vitamin D deficiency, with low 25-hydroxyvitamin D being a key finding. Of note, serum levels of 1,25-dihydroxyvitamin D are regulated primarily by PTH and have little or no relationship to vitamin D stores. 1,25-Dihdyroxyvitamin D can thus be elevated in vitamin D deficiency due to secondary hyperparathyroidism.

The pattern in Answer B is typical of vitamin D–dependent rickets type 1A, in which patients are unable to convert 25-hydroxyvitamin D to 1,25-dihydroxyvitamin D. Patients with vitamin D–dependent rickets type 1A have pathogenic variants in the *CYP27B1* gene that encodes the 25-hydroxyvitamin D_3-1α-hydroxylase. These patients respond well to treatment with exogenous activated vitamin D metabolites but not as well to usual vitamin D supplementation (hence, they were considered "resistant" to vitamin D in the era before activated vitamin D supplements were available).

The pattern in Answer C is typical of vitamin D–dependent rickets type 2A, in which patients have loss-of-function pathogenic variants in the gene encoding the vitamin D receptor, resulting in a form of tissue resistance to vitamin D.

The pattern in Answer D is typical of hypoparathyroidism, with a PTH deficiency that results in hypocalcemia, hyperphosphatemia, and low 1,25-dihydroxyvitamin D.

EDUCATIONAL OBJECTIVE

Diagnose X-linked hypophosphatemic rickets.

REFERENCE(S)

Levine MA. Diagnosis and management of vitamin D dependent rickets. *Front Pediatr.* 2020;8:315. PMID: 32596195

Chanchlani R, Nemer P, Sinha R, et al. An overview of rickets in children. *Kidney Int Rep.* 2020;5(7):980-990. PMID: 32647755

8 ANSWER: B) Order thoracic and lumbar spine radiographs

Patients with primary hyperparathyroidism are at increased risk for vertebral fractures. The Fifth International Workshop on the Management of Primary Hyperparathyroidism would recommend that this patient be screened with a vertebral fracture assessment at the time of DXA, if available, or with radiographs or other imaging (*table*) (Answer B). In the absence of a vertebral fracture, she has mild, asymptomatic primary hyperparathyroidism and monitoring would be appropriate. The presence of a nontraumatic vertebral fracture would change her diagnosis from osteopenia to osteoporosis and from asymptomatic to symptomatic primary hyperparathyroidism, for which parathyroid surgery would be recommended.

Table. Recommendations for Parathyroid Surgery From the Fifth International Workshop on the Management of Asymptomatic Primary Hyperparathyroidism

Surgery to be recommended if 1 of the following is present:
A. Serum calcium >1 mg/dL (>0.25 mmol/L) above upper normal limit
B. Skeletal features:
a. Fracture by vertebral fracture assessment or vertebral x-ray or
b. BMD by T-score ≤ −2.5 at any site
C. Kidney features:
a. Estimated glomerular filtration rate or creatinine clearance <60 cc/min or
b. Nephrocalcinosis or nephrolithiasis on x-ray, ultrasonography, or other imaging modality or
c. Urinary calcium excretion >250 mg/24 h (women) or >300 mg/24 h (men)
D. Age <50 years
Surgery to be recommended if 1 of the following occurs in follow-up:
A. Serum calcium consistently is measured >1 mg/dL (>0.25 mmol/L) above upper normal limit
B. Fracture
C. Kidney stone
D. Significant reduction in bone mineral density to a T-score of ≤ −2.5
E. Significant reduction in creatinine clearance

She has had a height loss of 2 in (5.1 cm). Based on recommendations from the American Association of Clinical Endocrinology and International Society for Clinical Densitometry, she should be screened for vertebral fracture due to height loss greater than 1.5 in (>3.8 cm), regardless of the diagnosis of primary hyperparathyroidism.

There is no indication to order parathyroid sestamibi (Answer A) for diagnosis of primary hyperparathyroidism, and imaging should only be performed in anticipation of parathyroid surgery.

There is no indication to restrict calcium and vitamin D intake (Answer C) in patients with primary hyperparathyroidism. The recommendations are for calcium intake/supplementation to follow the Institute of Medicine nutritional guidelines: 800 mg daily for women younger than 50 years and men younger than 70 years; 1000 mg daily for women older than 50 years and men older than 70 years; and to maintain the 25-hydroxyvitamin D concentration between 30 and 50 ng/mL (74.9-124.8 nmol/L).

Cinacalcet (Answer E) may be indicated for patients with primary hyperparathyroidism and severe hypercalcemia who are unable to undergo parathyroidectomy. This patient's serum calcium value remains within 1 mg/dL above the upper normal limit.

Alendronate (Answer D) may be considered for patients with osteoporosis or osteopenia at elevated fracture risk who are unable to undergo parathyroidectomy. In the absence of a vertebral fracture, she does not need osteoporosis therapy.

EDUCATIONAL OBJECTIVE

Recommend screening for vertebral fracture in patients with primary hyperparathyroidism.

REFERENCE(S)

Bilezikian JP, Silverberg SJ, Bandeira F, et al. Management of primary hyperparathyroidism. *J Bone Miner Res.* 2022;37(11):2391-2403. PMID: 36054638

Cusano NE. Challenges in screening and diagnosis of osteoporosis. In: Cusano NE, ed. *Osteoporosis: A Clinical Casebook.* Springer; 2021:1-15.

9 ANSWER: A) Age

Bone strength, which is what determines fracture risk, depends on bone density (easily measured by DXA) and bone quality (not so easily measured). Bone density is a powerful predictor of fracture risk, and for each standard deviation decrease in bone density, fracture risk increases 1.5- to 2.6-fold. Bone quality can be determined from a bone biopsy specimen, or noninvasively using high-resolution peripheral quantitative CT or trabecular bone score, although these measurements require specialized machinery and/or specialized software. The Fracture Risk Assessment Tool (FRAX) is a free online tool for estimation of 10-year major osteoporotic fracture and hip fracture risk. FRAX uses risk factors for fracture independent of bone density measurement. These risk factors are thought to indirectly assess bone quality, in addition to any effects they may have on bone density.

For any given T-score, the fracture risk is higher with advancing age (Answer A).

For the purposes of FRAX, previous factures denote low-trauma adult fractures; this patient's ankle fracture (Answer C) occurred in the setting of trauma and should not be included in the FRAX calculator.

A family history of hip fracture, but not vertebral fracture, should be included in the FRAX calculator. This patient's family history (Answer B) does not include hip fracture.

Current, but not history of, tobacco use (Answer E) is a risk factor in the FRAX calculator.

Causes of secondary osteoporosis (Answer D) for FRAX include type 1 diabetes, osteogenesis imperfecta in adults, untreated longstanding hyperthyroidism, hypogonadism or premature menopause (age <45 years), chronic malnutrition, malabsorption, and chronic liver disease. It is important to note that the "secondary osteoporosis" input affects FRAX calculations in the absence of a bone mineral density value, but not when bone density is included.

EDUCATIONAL OBJECTIVE

Differentiate among the risk factors for fracture used in the Fracture Risk Assessment Tool (FRAX).

REFERENCE(S)

Kanis JA, Johnell O, Oden A, Dawson A, De Laet C, Jonsson B. Ten year probabilities of osteoporotic fractures according to BMD and diagnostic thresholds. *Osteoporos Int.* 2001;12(12):989-995. PMID: 11846333

Siris ES, Chen YT, Abbott TA, et al. Bone mineral density thresholds for pharmacological intervention to prevent fractures. *Arch Intern Med.* 2004;164(10):1108-1112. PMID: 15159268

Kanis JA, Johnell O, Oden A, et al. Smoking and fracture risk: a meta-analysis. *Osteoporos Int.* 2005;16(2):155-162. PMID: 15175845

Kanis JA, Johansson H, Harvey NC, McCloskey EV. A brief history of FRAX. *Arch Osteoporos.* 2018;13(1):118. PMID: 30382424

10 ANSWER: D) +9% improvement in lumbar spine bone density and 70% vertebral fracture risk reduction

Denosumab is a monoclonal antibody against RANKL that has been approved for treatment of postmenopausal women and men with osteoporosis, as well as glucocorticoid-induced osteoporosis. In the pivotal clinical trial in postmenopausal women, treatment with denosumab resulted in improvements in bone density of 9.2% (95% CI, 8.2%-10.1%) at the lumbar spine and 6.0% at the total hip (95% CI, 5.2%-6.7%) compared with placebo at 36 months ($P < .001$ for both). Vertebral fracture risk was 68% lower in the denosumab arm than in the placebo arm (incidence 2.3% [86 of 3702 patients]) in the denosumab group vs 7.2% (264 of 3691 patients) in the placebo group. Answer D correctly gives the correct approximate expected changes for improvement in bone density and vertebral fracture risk reduction.

Data through up to 10 years of denosumab treatment demonstrated improvement in bone density of 21.7% at the lumbar spine and 9.2% at the total hip in postmenopausal women compared with values at baseline ($P < .05$ for both). Cessation of denosumab results in an increase in bone resorption markers above pretreatment values for approximately 24 months after the last dose. Abrupt discontinuation of denosumab therapy has been associated with increased risk of multiple vertebral fractures, as early as 7 months from the last dose. Transition to oral or intravenous bisphosphonate therapy is recommended before discontinuation of denosumab.

EDUCATIONAL OBJECTIVE

Describe densitometric changes and vertebral fracture risk reduction with denosumab therapy.

REFERENCE(S):

Cummings SR, San Martin J, McClung MR, et al; FREEDOM Trial. Denosumab for prevention of fractures in postmenopausal women with osteoporosis. *N Engl J Med.* 2009;361(8):756-765. PMID: 19671655

Bone HG, Wagman RB, Brandi ML, et al. 10 years of denosumab treatment in postmenopausal women with osteoporosis: results from the phase 3 randomised FREEDOM trial and open-label extension. *Lancet Diabetes Endocrinol.* 2017;5(7):513-523. PMID: 28546097

11 ANSWER: A) Calculate her FRAX score

A "low-trauma" or "fragility" fracture is defined by the World Health Organization as a fracture resulting from trauma equivalent to a fall from standing height or less. While low-trauma rib fractures are considered to be fragility fractures, most experts do not consider rib fractures to be osteoporosis-defining. Thus, starting alendronate (Answer C) is incorrect. There is general consensus, including guidelines from the Endocrine Society, that a low-trauma hip fracture is an osteoporosis-defining fracture. Many experts also consider low-trauma vertebral, proximal humerus, pelvis, and distal forearm fractures in the setting of osteopenia as diagnostic of osteoporosis; the American Association of Clinical Endocrinology uses this definition. A fragility fracture outside of these sites in a patient with osteopenia by bone density measurement should prompt use of the FRAX calculator (Answer A) to determine fracture risk and help guide consideration of treatment. Pharmacologic osteoporosis therapy would be recommended for patients with a T-score of −1 to −2.5 and a 10-year probability of 20% or higher for major osteoporotic fractures or 3% or higher for hip fractures based on the US-adapted FRAX tool.

Repeating bone mineral density assessment in 2 years (Answer B) without calculation of her FRAX score to determine whether therapy is needed is incorrect.

Hormone therapy (Answer E) can be considered for symptomatic relief of vasomotor symptoms in some women, but it is not indicated as specific therapy for osteoporosis unless a bisphosphonate or denosumab is not appropriate.

Increasing her calcium and vitamin D intake (Answer D) is not correct since her calcium intake is sufficient by history and her 25-hydroxyvitamin D level is within the sufficient range.

EDUCATIONAL OBJECTIVE

Diagnose low-trauma fractures and determine a treatment plan.

REFERENCE(S)

Siris ES, Adler R, Bilezikian J, et al. The clinical diagnosis of osteoporosis: a position statement from the National Bone Health Alliance Working Group. *Osteoporos Int.* 2014;25(5):1439-1443. PMID: 24577348

Camacho PM, Petak SM, Binkley N, et al. American Association of Clinical Endocrinologists/American College of Endocrinology clinical practice guidelines for the diagnosis and treatment of postmenopausal osteoporosis-2020 update. *Endocr Pract.* 2020;26(Suppl 1):1-46. PMID: 32427503

Shoback D, Rosen CJ, Black DM, Cheung AM, Murad MH, Eastell R. Pharmacological management of osteoporosis in postmenopausal women: an Endocrine Society guideline update. *J Clin Endocrinol Metab.* 2020;105(3):dgaa048. PMID: 32068863

12 ANSWER: C) Parathyroidectomy in the second trimester

This patient has an elevated serum calcium concentration with concurrently elevated PTH, consistent with primary hyperparathyroidism. Her elevated 24-hour urinary calcium excretion excludes familial hypocalciuric hypercalcemia. Primary hyperparathyroidism in pregnancy is associated with several maternal complications, including hyperemesis gravidarum, nephrolithiasis, pancreatitis, miscarriage, and preeclampsia. Parathyroidectomy in the second trimester (Answer C) has been associated with favorable outcomes in patients with moderate to severe hypercalcemia during pregnancy in several case reports and case series. Surgery should be avoided in the first trimester (Answer D) if possible.

Cinacalcet (Answer A) is pregnancy category C because it has been shown to cross the placenta, and there are no long-term safety data in pregnancy. However, a few case reports have been published.

Bisphosphonates and denosumab (Answer B) are pregnancy category D drugs and should be avoided in pregnancy because of adverse fetal skeletal outcomes in animal studies.

Calcitriol levels increase 2- to 5-fold in euparathyroid women in the first trimester of pregnancy to increase intestinal absorption of calcium. This patient's high 1,25-dihydroxyvitamin D level is due to increased production during pregnancy and activation of 1α-hydroxylase activity by PTH. Thus, prednisone (Answer E) is not indicated.

EDUCATIONAL OBJECTIVE

Manage primary hyperparathyroidism in pregnancy.

REFERENCE(S)

Ali DS, Dandurand K, Khan AA. Primary hyperparathyroidism in pregnancy: literature review of the diagnosis and management. *J Clin Med.* 2021;10(13):2956. PMID: 34209340

Bilezikian JP, Khan AA, Silverberg SJ, et al; International Workshop on Primary Hyperparathyroidism. Evaluation and management of primary hyperparathyroidism: summary statement and guidelines from the Fifth International Workshop. *J Bone Miner Res.* 2022;37(11):2293-2314. PMID: 36245251

13 ANSWER: C) Increased bone formation; decreased bone resorption

Bone formation and resorption are tightly linked processes. Romosozumab is a monoclonal antibody against sclerostin that has been approved for treatment of postmenopausal women with osteoporosis who are at high risk for fracture. Romosozumab results in an uncoupling of the bone remodeling cycle, with an increase in bone formation markers and a decrease in bone resorption markers (Answer C). Of note, romosozumab has been approved by the US FDA with a boxed warning that therapy should not be initiated in patients who have had a myocardial infarction or stroke within the preceding year.

Osteoanabolic therapy with teriparatide and abaloparatide initially increases bone formation markers with little effect on bone resorption (Answer A); however, because bone formation and resorption are tightly linked, bone resorption markers also rise during therapy (Answer B). The period when bone formation exceeds resorption is termed the "anabolic window." Antiresorptive medications, including bisphosphonates and denosumab, decrease markers of both bone resorption and formation (Answer E). There is no current osteoporosis drug therapy with antiresorptive properties that has no effect on bone formation (Answer D).

EDUCATIONAL OBJECTIVE

Describe romosozumab's mechanism of action in the management of osteoporosis.

REFERENCE(S)

Cosman F, Crittenden DB, Adachi JD, et al. Romosozumab treatment in postmenopausal women with osteoporosis. *N Engl J Med.* 2016;375(16):1532-1543. PMID: 27641143

14 ANSWER: C) McCune-Albright syndrome

The radiograph demonstrates irregular, marginated, ground-glass lucencies surrounded by reactive bone. The shaft has an appearance that has been described as a soap bubble. This x-ray is characteristic of fibrous dysplasia, a benign skeletal lesion, most commonly monostotic with a predilection for long bones, ribs, and craniofacial bones. Fibrous dysplasia and McCune-Albright syndrome (Answer C) (OMIM#174800) are skeletal diseases caused by pathogenic postzygotic somatic activating or gain-of-function *GNAS* variants. The fibrous dysplasia/McCune-Albright Syndrome International Consortium defines McCune-Albright syndrome as a combination of fibrous dysplasia and 1 or more extraskeletal feature, or the presence of 2 or more extraskeletal features. Extraskeletal features include:

1. Café-au-lait skin macules with characteristic appearance of jagged, irregular borders (coast of Maine) and a distribution showing the so-called respect of the midline of the body
2. Gonadotropin-independent sex steroid production resulting in precocious puberty, recurrent ovarian cysts in girls and women, or autonomous testosterone production in boys and men
3. Thyroid lesions consistent with fibrous dysplasia/McCune-Albright syndrome with or without nonautoimmune hyperthyroidism
4. GH excess
5. Neonatal hypercortisolism

This patient has evidence of fibrous dysplasia on radiographs and toxic multinodular goiter, meeting the criteria for McCune-Albright syndrome. Given the presence of extraskeletal features, monostotic fibrous dysplasia (Answer D) is incorrect. The remaining answers are not consistent with the patient's radiographic, physical examination, or laboratory findings.

Albright hereditary osteodystrophy (Answer A) is associated with pseudohypoparathyroidism and pseudopseudohypoparathyroidism. It is characterized by brachydactyly (classically described as shortening of the third, fourth, and fifth metacarpals), round facies, short stature, obesity, developmental delay, and subcutaneous calcifications.

Oncogenic osteomalacia (tumor-induced osteomalacia) (Answer E) is caused by small mesenchymal tumors that secrete high levels of FGF-23, producing renal tubular loss of phosphorus.

Fibrodysplasia ossificans progressiva (Answer B) is a disorder in which muscle and connective tissue are gradually replaced by bone (ossified), forming extraskeletal or heterotopic bone that can constrain movement.

EDUCATIONAL OBJECTIVE

Diagnose McCune-Albright syndrome.

REFERENCE(S)

Javaid MK, Boyce A, Appelman-Dijkstra N, et al. Best practice management guidelines for fibrous dysplasia/McCune-Albright syndrome: a consensus statement from the FD/MAS international consortium. *Orphanet J Rare Dis.* 2019;14(1):139. PMID: 31196103

15 ANSWER: D) 8 to 12 months

Vitamin D toxicity is not a common cause of hypercalcemia. The liver converts almost all vitamin D to 25-hydroxyvitamin D through the action of several loosely regulated substrate-dependent cytochrome P450-linked oxidases. High concentrations of 25-hydroxyvitamin D may saturate vitamin D–binding protein, resulting in greater availability of 1,25-dihydroxyvitamin D at tissue sites. In addition, high concentrations of 25-hydroxyvitamin D may compete to bind at vitamin D receptor sites, producing similar effects as 1,25-dihydroxyvitamin D by initiating translation of vitamin D receptor–responsive genes. The kidney 1α-hydroxylase enzyme is under strict control and limits the production of 1,25-dihydroxyvitamin D, even if large amounts of 25-hydroxyvitamin D are available. In addition to the kidney, however, several other tissues express 1α-hydroxylase, and local paracrine conversion of 25-hydroxyvitamin D to 1,25-dihydroxyvitamin D may also have contributed to this patient's hypercalcemia. In a series of 9 patients with vitamin D intoxication due to an over-the-counter vitamin supplement called Soladek, including the patient in this vignette, there were often other reasons for hypercalcemia (such as lymphoma, granulomatous disease, etc), so that the homeostatic and detoxifying mechanisms were overwhelmed.

The biological half-life of 1,25-dihydroxyvitamin D is only approximately 15 hours, and toxicity due to calcitriol or other active vitamin D concentrations is short-lived. In contrast, vitamin D is highly lipophilic and the half-life of vitamin D ranges from 20 days to months. In this patient with an initial 25-hydroxyvitamin D concentration of 525 ng/mL (1310 nmol/L), it took 12 months (Answer D) for it to drop to 32 ng/mL (79.9 nmol/L) (*figure, next page*).

Figure. Change in 25-Hydroxyvitamin D Over Time

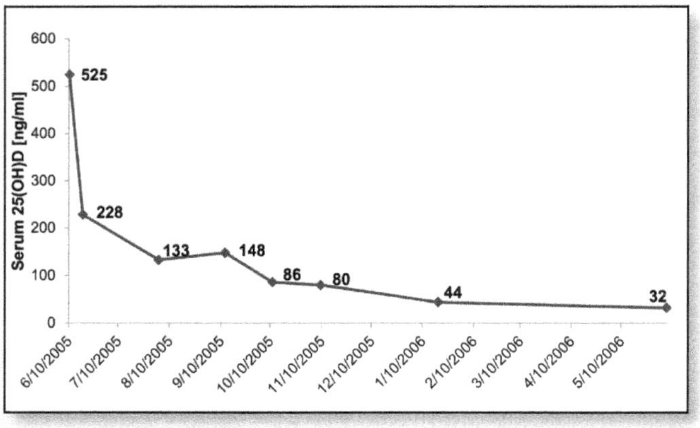

Reprinted from Lowe H et al. *J Clin Endocrinol Metab*, 2011; 96(2):291-295. © The Endocrine Society.

Treatment of vitamin D intoxication includes vigorous intravenous hydration, bisphosphonates, and glucocorticoids, with the caveat that resolution of the high 25-hydroxyvitamin D levels may take weeks or months.

EDUCATIONAL OBJECTIVE

Identify the timeframe for resolution of vitamin D toxicity.

REFERENCE(S)

Lowe H, Cusano NE, Binkley N, Blaner WS, Bilezikian JP. Vitamin D toxicity due to a commonly available "over the counter" remedy from the Dominican Republic. *J Clin Endocrinol Metab.* 2011;96(2):291-295. PMID: 21123442

Cusano NE, Thys-Jacobs S, and Bilezikian, JP. Hypercalcemia due to vitamin D toxicity. In: Feldman D, Pike JW, Glorieux FH, eds. *Vitamin D.* 3rd ed. Academic Press; 2011:1381-1402.

16 ANSWER: C) Decreased serum calcium, decreased PTH, no change in bone density

Cinacalcet is a calcimimetic that increases the sensitivity of the calcium-sensing receptor on the parathyroid gland. Cinacalcet is approved by the US FDA for treatment of hypercalcemia in adults with primary hyperparathyroidism for whom parathyroidectomy is indicated on the basis of serum calcium levels, but who are unable to undergo surgery. Cinacalcet has been demonstrated to significantly decrease serum calcium levels; therapy can also decrease PTH concentrations to a lesser extent in patients with primary hyperparathyroidism. Cinacalcet has no demonstrated effect on bone density. Answer C correctly lists the expected effects on biochemical and bone density parameters in patients with primary hyperparathyroidism treated with cinacalcet. Alendronate significantly improves bone density in patients with primary hyperparathyroidism, similar to its effects in euparathyroid patients, and it is routinely used in patients with primary hyperparathyroidism who have low bone density. Clinical trial data show that denosumab also improves bone density in patients with primary hyperparathyroidism. It is important to note there are no fracture data in patients with primary hyperparathyroidism treated with antiresorptive therapy.

EDUCATIONAL OBJECTIVE

Explain the mechanism of action of cinacalcet in primary hyperparathyroidism.

REFERENCE(S)

Peacock M, Bolognese MA, Borofsky M, et al. Cinacalcet treatment of primary hyperparathyroidism: biochemical and bone densitometric outcomes in a five-year study. *J Clin Endocrinol Metab.* 2009;94(12):4860-4867. PMID: 19837909

Marcocci C, Bollerslev J, Khan AA, Shoback DM. Medical management of primary hyperparathyroidism: proceedings of the fourth International Workshop on the Management of Asymptomatic Primary Hyperparathyroidism. *J Clin Endocrinol Metab.* 2014;99(10):3607-3618. PMID: 25162668

Leere JS, Karmisholt J, Robaczyk M, et al. Denosumab and cinacalcet for primary hyperparathyroidism (DENOCINA): a randomised, double-blind, placebo-controlled, phase 3 trial. *Lancet Diabetes Endocrinol.* 2020;8(5):407-417. PMID: 32333877

17 ANSWER: D) Kidney ultrasonography

Preservation of kidney function is critically important in patients with hypoparathyroidism. In a large Danish study of postoperative patients, risk of kidney calcification was increased 4.8-fold and risk of kidney insufficiency was increased 5-fold compared with observations in healthy control participants. International and European guidelines recommend routine monitoring of 24-hour urinary calcium excretion, at least annually or every 2 years. International guidelines recommend kidney imaging at baseline and if clinical symptoms arise or if there is unstable kidney function, such as this patient with a rising creatinine concentration. The European guidelines recommend kidney imaging if the patient develops kidney stones or if serum creatinine levels increase. In a direct comparison of ultrasonography and CT in 22 patients with hypoparathyroidism, ultrasonography was found to be superior to CT for detecting nephrocalcinosis. This patient has elevated creatinine, and kidney ultrasonography (Answer D) is recommended by both guidelines.

Patients with hypoparathyroidism have an increased risk of other complications, including cataracts and basal ganglia calcification. Slit-lamp examination for cataracts (but not measurement of intraocular pressure [Answer E]) may be indicated.

Head imaging (Answer C) is indicated for patients with neurologic symptoms.

Bone density assessment (Answer A) is recommended in the international guidelines if a patient otherwise meets criteria for measurement. The European guidelines recommend against routine monitoring of bone density.

While altered tooth morphology may be seen in very young patients with hypoparathyroidism, there are no apparent dental manifestations in adult patients. Routine dental examination (Answer B) can be recommended, but it is not as important as kidney imaging in this patient.

EDUCATIONAL OBJECTIVE

Manage chronic hypoparathyroidism in a patient who is at risk for kidney complications.

REFERENCE(S)

Khan AA, Bilezikian JP, Brandi ML, et al.; International Workshop on Primary Hyperparathyroidism. The Second International Workshop on the Evaluation and Management of Hypoparathyroidism. *J Bone Miner Res.* 2022;37(12):2566-2567. PMID: 36375811

Bilezikian JP, Brandi ML, Cusano NE, et al. Management of hypoparathyroidism: present and future. *J Clin Endocrinol Metab.* 2016;101(6):2313-2324. PMID: 26938200

Bollerslev J, Rejnmark L, Marcocci C, et al; European Society of Endocrinology. European Society of Endocrinology clinical guideline: treatment of chronic hypoparathyroidism in adults. *Eur J Endocrinol.* 2015;173(2):G1-G20. PMID: 26160136

Underbjerg L, Sikjaer T, Mosekilde L, Rejnmark L. Cardiovascular and renal complications to postsurgical hypoparathyroidism: a Danish nationwide controlled historic follow-up study. *J Bone Miner Res.* 2013;28(11):2277-2285. PMID: 23661265

18 ANSWER: C) Serum morning cortisol

This patient has autoimmune polyendocrine syndrome type 1 (APS type 1) due to a pathogenic variant in the autoimmune regulator gene (*AIRE*) and presents with symptoms and signs of Addison disease. APS type 1 is also known by the acronym APECED (autoimmune polyendocrinopathy-candidiasis-ectodermal dystrophy). The classic presentation includes at least 2 of the following 3 major clinical components: chronic mucocutaneous candidiasis, primary hypoparathyroidism, and autoimmune adrenal insufficiency. In this vignette, ectodermal dystrophy of the fingernails is noted on physical examination. Hyperpigmentation from adrenal insufficiency would also be expected on exam. Primary adrenal insufficiency may be diagnosed before clinical symptoms by checking for antibodies against the 21-hydroxylase enzyme, but in this case, serum morning cortisol (Answer C) must be measured immediately. Given the physical examination findings, one would expect to find hyponatremia, hyperkalemia, and elevated ACTH, along with a low or "normal" serum cortisol value (which is being maximally stimulated). Pending the results, a formal cosyntropin-stimulation test should be done.

Serum ceruloplasmin measurement (Answer A) is used to diagnose Wilson disease, a genetic syndrome in which copper accumulates in tissues, including the parathyroid glands. Classic findings include Kayser-Fleischer rings, liver damage, and neuropsychiatric symptoms.

Serum ferritin, iron, and total iron-binding capacity (Answer B) can be used to screen for hemochromatosis ("bronze diabetes"), but that would not fit the clinical picture.

Transglutaminase antibodies (Answer E) can be used to diagnose celiac disease. While up to 80% of patients with APECED have malabsorption or other gastrointestinal illness, celiac disease is not typical.

Hypothyroidism can occur with APECED, although this patient's symptoms are more consistent with adrenal insufficiency and prompt diagnosis of adrenal insufficiency is critical. Therefore, TSH measurement (Answer D) is not the best next step.

EDUCATIONAL OBJECTIVE
Diagnose Addison disease as part of autoimmune polyendocrine syndrome type 1.

REFERENCE(S)

Weiler FG, Dias-da-Silva MR, Lazaretti-Castro M. Autoimmune polyendocrine syndrome type 1: case report and review of literature. *Arq Bras Endocrinol Metabol.* 2012;56(1):54-66. PMID: 22460196

Akirav EM, Ruddle NH, Herold KC. The role of AIRE in human autoimmune disease. *Nat Rev Endocrinol.* 2011;7(1):25-33. PMID: 21102544

Eisenbarth GS, Gottlieb PA. Autoimmune polyendocrine syndromes. *N Engl J Med.* 2004;350(20):2068-2079. PMID: 15141045

Ferre EMN, Rose SR, Rosenzweig SD, et al. Redefined clinical features and diagnostic criteria in autoimmune polyendocrinopathy-candidiasis-ectodermal dystrophy. *JCI Insight.* 2016;1(13):e88782. PMID: 27588307

19 **ANSWER: A) Begin alendronate**

This man has a symptomatic, acute vertebral compression fracture at L1. This warrants intervention with antiresorptive therapy regardless of the DXA results because vertebral fractures are strong independent predictors of both future vertebral and nonvertebral fractures. Repeating DXA now (Answer D) is unlikely to be helpful given his degenerative arthritis at the spine, and the results will not change recommended therapy. The correct answer is to begin alendronate (Answer A) because it is an approved and effective therapy in this setting.

Teriparatide (Answer B) is contraindicated in a man who has received pelvic irradiation.

Invasive procedures, such as bone biopsy and kyphoplasty (Answer E), are not indicated in the acute setting given the absence of clinical or biochemical evidence (ie, his alkaline phosphatase level is normal) of recurrent bladder cancer or other malignancy. Patients with acute vertebral fractures from osteoporosis should generally not be referred for vertebral augmentation (kyphoplasty or vertebroplasty) unless severe pain has not responded to medical therapies.

Because there are no large randomized controlled trials showing antifracture efficacy for testosterone in men with osteoporosis, testosterone therapy (Answer C) should be considered only for hypogonadal men who are symptomatic, have an organic cause for the hypogonadism, have testosterone concentrations less than 200 ng/dL (<6.9 nmol/L), and/or are not candidates for other therapies. In hypogonadal men with benign prostatic hypertrophy, testosterone therapy, along with a 5α-reductase inhibitor such as finasteride, has been given without exacerbating benign prostatic hypertrophy. However, even men with marked hypogonadism have good skeletal responses to bisphosphonate therapy without correction of hypogonadism. Of note, a subtrial of the TRAVERSE study (Testosterone Replacement Therapy for Assessment of Long-term Vascular Events and Efficacy Response in Hypogonadal Men) demonstrated a fracture incidence that was numerically higher among men who received testosterone than among those who received placebo, which requires further study.

EDUCATIONAL OBJECTIVE

Manage an acute vertebral fracture in an elderly man.

REFERENCE(S)

Watts NB, Adler RA, Bilezikian JP, et al; Endocrine Society. Osteoporosis in men: an Endocrine Society clinical practice guideline. *J Clin Endocrinol Metab.* 2012;97(6):1802-1822. PMID: 22675062

Cosman F, de Beur SJ, LeBoff MS, et al; National Osteoporosis Foundation. Clinician's guide to prevention and treatment of osteoporosis. *Osteoporos Int.* 2014;25(10):2359-2381. PMID: 25182228

McConnell CT Jr, Wippold FJ 2nd, Ray CE Jr, et al. ACR appropriateness criteria for management of vertebral compression fractures. *J Am Coll Radiol.* 2014;11(8):757-763. PMID: 24935074

20 ANSWER: E) Worsening arthritis in the hip

Zoledronic acid should improve pain arising from the pagetic involvement of the patient's left hip, but it is not expected to help the pain due to degenerative arthritis and may not prevent arthritis progression (thus, Answer E is correct and Answer D is incorrect).

Paget disease does not extend across joint spaces and has never been reported to develop in new bones not involved at diagnosis (thus, Answer C is incorrect).

Since she does not have Paget disease in her skull, it will not cause hearing loss (Answer A).

Osteonecrosis of the femoral neck (Answer B) is not more likely after treatment with zoledronic acid in patients with Paget disease of the hip.

Whether all patients with Paget disease should be treated is controversial. Indications for treatment in asymptomatic patients include the following:

- Involvement of a weight-bearing bone (eg, spine or leg)
- Involvement near a joint
- Involvement of the skull
- Serum alkaline phosphatase level greater than 3 times the upper normal limit

Zoledronic acid is clearly the most effective treatment for Paget disease. It normalizes bone turnover markers and maintains normal values for the longest duration of any medication. Normal turnover markers are associated with normalization of pagetic woven bone to lamellar bone and can eliminate pain arising from pagetic bone. A single dose of zoledronic acid results in many years of disease inactivity in most patients.

EDUCATIONAL OBJECTIVE

Counsel patients that treating Paget disease should effectively eliminate pain attributable to pagetic bone, but it is not expected to resolve pain due to degenerative arthritis.

REFERENCE(S)

Reid IR, Lyles K, Su G, et al. A single infusion of zoledronic acid produces sustained remissions in Paget disease: data to 6.5 years. *J Bone Miner Res.* 2011;26(9):2261-2270. PMID: 21638319

Langston AL, Campbell MK, Fraser WD, et al; PRISM Trial Group. Randomized trial of intensive bisphosphonate treatment versus symptomatic management in Paget's disease of bone. *J Bone Miner Res.* 2010;25(1):20-31. PMID: 19580457

Ralston SH. Clinical practice. Paget's disease of bone. *N Engl J Med.* 2013;368(7):644-650. PMID: 23406029

21 ANSWER: B) 25-Hydroxyvitamin D

The radiograph shows a Looser zone, which is characteristic of osteomalacia. Mechanical stress of blood vessels overlying the uncalcified cortical bone affected by osteomalacia is thought to cause "pseudofractures" that appear as transverse zones of rarefaction, sometimes as wide as 1 cm, often multiple, and generally symmetric. Typical locations are the ischium, ilium, pubis, femur, tibia, radius, fibula, lower ribs, and scapula.

This patient had malabsorption of both vitamin D and calcium after bariatric surgery, and she did not adhere to calcium and vitamin D supplementation. Her serum 25-hydroxyvitamin D level (Answer B) was undetectable (<7 ng/mL [<17.5 nmol/L]). High-dosage vitamin D_3, 50,000 international units daily, did not correct the vitamin D deficiency, but ultraviolet light (increased sun exposure) was successful.

Chemical clues to osteomalacia include hypocalcemia, hypophosphatemia, and elevated alkaline phosphatase.

Measuring FGF-23 (Answer D), 1,25-dihydroxyvitamin D (Answer A), intact PTH (Answer E), and C-telopeptide (Answer C) would not clarify the diagnosis.

EDUCATIONAL OBJECTIVE

Identify clinical and radiographic findings of osteomalacia after gastric bypass (severe vitamin D deficiency).

REFERENCE(S)

Karefylakis C, Näslund I, Edholm D, Sundbom M, Karlsson FA, Rask E. Vitamin D status 10 years after primary gastric bypass: gravely high prevalence of hypovitaminosis D and raised PTH levels. *Obes Surg.* 2014;24(3):343-348. PMID: 24163201

Bal BS, Finelli FC, Shope TR, Koch TR. Nutritional deficiencies after bariatric surgery. *Nat Rev Endocrinol.* 2012;8(9):544-556. PMID: 22525731

Reginato AJ, Falasca GF, Pappu R, McKnight B, Agha A. Musculoskeletal manifestations of osteomalacia: report of 26 cases and literature review. *Semin Arthritis Rheum.* 1999;28(5):287-304. PMID: 10342386

Thacher TD, Clarke BL. Vitamin D insufficiency. *Mayo Clin Proc.* 2011;86(1):50-60. PMID: 21193656

Bhan A, Rao AD, Rao DS. Osteomalacia as a result of vitamin D deficiency. *Endocrinol Metab Clin North Am.* 2010;39(2):321-331. PMID: 20511054

22 ANSWER: D) Zoledronic acid

The 2022 guidelines from the American College of Rheumatology recommend some type of pharmacologic treatment for adults 40 years and older with a moderate fracture risk, defined as a glucocorticoid-adjusted FRAX risk of 10% to 19% for major osteoporotic fracture or 1.1% to 2.9% for hip fracture.

Alendronate, risedronate, zoledronic acid (Answer D), teriparatide (Answer C), and denosumab (Answer A) (but not ibandronate [Answer B]) are all FDA approved for management of glucocorticoid-induced osteoporosis. Because there is still controversy about the link between esophageal cancer and oral bisphosphonate use, it may be preferable to start with intravenous zoledronic acid (Answer D) rather than an oral bisphosphonate in a patient with Barrett esophagus.

Teriparatide (Answer C) is usually reserved for patients with prevalent vertebral fractures or much lower vertebral T-scores—in the frankly osteoporotic range.

Given limited safety data, denosumab (Answer A) is generally not recommended as first-line therapy in patients taking multiple immunosuppressive drugs or biologic drugs.

Finally, the low FRAX scores underestimate the fracture risk in patients on long-term glucocorticoid therapy. FRAX does not account for the disproportionate negative effects of glucocorticoids on spinal trabecular bone and does not include spinal bone mineral density in the calculation. Therefore, recommending no therapeutic intervention (Answer E) is incorrect despite the patient's low FRAX scores.

EDUCATIONAL OBJECTIVE

Determine whether pharmacologic treatment to reduce fracture risk is necessary in a patient taking glucocorticoids.

REFERENCE(S)

Humphrey MB, Russell L, Danila MI, et al. 2022 American College of Rheumatology guideline for the prevention and treatment of glucocorticoid-induced osteoporosis. *Arthritis Rheumatol.* 2023;75(12):2088-2102. PMID: 37845798

Venuturupalli SR, Sacks W. Review of new guidelines for the management of glucocorticoid induced osteoporosis. *Curr Osteoporos Rep.* 2013;11(4):357-364. PMID: 24114241

Leib ES, Saag KG, Adachi JD, et al; FRAX(®) Position Development Conference Members. Official Positions for FRAX(®) clinical regarding glucocorticoids: the impact of the use of glucocorticoids on the estimate by FRAX(®) of the 10 year risk of fracture from Joint Official Positions Development Conference of the International Society for Clinical Densitometry and International Osteoporosis Foundation on FRAX(®). *J Clin Densitom.* 2011;14(3):212-219. PMID: 21810527

23 ANSWER: B) Increased fluid intake

According to a comprehensive meta-analysis in patients who had a single kidney stone, increased fluid intake (Answer B) was the one intervention that was clearly shown to reduce recurrent stone disease. Of interest, reducing phosphate-containing soft drink consumption (not an answer option above) was moderately helpful. In patients with multiple stone episodes—most of whom had already increased their fluid intake—thiazide diuretics (Answer A) and citrate supplements (Answer C) were similarly effective in patients with hypercalciuria, as well as in unselected patients. Hydrochlorothiazide acts to enhance kidney calcium reabsorption to reduce urinary calcium excretion and might be an additional measure to consider if he has more stones.

Hypercalciuria may be caused by increased sodium intake, which leads to increased sodium excretion and an obligatory loss of calcium in the urine. However, this patient's normal urinary sodium excretion indicates that is not the case here and reducing his dietary sodium (Answer E) is incorrect.

His urinary oxalate level is not elevated, so there would be no benefit in reducing his dietary oxalate intake (Answer D).

EDUCATIONAL OBJECTIVE

Recommend increased fluid intake to reduce the risk of a second kidney stone.

REFERENCE(S)

Fink HA, Wilt TJ, Eldman KE, et al. Medical management to prevent recurrent nephrolithiasis in adults: a systematic review for an American College of Physicians Clinical Guideline [published correction appears in *Ann Intern Med.* 2013;159(3):230-232]. *Ann Intern Med.* 2013;158(7):535-543. PMID: 23546565

Vigen R, Weideman RA, Reilly RF. Thiazides diuretics in the treatment of nephrolithiasis: are we using them in an evidence-based fashion? *Int Urol Nephrol.* 2011;43(3):813-819. PMID: 20737209

Borghi L, Schianchi T, Meschi T, et al. Comparison of two diets for the prevention of recurrent stones in idiopathic hypercalciuria. *N Engl J Med.* 2002;346(2):77-84. PMID: 11784873

24 ANSWER: C) Intravenous bolus of 150 mg calcium gluconate followed by a continuous calcium gluconate infusion of 1 mg/kg per h

Intravenous calcium should be considered for patients presenting with clinical features of hypocalcemia, including symptoms of paresthesias, carpopedal spasm, bronchospasm or laryngospasm, tetany, seizures, mental status changes, positive Chvostek or Trousseau signs, bradycardia, impaired cardiac contractility, and prolonged QT interval. While some patients with marked hypocalcemia (ie, corrected calcium <7.0 mg/dL [<1.8 mmol/L]) may not be symptomatic, intravenous therapy may be indicated because at those levels, life-threatening features such as laryngeal spasm and seizures can appear acutely. This patient needs rapid correction of hypocalcemia. Calcium gluconate is preferred over calcium chloride because the latter is more likely to cause vein sclerosis and tissue necrosis if extravasated (thus, Answers A and B are incorrect). Dosing at 1 mg/kg per h would be a total dose of 1680 mg daily for a 70-kg patient (thus, Answer C is correct); a higher rate might be required for patients with profound calcium deficiency. The dose of intravenous calcium is dangerously high in Answer E. There are case reports using teriparatide (PTH [1-34]) in acute hypocalcemia (Answer D) as an off-label therapy; however, the listed dosage is very high. In addition, teriparatide typically requires multiple daily doses to maintain serum calcium in patients with hypoparathyroidism.

Ordering intravenous calcium can be confusing. For intravenous use, a 10-mL ampule of calcium gluconate contains 93 mg of calcium, and a 10-mL ampule of 10% calcium chloride contains 272 mg of calcium. In some situations, adding a calcium salt to an intravenous liter bag of 0.9% saline or 5% dextrose requires removing some of the fluid to allow space for the added calcium salt.

EDUCATIONAL OBJECTIVE

Manage acute, severe hypocalcemia.

REFERENCE(S)

Zalonga GP, Chernow B. Hypocalcemia in critical illness. *JAMA*. 1986;256(14):1924-1929. PMID: 3531557

Vetter T, Lohse MJ. Magnesium and the parathyroid. *Curr Opin Nephrol Hypertens*. 2002;11(4):403-410. PMID: 12105390

al-Ghamdi SM, Cameron EC, Sutton RA. Magnesium deficiency: pathophysiologic and clinical overview. *Am J Kidney Dis*. 1994;24(5):737-752. PMID: 7977315

25 ANSWER: C) FGF-23 measurement

This patient has tumor-induced osteomalacia caused by a benign mesenchymal tumor that is secreting FGF-23 (Answer C). This causes renal tubular loss of phosphate and inhibits 1α-hydroxylase, resulting in low 1,25-dihydroxyvitamin D levels. These tumors are typically located in the skin, bones, or connective tissue (eg, sinuses) and may be difficult to localize. Imaging to localize the tumor includes nuclear medicine techniques such as bone scan, octreotide scan, or PET. In difficult cases, serum FGF-23 measurement in selective venous sampling may be used to localize the extremity from which FGF-23 is being secreted. Tumor removal (if it can be located and removed) normalizes kidney phosphate handling within hours to days.

Hypophosphatemia induced by tenofovir (and adefovir) is part of a more generalized syndrome known as Fanconi syndrome in which multiple substances such as bicarbonate, glucose, uric acid, potassium, and phosphate are "wasted" in the urine (Answer A). This patient has no evidence of this syndrome.

Low levels of 24,25-dihydroxyvitamin D (Answer B) can be useful to diagnose patients with hypercalcemia and kidney stones who have pathogenic variants in the *CYP24A1* gene.

While the severity of X-linked hypophosphatasia caused by pathogenic variants in *PHEX* (Answer D) varies widely, even among members of the same family, the disease is completely penetrant and not expected to present later in life.

A sestamibi scan (Answer E) is not helpful in diagnosing tumor-induced osteomalacia.

EDUCATIONAL OBJECTIVE

Diagnose tumor-induced osteomalacia by measuring FGF-23.

REFERENCE(S)

Ruppe MD, Jan de Beur SM. Disorders of phosphate homeostasis. In: Rosen CJ, Compston JE, Lian JB, eds. *Primer on the Metabolic Bone Diseases and Disorders of Mineral Metabolism*. Washington, DC: The American Society for Bone and Mineral Research; 2008:601-612.

Jan de Beur SM. Tumor-induced osteomalacia. *JAMA*. 2005;294(10):1260-1267. PMID: 16160135

Andreopoulou P, Dumitrescu CE, Kelly MH, et al. Selective venous catheterization for the localization of phosphaturic mesenchymal tumors. *J Bone Miner Res*. 2011;26(6):1295-1302. PMID: 21611969

26 ANSWER: E) Working with a dietician to resolve energy deficiency

Relative energy deficiency in sport (RED-S) is a syndrome consisting of disordered eating (or low energy availability), oligomenorrhea/amenorrhea, and decreased bone mineral density. RED-S is a more inclusive and comprehensive term for what was formally referred to as the "female athletic triad."

While this patient's BMI is normal, she has evidence of functional amenorrhea and relative energy deficiency. The Endocrine Society guidelines for functional hypothalamic amenorrhea recommend correcting the energy imbalance (Answer E) to improve function of her hypothalamic-pituitary-ovarian axis, which should also improve bone mineral density.

The guidelines recommend against use of oral contraceptive pills (Answer B) for the sole purpose of regaining menses or improving bone mineral density. There has been lack of clear benefit in studies evaluating bone density effects of oral contraceptive pills vs placebo in women with functional amenorrhea. There are some data that transdermal estrogen with progesterone may be of benefit in women who have not had return of menses after a trial of nutritional, psychological, and/or modified exercise intervention. Transdermal estrogen may improve bone density more than oral contraceptive pills because it does not affect IGF-1 secretion, a bone-trophic hormone that oral contraceptive pills down-regulate.

The guidelines recommend against using bisphosphonates (Answer A), denosumab (Answer C), testosterone, or leptin to improve bone mineral density in women with functional amenorrhea.

Short-term teriparatide therapy (Answer D) can be considered in rare cases of women with functional amenorrhea in the setting of delayed fracture healing and very low bone mineral density. This patient has had good fracture healing, and treatment with teriparatide is not indicated.

EDUCATIONAL OBJECTIVE

Treat low bone density in a patient with functional hypothalamic amenorrhea/relative energy deficiency in sport.

REFERENCE(S)

Ackerman KE, Singhal V, Slattery M, et al. Effects of estrogen replacement on bone geometry and microarchitecture in adolescent and young adult oligoamenorrheic athletes: a randomized trial. *J Bone Miner Res.* 2020;35(2):248-260. PMID: 31603998

Gordon CM, Ackerman KE, Berga SL, et al. Functional hypothalamic amenorrhea: an Endocrine Society clinical practice guideline. *J Clin Endocrinol Metab.* 2017;102(5):1413-1439. PMID: 28368518

27 ANSWER: D) Decrease the cinacalcet dosage

This patient's PTH concentration is lower than the goal in patients undergoing dialysis and may indicate underlying adynamic bone disease. Because of the low PTH and hypocalcemia, the cinacalcet dosage should be decreased (Answer D). Adynamic bone disease, a type of chronic kidney disease–mineral bone disorder (CKD-MBD), is present in at least one-third of patients receiving dialysis. The term "renal osteodystrophy" which was previously used generally for kidney bone disease is now used exclusively for definition of particular alterations in bone histomorphology associated with CKD based on bone biopsy evaluation. Adynamic bone disease is characterized by markedly low bone turnover, no accumulation of osteoid, and high fracture risk. Serum PTH levels in adynamic bone disease are relatively low (usually <100 pg/mL [<10.6 pmol/L]) compared with levels in patients undergoing dialysis who have other forms of CKD-MBD.

In patients with end-stage kidney disease, there is resistance to PTH due at least in part to increased N-terminal truncated PTH (7-84), which counteracts the effect of the 1-84 whole molecule on bone. This can be exacerbated by the use of cinacalcet, as well as overly aggressive treatment with calcitriol, both of which reduce PTH secretion. This patient's low alkaline phosphatase level is also consistent with a low bone turnover state.

Increasing the calcitriol dosage (Answer E) would further suppress PTH, which is not a desired outcome. Decreasing the calcitriol dosage (Answer C) may worsen the hypocalcemia.

Teriparatide (Answer B) has been used anecdotally in some patients with end-stage kidney disease, low bone turnover, and fractures, but it is not an approved therapy in this context.

Although denosumab (Answer A) can be used in patients receiving dialysis, it would be inappropriate to administer it now in the face of hypocalcemia, vitamin D deficiency, and probable adynamic bone disease. A potent antiresorptive agent would theoretically worsen the adynamic bone disease and increase fracture risk.

Impaired mineralization, osteitis fibrosa cystica, and mixed renal osteodystrophy are other forms of CKD-MBD, but these diagnoses are unlikely given the laboratory findings. Osteitis fibrosa cystica and high bone turnover are associated with elevated PTH, osteomalacia is associated with very low 25-hydroxyvitamin D, and mixed renal osteodystrophy is associated with both findings.

EDUCATIONAL OBJECTIVE

Diagnose and manage adynamic bone disease in a patient undergoing dialysis.

REFERENCE(S)

Cannata-Andía JB, Rodriguez García M, Gómez Alonso C. Osteoporosis and adynamic bone in chronic kidney disease. *J Nephrol.* 2013;26(1):73-80. PMID: 23023723

Hruska KA, Mathew S. Chronic kidney disease mineral bone disorder (CKD-MBD). In: Rosen CJ, Compston JE, Lian JB, eds. *Primer on the Metabolic Bone Diseases and Disorders of Mineral Metabolism.* Washington, DC: The American Society for Bone and Mineral Research; 2008:343-349.

Brandenburg VM, Floege J. Adynamic bone disease: bone and beyond. *NDT Plus.* 2008;1(3):135-147. PMID: 25983860

Kidney Disease: Improving Global Outcomes (KDIGO) CKD-MBD Work Group. KDIGO clinical practice guideline for the diagnosis, evaluation, prevention, and treatment of chronic kidney disease-mineral and bone disorder (CKD-MBD). *Kidney Int Suppl.* 2009;(Suppl 113):S1-S130. PMID: 19644521

28 ANSWER: D) Genetic testing for pathogenic variants in the multiple endocrine neoplasia type 1 gene (*MEN1*)

It is critical to think about and screen for *MEN1* pathogenic variants (Answer D) in all young patients (<30 years) who present with primary hyperparathyroidism. Up to 10% of patients with primary hyperparathyroidism have a familial (germline) pathogenic variant. Hereditary syndromes should be suspected in anyone with a personal history of other endocrine tumors (especially pancreatic or pituitary) or a family history of parathyroid disease, kidney stones, or pancreatic/pituitary tumors in first-degree relatives. These syndromes should also be suspected and screened for in patients presenting with atypical or multigland parathyroid adenomas at any age. Only 2% to 4% of all patients with primary hyperparathyroidism present with multigland adenomas.

In addition to multiple endocrine neoplasia type 1, other more rare causes of multiorgan syndromic primary hyperparathyroidism include multiple endocrine neoplasia type 2, multiple endocrine neoplasia type 4, and hyperparathyroidism–jaw tumor syndrome. Familial idiopathic primary hyperparathyroidism may be a subtype of hyperparathyroidism–jaw tumor syndrome.

The presence of kidney stones and high urinary calcium excretion excludes familial hypocalciuric hypercalcemia caused by an inactivating variant in the gene encoding the calcium sensing receptor (*CASR*) (Answer C).

Although a 4D CT of the neck (Answer A) would be reasonable in an older patient with persistent primary hyperparathyroidism, in this young man it is mandatory to screen for multiple endocrine neoplasia first because that diagnosis would alter the surgical management and medical follow-up.

Another sestamibi scan (Answer E) looking for a second adenoma would not be indicated when all 4 glands may be involved.

Calcium supplementation would not be responsible for these laboratory findings, so cessation of this treatment (Answer B) is not necessary.

EDUCATIONAL OBJECTIVE

Pursue the diagnosis of multiple endocrine neoplasia type 1 in young patients presenting with primary hyperparathyroidism.

REFERENCE(S)

Thakker RV, Newey PJ, Walls GV, et al; Endocrine Society. Clinical practice guidelines for multiple endocrine neoplasia 1 (MEN1). *J Clin Endocrinol Metab.* 2012;97(9):2990-3011. PMID: 22723327

Eastell R, Brandi ML, Costa AG, D'Amour P, Shoback DM, Thakker RV. Diagnosis of asymptomatic primary hyperparathyroidism: proceedings of the Fourth International Workshop. *J Clin Endocrinol Metab.* 2014;99(10):3570-3579. PMID: 25162666

Lassen T, Friis-Hansen L, Rasmussen AK, Knigge U, Feldt-Rasmussen U. Primary hyperparathyroidism in young people. When should we perform genetic testing for multiple endocrine neoplasia 1 (MEN-1)? *J Clin Endocrinol Metab.* 2014;99(11):3983-3987. PMID: 24731012

29 ANSWER: C) Calcium citrate, 600 mg 4 times daily

Absorption of calcium carbonate is pH dependent. In one experiment, only 1% of 500 mg of calcium carbonate was dissolved in 500 mL of water after 1 hour at 98.6°F (37°C) at a neutral pH, with 100% dissolving at a pH of 2.5, similar to that observed in the stomach. Proton-pump inhibitors inhibit the parietal cell H+ K+ATPase pump, leading to suppressed acid secretion and increased stomach pH. There have been multiple case reports of acute hypocalcemia in patients with hypoparathyroidism on calcium carbonate subsequently treated with a proton-pump inhibitor. Absorption of calcium citrate is not pH dependent, and patients with hypoparathyroidism who will be starting a proton-pump inhibitor should be transitioned to a regimen of calcium citrate (Answer C) since calcium carbonate (Answers A, B, D, and E) is not well absorbed in this setting.

rhPTH (1-84) (Answer E) has not been studied in patients with acute hypocalcemia.

While there are case reports of use of PTH (1-34) (Answer D) in acute hypocalcemia, it is not standard treatment.

Hydrochlorothiazide (Answer B) can be used to treat hypercalciuria, but it is not used for acute hypocalcemia.

Of note, there are also multiple cases of euparathyroid individuals developing functional hypoparathyroidism caused by hypomagnesemia related to proton-pump inhibitor use, since the secretion of PTH is magnesium dependent.

EDUCATIONAL OBJECTIVE

Describe problems with calcium absorption in the setting of proton-pump inhibitor use.

REFERENCE(S)

Bilezikian JP, Brandi ML, Cusano NE, et al. Management of hypoparathyroidism: present and future. *J Clin Endocrinol Metab.* 2016;101(6):2313-2324. PMID: 26938200

Epstein M, McGrath S, Law F. Proton-pump inhibitors and hypomagnesemic hypoparathyroidism. *N Engl J Med.* 2006;355(17):1834-1836. PMID: 17065651

Milman S, Epstein EJ. Proton pump inhibitor-induced hypocalcemic seizure in a patient with hypoparathyroidism. *Endocr Pract.* 2011;17(1):104-107. PMID: 21041166

Vallejo F, Sum M. Acute hypocalcemia from proton pump inhibitor use. In: *Hypoparathyroidism: A Clinical Casebook.* Cusano NE, ed. Switzerland: Springer; 2020:9-15.

30 ANSWER: E) Type 1 collagen α1 and 2 genes (*COL1A1/COL1A2*)

This patient has the mildest form of osteogenesis imperfecta, known as type 1. Inheritance is autosomal dominant, but pathogenic variants can occur de novo, so the family history may be negative. Persons with osteogenesis imperfecta type 1 have normal stature and little or no skeletal deformity. Fractures occur in childhood or adolescence and their incidence decreases markedly after puberty. As is the case in this vignette, affected patients may then present in middle age with "osteoporosis." In 50% of patients, there is early-onset hearing loss before age 40 years. On physical examination, there may be blue sclerae and easy bruising. Joint laxity may be present, but dentinogenesis imperfecta is usually absent.

The diagnosis is made by sequencing the genes that encode type 1 collagen (α1 and α2) (*COL1A1/COL1A2*) (Answer E). Pathogenic variants in *COL1A1* or *COL1A2* cause decreased amounts of normal collagen and lead to the mild phenotype seen in patients with osteogenesis imperfecta type 1. Pathogenic variants that disrupt the formation of the normal type I collagen triple helix cause the lethal phenotype seen in type IIA. Posttranslational defects in the interferon-induced transmembrane protein 5 gene (*IFITM5*), FK506-binding protein 10 gene (*FKBP10* [*FKBP65*]), and cartilage-associated protein gene (*CRTAP*) are among the causes of osteogenesis imperfecta in the 10% patients without pathogenic variants in *COL1A1* or *COL1A2*.

The main therapy for osteogenesis imperfecta remains bisphosphonates (intravenous pamidronate and zoledronic acid and oral bisphosphonates). Denosumab has been used in rare case reports. Teriparatide does not dramatically change clinical outcomes. It is hoped that the sclerostin inhibitor romosozumab may have some effectiveness in decreasing fractures in osteogenesis imperfecta, but this awaits clinical trials.

Osteoprotegerin (Answer B) is a cytokine and decoy receptor for the receptor activator of nuclear factor kappa B ligand (RANKL). By binding to RANKL, it reduces differentiation of precursors to osteoclasts and blocks osteoclast production and proliferation, thus reducing bone resorption. Pathogenic variants in this gene have been associated with osteoarthritis but not with the phenotype illustrated in this vignette.

Pathogenic variants in the gene encoding the LDL receptor-related protein 5 (Answer A) are involved with the canonical Wnt pathway. Loss-of-function variants can cause osteoporosis-pseudoglioma syndrome, while gain-of-function variants result in a high bone mass phenotype.

X-linked hypophosphatemia with its characteristic hypophosphatemia (not seen in this patient) is caused by a defective *PHEX* gene product (phosphate-regulating gene with homology to endopeptidases on the X chromosome) (Answer C), which results in elevated FGF-23 levels and impaired renal proximal tubule phosphate reabsorption.

Sclerostin, produced by the *SOST* gene (Answer D), is produced by osteocytes and has antianabolic effects on bone formation by suppressing Wnt signaling. Inactivating variants in the *SOST* gene cause syndromes of high bone mass (sclerosteosis and van Buchem disease).

EDUCATIONAL OBJECTIVE

Diagnose osteogenesis imperfecta type 1 (the mildest form).

REFERENCE(S)

Van Dijk FS, Sillence DO. Osteogenesis imperfecta: clinical diagnosis, nomenclature and severity assessment [published correction appears in *Am J Med Genet A.* 2015;167A(5):1178]. *Am J Med Genet A.* 2014;164A(6):1470-1481. PMID: 24715559

Thomas IH, DiMeglio LA. Advances in the classification and treatment of osteogenesis imperfecta. *Curr Osteoporos Rep.* 2016;14(1):1-9. PMID: 26861807

Shapiro JR, Thompson CB, Wu Y, Nunes M, Gillen C. Bone mineral density and fracture rate in response to intravenous and oral bisphosphonates in adult osteogenesis imperfecta. *Calcif Tissue Int.* 2010;87(2):120-129. PMID: 20544187

31 ANSWER: B) 25-Hydroxyvitamin D measurement

Although this patient may have Paget disease, other causes of elevated alkaline phosphatase must be considered before proceeding to bone scan, including vitamin D deficiency and/or secondary hyperparathyroidism, particularly given his age and chronic kidney disease. This patient was indeed found to have vitamin D deficiency with secondary hyperparathyroidism. Thus, measurement of 25-hydroxyvitamin D (Answer B) is the correct next step. Although he has been taking 2000 international units of vitamin D daily, this is not enough to maintain a normal 25-hydroxyitamin D level in some patients after bariatric surgery.

Serum levels of 1,25-dihydroxyvitamin D are regulated primarily by PTH levels, which in turn are regulated by calcium and/or vitamin D. 1,25-Dihydroxyvitamin D levels do not reflect vitamin D stores, and in vitamin D deficiency, 1,25-dihydroxyvitamin D levels are normal or even elevated due to secondary hyperparathyroidism. Thus, measuring 1,25-dihydroxyvitamin D (Answer A) is incorrect.

In this patient, a whole-body bone scan (Answer E) may be spuriously abnormal, showing multiple areas of uptake due to increased bone turnover.

Serum C-telopeptide (Answer C) may be elevated, but its measurement would not help to determine the cause of his elevated alkaline phosphatase.

A skeletal survey (Answer D) would be helpful if multiple myeloma were the suspected diagnosis, which is not the case.

EDUCATIONAL OBJECTIVE

Rule out vitamin D deficiency and secondary hyperparathyroidism before evaluating for Paget disease.

REFERENCE(S)

Karefylakis C, Näslund I, Edholm D, Sundbom M, Karlsson FA, Rask E. Vitamin D status 10 years after primary gastric bypass: gravely high prevalence of hypovitaminosis D and raised PTH levels. *Obes Surg.* 2014;24(3):343-348. PMID: 24163201

32 ANSWER: B) Genetic testing for *GNA11* and *AP2S1* pathogenic variants

Familial hypocalciuric hypercalcemia (FHH) is a rare disease resulting in a rightward shift of a patient's calcium-sensing curve. Patients with FHH do not shut off production of PTH in response to a serum calcium value that for the general population would be considered hypercalcemic. There are 3 variants of the disease: type 1 due to pathogenic variants in the calcium-sensing receptor gene (*CASR*), type 2 caused by pathogenic variants in the guanine nucleotide–binding protein (G-protein) subunit α_{11} gene (*GNA11*), and type 3 due to pathogenic variants in the adaptor-related protein complex 2, sigma 1 subunit gene (*AP2S1*). Patients with FHH have low urinary calcium excretion, calculated with the following formula:

[urine calcium (mg/24 h) × serum creatinine (mg/dL)] / [urine creatinine (mg/24 h) × serum calcium (mg/dL)]

A urinary calcium-to-creatinine ratio less than 0.01 is consistent with a diagnosis of FHH, although patients must be vitamin D replete (>20 ng/mL [>49.9 mmol/L]) with good kidney function for the collection to be interpretable. A patient with no identifiable *CASR* pathogenic variants and clinical concern for FHH should have *GNA11* and *AP2S1* genetic testing (Answer B). This patient was documented to have a pathogenic variant in *AP2S1*.

While FHH is a benign disease that does not carry an increased risk of nephrolithiasis or osteoporosis as does primary hyperparathyroidism, patients with FHH type 3 may have significant hypercalcemia and clinical symptoms related to high serum calcium. A case series demonstrated successful cinacalcet therapy for 3 patients with FHH type 3.

It is important to distinguish between FHH and primary hyperparathyroidism, as surgical treatment is not indicated in patients with FHH. Thus, preoperative localization studies (Answers A and D) or referral to a parathyroid surgeon (Answer E) is incorrect.

Pathogenic variants in the *PHEX* gene (Answer C) result in X-linked hypophosphatasia, a genetic disorder causing rickets and phosphate wasting.

EDUCATIONAL OBJECTIVE

Distinguish familial hypocalciuric hypercalcemia from primary hyperparathyroidism.

REFERENCE(S)

Eastell R, Brandi ML, Costa AG, D'Amour P, Shoback DM, Thakker RV. Diagnosis of asymptomatic primary hyperparathyroidism: proceedings of the Fourth International Workshop. *J Clin Endocrinol Metab.* 2014;99(10):3570-3579. PMID: 25162666

Howles SA, Hannan FM, Babinsky VN, et al. Cinacalcet for symptomatic hypercalcemia caused by AP2S1 mutations. *N Engl J Med.* 2016;374(14):1396-1398. PMID: 27050234

33 ANSWER: E) Primary hyperparathyroidism

Primary hyperparathyroidism (Answer E) is one of the most common endocrine disorders and is diagnosed in the setting of hypercalcemia with an elevated or inappropriately normal PTH. This patient's PTH concentration, although technically within normal limits, is inappropriate in the setting of hypercalcemia. In primary hyperparathyroidism, PTH facilitates the conversion of 25-hydroxyvitamin D to 1,25-dihydroxyvitamin D, and up to 25% of patients have frankly elevated 1,25-dihydroxyvitamin D levels.

Familial hypocalciuric hypercalcemia (FHH) (Answer B) is a rare, benign disorder caused by loss-of-function pathogenic variants in the gene encoding the calcium-sensing receptor. Patients with FHH usually have a positive family history, although a given patient could represent an index case. The extremely high penetrance of FHH ensures that virtually all patients develop hypercalcemia by their third decade. In FHH, 24-hour urinary calcium excretion is typically less than 100 mg with a calcium-to-creatinine clearance ratio less than 0.01, while the ratio is typically greater than 0.02 in patients with primary hyperparathyroidism. It can be difficult to distinguish between FHH and primary hyperparathyroidism when the ratio is between 0.01 and 0.02; however, patients must be vitamin D replete (>20 ng/mL [>49.9 mmol/L]) with good kidney function for the collection to be interpretable. In younger patients, genetic testing may assist with making the diagnosis.

In granulomatous disease (Answer C), while 1,25-dihydroxyvitamin D is typically elevated because macrophages in the granulomas synthesize the active metabolite of vitamin D, PTH levels are also suppressed.

PTH levels would also be suppressed in the case of calcitriol toxicity (Answer A).

In humoral hypercalcemia of malignancy (Answer D), PTH levels are classically undetectable because endogenous PTH is suppressed and PTHrP, a major cause of humoral hypercalcemia of malignancy, is not detected by immunoassays for PTH.

EDUCATIONAL OBJECTIVE

Diagnose primary hyperparathyroidism.

REFERENCE(S)

Cusano NE, Bilezikian JP. Parathyroid hormone in the evaluation of hypercalcemia. *JAMA.* 2014;312(24):2680-2681. PMID: 25536261

Eastell R, Brandi ML, Costa AG, D'Amour P, Shoback DM, Thakker RV. Diagnosis of asymptomatic primary hyperparathyroidism: proceedings of the Fourth International Workshop. *J Clin Endocrinol Metab.* 2014;99(10):3570-3579. PMID: 25162666

Diabetes Mellitus, Section 1 Board Review

Anne Peters, MD

1 **ANSWER: B) 150 mg/dL (8.3 mmol/L)**

Reducing the glucose concentration too quickly in people with chronically elevated glucose can worsen diabetic retinopathy. This phenomenon was first documented in the Diabetes Control and Complications Trial, in which rapid decreases in glucose levels led to worsening retinopathy. However, long-term better glycemic control slowed the progression of retinopathy in patients in the treatment arm of the study. This was also seen in randomized controlled trials using GLP-1 receptor agonists. There are data that rapid decreases in glucose levels can also precipitate symptoms of diabetic neuropathy. Additionally, people who have chronically high glucose levels often feel as though they are hypoglycemic when their glucose levels are lowered too quickly.

A glycemic target below 150 mg/dL (<8.3 mmol/L) is likely to lower her glucose too quickly, especially since her values have been higher for a long period. Starting at 150 mg/dL (8.3 mmol/L) (Answer B) will allow for more gradual lowering of glucose levels, and the targets can be reduced as her glucose levels decrease.

A target of 110 mg/dL (6.1 mmol/L) (Answer A) is most often used by people whose glycemic control is stable using an AID system, and it is associated with the best hemoglobin A_{1c} levels and time-in-range. However, it is the target level achieved over time. At a target of 110 mg/dL (6.1 mmol/L), the patient would be getting too much insulin, which would decrease her glucose levels quickly.

Neither 180 mg/dL (10.0 mmol/L) (Answer C) nor 220 mg/dL (12.1 mmol/L) (Answer D) is a target glucose value on the tubeless AID system. A "correct above" setting can be set at 180 mg/dL (10.0 mmol/L) but not a target level.

EDUCATIONAL OBJECTIVE

Explain the risk of rapidly decreasing glucose concentrations in patients with diabetes who have preexisting retinopathy.

REFERENCE(S)

Yoshida Y, Joshi P, Barri S, et al. Progression of retinopathy with glucagon-like peptide-1 receptor agonists with cardiovascular benefits in type 2 diabetes - a systematic review and meta-analysis. *J Diabetes Complications.* 2022;36(8):108255. PMID: 35817678.

Gibbons CH. Treatment induced neuropathy of diabetes-long term implications in type 1 diabetes. *J Diabetes Complications.* 2017;31(4):715-720. PMID: 28159476

Early worsening of diabetic retinopathy in the Diabetes Control and Complications Trial. *Arch Ophthalmol.* 1998;116(7):874-886. PMID: 9682700

2 **ANSWER: C) Has no significant difference in the time to a beneficial response**

Understanding glucagon use to treat severe hypoglycemia is very important for patients with diabetes and their families. Many people have the misperception that consciousness is regained immediately after glucagon administration, but it takes time. This can cause panic if family members are not educated about the timeframe. Additionally, people sometimes think that intranasal glucagon acts more quickly than intramuscular glucagon, but it actually does not (thus, Answer C is correct and Answer A is incorrect). In clinical trials, the mean time to success was 16 minutes for intranasal glucagon and 13 minutes for intramuscular glucagon. Both forms of glucagon have very similar pharmacokinetic/pharmacodynamic profiles, but bystanders are much more likely to successfully use intranasal glucagon instead of glucagon that requires reconstitution before injection.

Both forms of glucagon have similar adverse effects in terms of nausea, vomiting, and headache, among others (thus, Answer B is incorrect). Intranasal glucagon can cause additional adverse effects in terms of nose, throat, and/or sinus irritation and pain.

For adults, the dose of intranasal glucagon is 3 mg, while the dose of intramuscular glucagon is 1 mg (thus, Answer D is incorrect).

EDUCATIONAL OBJECTIVE

List the similarities and differences between intranasal and intramuscular glucagon.

REFERENCE(S)

Pontiroli AE, Tagliabue E. Intranasal versus injectable glucagon for hypoglycemia in type 1 diabetes: systematic review and meta-analysis. *Acta Diabetol.* 2020;57(6):743-749. PMID: 32025860

Singh-Franco D, Moreau C, Levin AD, Rosa D, Johnson M. Efficacy and usability of intranasal glucagon for the management of hypoglycemia in patients with diabetes: a systematic review. *Clin Ther.* 2020;42(9):e177-e208. PMID: 32873417

Rickels MR, Ruedy KJ, Foster NC, et al; T1D Exchange Intranasal Glucagon Investigators. Intranasal glucagon for treatment of insulin-induced hypoglycemia in adults with type 1 diabetes: a randomized crossover noninferiority study. *Diabetes Care.* 2016;39(2):264-270. PMID: 26681725

3 ANSWER: D) Bicarbonate and plasma/capillary ketone concentrations

The most recent American Diabetes Association/European Association for the Study of Diabetes guidelines state that venous pH *and/or* bicarbonate value and β-hydroxybutyrate value are the indicators for resolution of diabetic ketoacidosis (DKA). Resolution of DKA is defined as a venous pH value greater than 7.3 *or* a bicarbonate concentration greater than 18 mEq/L (>18 mmol/L) *and* a plasma/capillary ketone concentration less than 0.6 mmol/L (Answer D). The use of the anion gap (Answers A, B, and C) for this purpose is no longer recommended. The patient's clinical status is also important; when transitioning from intravenous to subcutaneous insulin, overlapping the 2 modes of insulin delivery is important to avoid recurrent DKA.

EDUCATIONAL OBJECTIVE

Determine whether diabetic ketoacidosis has resolved in a patient with diabetes.

REFERENCE(S)

Umpierrez GE, Davis GM, ElSayed NA, et al. Hyperglycaemic crises in adults with diabetes: a consensus report. *Diabetologia.* 2024 [Online ahead of print]

4 ANSWER: D) Vitamin C

Continuous glucose monitors are subject to interference by a variety of substances, including those listed in the *table (following page)* from the American Diabetes Association 2024 Standards of Care.

Vitamin C (Answer D), a commonly used vitamin for "wellness," is known to interfere with continuous glucose monitoring (Libre devices), and it is the supplement that is most likely to be causing an increase in this patient's glucose readings.

Acetaminophen (Answer A) interferes with some continuous glucose monitoring devices (Dexcom and Medtronic).

Neither biotin (Answer B) nor vitamin B_{12} (Answer C) interferes with continuous glucose monitoring.

EDUCATIONAL OBJECTIVE

Identify substances that interfere with continuous glucose monitoring.

REFERENCE(S)

Heinemann L. Interferences with CGM systems: practical relevance? *J Diabetes Sci Technol.* 2022;16(2):271-274. PMID: 34911382

American Diabetes Association Professional Practice Committee. 7. Diabetes technology: standards of care in diabetes-2024. *Diabetes Care.* 2024;47(Suppl 1):S126-S144. PMID: 38078575

Table 7.4—Continuous glucose monitoring devices interfering substances

Medication	Systems affected	Effect
Acetaminophen		
>4 g/day	Dexcom G6, Dexcom G7	Higher sensor readings than actual glucose
Any dose	Medtronic Guardian	Higher sensor readings than actual glucose
Ascorbic acid (vitamin C), >500 mg/day	FreeStyle Libre 14 day, FreeStyle Libre 2, FreeStyle Libre 3	Higher sensor readings than actual glucose
Hydroxyurea	Dexcom G6, Dexcom G7, Medtronic Guardian	Higher sensor readings than actual glucose
Mannitol (intravenously or as peritoneal dialysis solution)	Senseonics Eversense	Higher sensor readings than actual glucose
Sorbitol (intravenously or as peritoneal dialysis solution)	Senseonics Eversense	Higher sensor readings than actual glucose

Basu A, Veettil S, Dyer R, Peyser T, Basu R. Direct evidence of acetaminophen interference with subcutaneous glucose sensing in humans: a pilot study. *Diabetes Technol Ther.* 2016;18(Suppl 2):S243-S247. PMID: 26784129

5 ANSWER: D) Greater time-in-range with nighttime glucose values than with daytime glucose values

The American Diabetes Association currently recommends automated insulin delivery (AID) systems for the management of type 1 diabetes in adults and youth who are capable of using the device safely (either by themselves or with a caregiver). When discussing the benefits of AID systems, it is important for patients know what to expect, so they can make informed decisions as to which management approach is best for them. The American Diabetes Association recommendations state throughout: "the choice of devices should be made based on the individual's circumstances, preferences, and needs."

In randomized controlled trials and observational studies, nighttime glycemic control with AID systems is generally better (when people are not eating), with more time-in-range, compared with daytime glucose values (Answer D).

AID systems still require premeal bolus insulin doses to be given, generally 15 to 30 minutes before eating (thus, Answer A is incorrect).

Only on AID system (Tandem) has basal rates that are set for use during automode. The other AID systems automatically calculate the basal rates (thus, Answer B is incorrect).

The risk of severe (level 3) hypoglycemia episodes has not been shown to be reduced by AID systems (thus, Answer C is incorrect).

EDUCATIONAL OBJECTIVE

Explain the clinical benefits of automated insulin delivery systems to help set patient expectations.

REFERENCE(S)

Sherr JL, Laffel LM, Liu J, et al. Severe hypoglycemia and impaired awareness of hypoglycemia persist in people with type 1 diabetes despite use of diabetes technology: results from a cross-sectional survey. *Diabetes Care.* 2024:dc231765. PMID: 38295397

Freckmann G, Waldenmaier D, Heinemann L. Head-to-head evaluation of continuous glucose monitoring and automated insulin delivery systems: why are they not used more systematically? *J Diabetes Sci Technol.* 2024 [Online ahead of print] PMID: 38293951

Lakshman R, Boughton C, Hovorka R. The changing landscape of automated insulin delivery in the management of type 1 diabetes. *Endocr Connect.* 2023;12(8):e230132. PMID: 37289734

6 ANSWER: B) Is not expected to influence to his response to insulin pump therapy

Insulin pump therapy, particularly with an automated insulin delivery system, has been increasing shown to be beneficial in insulin-requiring individuals with type 2 diabetes.

Although the total daily dose of insulin may be higher in people with type 2 diabetes and insulin resistance, this does not affect the pump's ability to function. Automated insulin delivery systems have been increasingly studied in people with type 2 diabetes, and no relationship has been found between the C-peptide level and response (thus, Answer B is correct). Many people with type 2 diabetes remain on their noninsulin therapies (excluding sulfonylurea agents) when they are on insulin therapy. Although Medicare has required documentation of a low C-peptide concentration for eligibility to use insulin pump therapy, there is no reason that this is clinically relevant. C-peptide concentrations do not predict response to or benefit of insulin pump therapy.

There is no documented relationship between C-peptide concentrations and rates of hypoglycemia (thus, Answer C is incorrect).

C-peptide levels do not directly relate to the risk of diabetes complications, which are most strongly related to glycemic control and duration of diabetes (thus, Answer D is incorrect).

The limited data available show that insulin pumps and automated insulin delivery systems work well in people with type 2 diabetes, regardless of C-peptide concentrations (thus, Answer A is incorrect).

EDUCATIONAL OBJECTIVE

Explain that benefits of insulin pump therapy exist regardless of measured C-peptide concentration.

REFERENCE(S)

Hankosky ER, Katz ML, Fan L, et al. Predictors of insulin pump initiation among people with type 2 diabetes from a US claims database using machine learning. *Curr Med Res Opin.* 2023;39(6):843-853. PMID: 37139823

Davis GM, Peters AL, Bode BW, et al. Safety and efficacy of the Omnipod 5 automated insulin delivery system in adults with type 2 diabetes: from injections to hybrid closed-loop therapy. *Diabetes Care.* 2023;46(4):742-750. PMID: 36787903

Gill M, Chhabra H, Shah M, Zhu C, Grunberger G. C-peptide and beta-cell autoantibody testing prior to initiating continuous subcutaneous insulin infusion pump therapy did not improve utliziation or medical costs among older adults with diabetes mellitus. *Endocr Pract.* 2018;24(7):634-645. PMID: 29848066

Vigersky RA, Huang S, Cordero TL, et al; OpT2mise Study Group. Improved HBA1C, totally daily insulin dose, and treatment satisfaction with insulin pump therapy compared to multiple daily insulin injections in patients with type 2 diabetes irrespective of baseline C-peptide levels. *Endocr Pract.* 2018;24(5):446-452. PMID: 29847166

Reznik Y, Huang S; OpT2mise Study Group. Reductions in A1C with pump therapy in type 2 diabetes are independent of C-peptide and anti-glutamic acid decarboxylase antibody concentrations. *Diabetes Technol Ther.* 2014;16(11):816-818. PMID: 25192407

7 ANSWER: B) Continue her current regimen

As adults with diabetes age, it is important to balance the benefits of tighter glycemic control with its risks. The American Diabetes Association has different targets for older individuals based on their comorbidities and functional status (*see table, following page*).

The risks in older individuals are more related to hypoglycemia than to hyperglycemia. Use of medications that can cause hypoglycemia should be avoided as much as possible. When insulin is prescribed, continuous glucose monitoring should also be used. The use of premeal insulin can be complicated and is often associated with an increased risk of hypoglycemia. Glycemic targets for older individuals are shown in the *figure* *(following page)*.

Changing this patient's therapy is likely to worsen her overall state of health by increasing complexity and, if premeal insulin is added, increase her risk for hypoglycemia. She is currently at glycemic target for her age; the presence of frailty and other medical comorbidities changes her targets. Her measured hemoglobin A_{1c} is 7.4% (57 mmol/mol), which is well within a target of

Table 13.1—Framework for considering treatment goals for glycemia, blood pressure, and dyslipidemia in older adults with diabetes

Characteristics and health status of person with diabetes	Rationale	Reasonable A1C goal*	Fasting or preprandial glucose	Bedtime glucose	Blood pressure	Lipids
Healthy (few coexisting chronic illnesses, intact cognitive and functional status)	Longer remaining life expectancy	<7.0–7.5% (<53–58 mmol/mol)	80–130 mg/dL (4.4–7.2 mmol/L)	80–180 mg/dL (4.4–10.0 mmol/L)	<130/80 mmHg	Statin, unless contraindicated or not tolerated
Complex/intermediate (multiple coexisting chronic illnesses† or two or more instrumental ADL impairments or mild to moderate cognitive impairment)	Variable life expectancy. Individualize goals, considering: • Severity of comorbidities • Cognitive and functional limitations • Frailty • Risk-to-benefit ratio of diabetes medications • Individual preference	<8.0% (<64 mmol/mol)	90–150 mg/dL (5.0–8.3 mmol/L)	100–180 mg/dL (5.6–10.0 mmol/L)	<130/80 mmHg	Statin, unless contraindicated or not tolerated
Very complex/poor health (LTC or end-stage chronic illnesses‡ or moderate to severe cognitive impairment or two or more ADL impairments)	Limited remaining life expectancy makes benefit minimal	Avoid reliance on A1C; glucose control decisions should be based on avoiding hypoglycemia and symptomatic hyperglycemia	100–180 mg/dL (5.6–10.0 mmol/L)	110–200 mg/dL (6.1–11.1 mmol/L)	<140/90 mmHg	Consider likelihood of benefit with statin

This table represents a consensus framework for considering treatment goals for glycemia, blood pressure, and dyslipidemia in older adults with diabetes. The characteristic categories are general concepts. Not every individual will clearly fall into a particular category. Consideration of individual and caregiver preferences is an important aspect of treatment individualization. Additionally, an individual's health status and preferences may change over time. ADL, activities of daily living; LTC, long-term care. *A lower A1C goal may be set for an individual if achievable without recurrent or severe hypoglycemia or undue treatment burden. †Coexisting chronic illnesses are conditions serious enough to require medications or lifestyle management and may include arthritis, cancer, heart failure, depression, emphysema, falls, hypertension, incontinence, stage 3 or worse chronic kidney disease, myocardial infarction, and stroke. "Multiple" means at least three, but many individuals may have five or more (74). ‡The presence of a single end-stage chronic illness, such as stage 3–4 heart failure or oxygen-dependent lung disease, chronic kidney disease requiring dialysis, or uncontrolled metastatic cancer, may cause significant symptoms or impairment of functional status and significantly reduce life expectancy. Adapted from Kirkman et al. (3).

Reprinted from *Standards of Care in Diabetes 2024*, Section 13: Older Adults. Diabetes Care, 2024; 47(Supplement_1): S244–S257 © The American Diabetes Association.

Figure. Glycemic Targets for Older Individuals

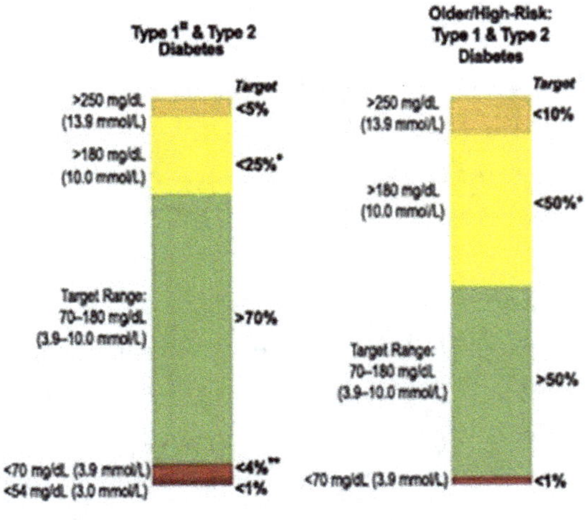

Reprinted from Battelino T et al. *Diabetes Care*, 2019; 42(8):1593–1603. © The American Diabetes Association.

less than 8.0% (<64 mmol/mol), with a time-below-range of 0% and a time-in-range of 55%. She has no complications of her longstanding diabetes. The patient should be reassured that she is doing well and does not need to focus on achieving lower postprandial glucose concentrations by administering mealtime insulin or restricting her caloric intake (Answer B).

Increasing her morning insulin glargine dose (Answer C) could reduce her overnight blood glucose levels, which should not be decreased any further. Her daytime postprandial glucose levels are elevated, not her overnight values.

Premeal insulin (Answer D) could increase her risk for low glucose values during the day, especially at a fixed dose given her variability of meal intake and activity.

Adding a GLP-1 receptor agonist (Answer A) to the regimen of this older woman with a BMI of 18.1 kg/m^2 and a poor appetite could cause weight loss, which would not be beneficial to her overall health. She needs to maintain her lean body mass and stay as physically active as possible.

EDUCATIONAL OBJECTIVE

List the risks and benefits of diabetes therapies in older adults.

REFERENCE(S)

Lipska KJ, Huang ES, Liu JY, et al. Glycemic control and diabetes complications across health status categories in older adults treated with insulin or insulin secretagogues: the Diabetes & Aging Study. *J Am Geriatr Soc.* 2023;71(12):3692-3700. PMID: 37638777

Huang ES, Sinclair A, Conlin PR, et al. The growing role of technology in the care of older adults with diabetes. *Diabetes Care.* 2023;46(8):1455-1463. PMID: 37471606

Battelino T, Danne T, Bergenstal RM, et al. Clinical targets for continuous glucose monitoring data interpretation: recommendations from the International Consensus on Time in Range. *Diabetes Care.* 2019;42(8):1593-1603. PMID: 31177185

Leung E, Wongrakpanich S, Munshi MN. Diabetes management in the elderly. *Diabetes Spectr.* 2018;31(3):245-253. PMID: 30140140

American Diabetes Association Professional Practice Committee. 13. Older adults: standards of care in diabetes-2024. *Diabetes Care.* 2024;47(Suppl 1):S244-S257. PMID: 38078575

8 ANSWER: C) Add semaglutide or tirzepatide as a weight-loss formulation

Incretin mimetics for weight loss, such as semaglutide and tirzepatide (Answer C), are recommended for use in people with a BMI greater than 30 kg/m^2. Obesity is associated with multiple comorbidities, and physicians should work with patients with overweight or obesity to lose weight through the available tools of lifestyle modification, weight-loss medications, and bariatric surgery, if needed. Treatment of obesity in people with type 2 diabetes is now highlighted in the American Diabetes Association Standards of Care, and many of the issues surrounding obesity are also relevant to those with type 1 diabetes. In the package inserts for the weight-loss forms of liraglutide (Saxenda), semaglutide (Wegovy), and tirzepatide (Zepbound), there are no contraindication to their use in people with type 1 diabetes. They are indicated for adults with obesity. Therefore, because of their weight-loss benefits and potential benefits in terms of cardiovascular disease and chronic kidney disease risk, these medications are being prescribed to patients with type 1 diabetes. However, prescribers must recognize that if people with type 1 diabetes eat less and lose weight, their insulin doses may need to be reduced to avoid hypoglycemia.

Automated insulin delivery (Answer D) is the preferred approach for managing this patient's diabetes, although her hemoglobin A_{1c} value is at target. This mode of insulin delivery would not help with weight loss.

In general, metformin (Answer B) does not cause weight loss in people with type 1 diabetes, but it can help maintain weight and reduce weight gain.

SGLT-2 inhibitors (Answer A) only lead to a small amount of weight loss (2-3 kg) and can cause diabetic ketoacidosis in patients with type 1 diabetes. Therefore, they are not recommended in this patient population.

EDUCATIONAL OBJECTIVE

Describe the potential use and adverse effects of incretin mimetics in people with obesity and type 1 diabetes.

REFERENCE(S)

Park J, Ntelis S, Yunasan E, et al. Glucagon-like peptide 1 analogues as adjunctive therapy for patients with type 1 diabetes: an updated systematic review and meta-analysis. *J Clin Endocrinol Metab.* 2023;109(1):279-292. PMID: 37561012

American Diabetes Association Professional Practice Committee. 8. Obesity and weight management for the prevention and treatment of type 2 diabetes. *Diabetes Care.* 2024;47(Suppl 1):S244-S257. PMID: 38078578

Steenackers N, Feldman AN, Mathieu C, et al. The double burden: navigating type 1 diabetes and obesity. *Clin Obes.* 2024:e12645 [Online ahead of print]. PMID: 38334191

Kueh MTW, Chew NWS, Al-Ozairi E, le Roux CW. The emergence of obesity in type 1 diabetes. *Int J Obes (Lond).* 2023;48(3):289-301. PMID: 38092958

Al-Ozairi E, Irshad M, Taghadom E, et al. Glucagon-like peptide-1 agonists combined with sodium-glucose cotransporter-2 inhibitors reduce weight in type 1 diabetes. *Obesity (Silver Spring).* 2023;31(3):716-723. PMID: 36811241

9 ANSWER: A) 10 units of rapid-acting insulin before meals with a correction dose

Transition from intravenous to subcutaneous insulin therapy is frequently accompanied by rebound hyperglycemia. Patients with type 1 diabetes on intravenous infusions who are transferring from the intensive care unit to a medical-surgical ward require transition to subcutaneous insulin management to meet basal, nutritional, and corrective (supplemental) insulin requirements. Subcutaneous insulin requirements can be calculated from the estimated total daily insulin dose while on stable intravenous insulin therapy, may be weight-based, or may be based on the preadmission insulin regimen if it was providing adequate glycemic control.

The first consideration in making this transition from intravenous to subcutaneous insulin is determination of appropriate basal insulin dosing. When the insulin drip rate is used as the basis for the determination of the total daily insulin requirement at the time of transition to subcutaneous insulin, several studies recommend starting at a daily insulin dose that is approximately 60% to 80% of the total number of units of intravenous insulin used in the preceding 12 to 24 hours. In this case, this represents the patient's basal insulin requirement, as he was not eating while in the intensive care unit, so it is 40 units of insulin glargine. This may be given once daily or split into 2 doses.

The second consideration in this case is determining an appropriate mealtime insulin dose. The meal dose of 10 units of insulin is calculated as 0.1 units/kg with each meal, and when it is administered as a rapid-acting insulin analogue, it should be given before the meal (Answer A).

A mealtime dose of 15 units of insulin lispro (Answers B and C) is high for this man, as it would lead to a skewed distribution of prandial to basal insulin, with more than 50% of his total daily dose being prandial, which would increase the risk for hypoglycemia. It is considered prudent to underestimate, rather than overestimate, the amount of insulin given with meals, especially when the patient is just beginning to eat. It is generally considered safe to limit the allocation of daily insulin given with meals or enteral feedings to 40% of the total daily insulin dose.

People with type 1 diabetes should be administering rapid-acting insulin before meals, not every 6 hours (Answer D), which may be discordant with their eating pattern.

EDUCATIONAL OBJECTIVE

Devise a rational plan for transitioning from intravenous insulin to a subcutaneous insulin regimen in hospitalized patients.

REFERENCE(S)

Dhatariya KK; Joint British Diabetes Societies for Inpatient Care. The management of diabetic ketoacidosis in adults-an updated guideline from the Joint British Diabetes Society for Inpatient Care. *Diabet Med.* 2022;39(6):e14788. PMID: 35224769

American Diabetes Association Professional Practice Committee. 16. Diabetes care in the hospital: standards of care in diabetes-2024. *Diabetes Care.* 2024;47(Suppl 1):S295-S306. PMID 38078585

10 ANSWER: C) Start a statin

The American College of Cardiology/American Heart Association Blood Cholesterol and the National Lipid Association guidelines recommend statin treatment (Answer C) for patients such as the one described in this vignette (ie, individuals with diabetes aged 40 to 75 years with LDL-cholesterol concentrations between 70 and 189 mg/dL [1.81-4.90 mmol/L] who do not have clinical atherosclerotic cardiovascular disease).

It is not clear whether a relatively minor reduction in hemoglobin A_{1c} from 7.2% (55 mmol/mol) to less than 7.0% (<53 mmol/mol) (Answer A) would have any effect on this patient's cardiovascular disease risk, given his 19-year history of diabetes. His previous degree of glycemic control is much more important.

Without clinical albuminuria, adding an ACE inhibitor (Answer D) would not be expected to result in a cardiovascular disease benefit in a normotensive, normoalbuminuric patient with type 1 diabetes.

His BMI of 28 kg/m^2 is modestly elevated, thus he is not expected to gain much benefit from weight loss (Answer B).

Because of potential harm (eg, bleeding) and minimal benefit, aspirin (Answer E) is no longer recommended for primary prevention of cardiovascular disease in patients at lower overall risk.

EDUCATIONAL OBJECTIVE

Recommend statin use as part of cardiovascular risk reduction in patients with type 1 diabetes.

REFERENCE(S)

American Diabetes Association Professional Practice Committee. 10. Cardiovascular disease and risk management: standards of care in diabetes-2024. *Diabetes Care.* 2024;47(Suppl 1):S179-S218. PMID: 38078592

Grundy SM, Stone NJ, Bailey AL, et al. 2018 AHA/ACC/AACVPR/AAPA/ABC/ACPM/ADA/AGS/APhA/ASPC/NLA/PCNA guideline on the management of blood cholesterol: a report of the American College of Cardiology/American Heart Association Task Force on Clinical Practice Guidelines. *Circulation.* 2019;139(25):e1082-e1143. PMID: 30586774

Nathan DM, Cleary PA, Backlund J-YC, et al; Diabetes Control and Complications Trial/Epidemiology of Diabetes Interventions and Complications (DCCT/EDIC) Study Research Group. Intensive diabetes treatment and cardiovascular disease in patients with type 1 diabetes. *N Engl J Med.* 2005;353(25):2643-2653. PMID: 16371630

ASCEND Study Collaborative Group, Bowman L, Mafham M, et al. Effects of aspirin for primary prevention in persons with diabetes mellitus. *N Engl J Med.* 2018;379(16):1529-1539. PMID: 30146931

11 ANSWER: D) Oral glucose tolerance test

Cystic fibrosis–related diabetes (CFRD) results from a primary defect in insulin secretion due in part to nonautoimmune destruction of β cells (mainly) and α cells in the pancreas. Thus, both insulin and glucagon secretion are defective. However, histologic studies have reported variability in the degree of islet-cell destruction. This indicates there are other factors contributing to insulin deficiency in CFRD, perhaps "collateral damage" from fibrosis and fatty infiltration or islet amyloid. The presence of CFRD strongly correlates with poorer clinical status, reflected by reduced pulmonary function and nutritional status, increased frequency of acute pulmonary exacerbations, and significant sputum pathogens. Annual screening for CFRD in all patients with cystic fibrosis is recommended beginning by age 10 years, consistent with guidelines from the American Diabetes Association, Cystic Fibrosis Foundation, Pediatric Endocrine Society, and International Society for Pediatric and Adolescent Diabetes. The best method to screen for and diagnose CFRD is oral glucose tolerance testing (Answer D).

Hemoglobin A_{1c} (Answer C) and fasting plasma glucose measurement (Answer A) should not be used for screening because they have low sensitivity for detecting CFRD. This has been confirmed in several studies. In these patients, hemoglobin A_{1c} is often normal, regardless of the degree of hyperglycemia. In 1 study, only 16% of patients with cystic fibrosis had elevated hemoglobin A_{1c} values at the time of CFRD diagnosis. In a population of pediatric patients with cystic fibrosis in Toronto, only 2.7% were clinically recognized as having CFRD, but with oral glucose tolerance testing of asymptomatic adolescents (aged 10 to 18 years), 17% were found to have impaired glucose tolerance and 13% had CFRD without fasting hyperglycemia. The recommended treatment of CFRD is insulin, albeit this is based on only a few clinical trials.

Fructosamine (Answer B) is not used for diabetes screening.

EDUCATIONAL OBJECTIVE

Recommend the best screening method for cystic fibrosis–related diabetes.

REFERENCE(S)

Moran A, Pillay K, Becker DJ, Acerini CL; International Society for Pediatric and Adolescent Diabetes. ISPAD Clinical Practice Consensus Guidelines 2014. Management of cystic fibrosis-related diabetes in children and adolescents. *Pediatr Diabetes.* 2014;15(Suppl 20):65-76. PMID: 25182308

O'Shea D, O'Connell J. Cystic fibrosis related diabetes. *Curr Diab Rep.* 2014;14(8):511. PMID: 24915888

Kelly A, Moran A. Update on cystic fibrosis-related diabetes [published correction appears in *J Cyst Fibros.* 2014;13(1):119]. *J Cyst Fibros.* 2013;12(4):318-331. PMID: 23562217

American Diabetes Association Professional Practice Committee. 2. Diagnosis and classification of Diabetes: standards of care in diabetes-2024. *Diabetes Care.* 2024;47(Suppl 1):S20-S42. PMID: 38078592

11 ANSWER: D) Oral glucose tolerance test

Cystic fibrosis–related diabetes (CFRD) results from a primary defect in insulin secretion due in part to nonautoimmune destruction of β cells (mainly) and α cells in the pancreas. Thus, both insulin and glucagon secretion are defective. However, histologic studies have reported variability in the degree of islet-cell destruction. This indicates there are other factors contributing to insulin deficiency in CFRD, perhaps "collateral damage" from fibrosis and fatty infiltration or islet amyloid. The presence of CFRD strongly correlates with poorer clinical status, reflected by reduced pulmonary function and nutritional status, increased frequency of acute pulmonary exacerbations, and significant sputum pathogens. Annual screening for CFRD in all patients with cystic fibrosis is recommended beginning by age 10 years, consistent with guidelines from the American Diabetes Association, Cystic Fibrosis Foundation, Pediatric Endocrine Society, and International Society for Pediatric and Adolescent Diabetes. The best method to screen for and diagnose CFRD is oral glucose tolerance testing (Answer D).

Hemoglobin A_{1c} (Answer C) and fasting plasma glucose measurement (Answer A) should not be used for screening because they have low sensitivity for detecting CFRD. This has been confirmed in several studies. In these patients, hemoglobin A_{1c} is often normal, regardless of the degree of hyperglycemia. In 1 study, only 16% of patients with cystic fibrosis had elevated hemoglobin A_{1c} values at the time of CFRD diagnosis. In a population of pediatric patients with cystic fibrosis in Toronto, only 2.7% were clinically recognized as having CFRD, but with oral glucose tolerance testing of asymptomatic adolescents (aged 10 to 18 years), 17% were found to have impaired glucose tolerance and 13% had CFRD without fasting hyperglycemia. The recommended treatment of CFRD is insulin, albeit this is based on only a few clinical trials.

Fructosamine (Answer B) is not used for diabetes screening.

EDUCATIONAL OBJECTIVE

Recommend the best screening method for cystic fibrosis–related diabetes.

REFERENCE(S)

Moran A, Pillay K, Becker DJ, Acerini CL; International Society for Pediatric and Adolescent Diabetes. ISPAD Clinical Practice Consensus Guidelines 2014. Management of cystic fibrosis-related diabetes in children and adolescents. *Pediatr Diabetes.* 2014;15(Suppl 20):65-76. PMID: 25182308

O'Shea D, O'Connell J. Cystic fibrosis related diabetes. *Curr Diab Rep.* 2014;14(8):511. PMID: 24915888

Kelly A, Moran A. Update on cystic fibrosis-related diabetes [published correction appears in *J Cyst Fibros.* 2014;13(1):119]. *J Cyst Fibros.* 2013;12(4):318-331. PMID: 23562217

American Diabetes Association Professional Practice Committee. 2. Diagnosis and classification of Diabetes: standards of care in diabetes-2024. *Diabetes Care.* 2024;47(Suppl 1):S20-S42. PMID: 38078592

12 ANSWER: B) Continue metformin at current dosage and add dulaglutide

Unless there is intolerance or a contraindication to its use, a combination of metformin plus lifestyle changes (eg, lifestyle counseling, weight-loss education, and exercise) is an initial treatment of type 2 diabetes if the patient does not have high-risk characteristics such as heart failure, chronic kidney disease, or cardiovascular disease (or high risk for cardiovascular disease). If a patient's hemoglobin A_{1c} level is not 7.0% or lower (≤53 mmol/mol) after approximately 3 months of the initial chosen therapy, an additional agent should be initiated. In the absence of high risk for or established cardiovascular disease and in the presence of a compelling need to minimize weight gain or promote loss, as is the case in this patient, a combination of metformin and GLP-1 receptor agonist or SGLT-2 inhibitor is recommended. Thus, because the patient has moderate to poor glycemic control on metformin monotherapy, the best course of action is to add the GLP-1 receptor agonist dulaglutide (Answer B) to her current regimen. Adding an SGLT-2 inhibitor would also be an option, but it is associated with less weight loss and less reduction in hemoglobin A_{1c}.

Stopping metformin and starting empagliflozin (Answer E) would result in monotherapy rather than the recommended dual therapy.

Continuing metformin at the current dosage (Answer A) or increasing the metformin dosage (Answer D) would not be adequate.

Adding sitagliptin (Answer C), a DPP-4 inhibitor, would not be as likely as a GLP-1 receptor agonist to help her achieve weight management or glucose-lowering goals.

EDUCATIONAL OBJECTIVE

Guide therapy for type 2 diabetes when initial management with lifestyle efforts and metformin fails to provide adequate glycemic control.

REFERENCE(S)

American Diabetes Association Professional Practice Committee. 9. Pharmacologic approaches to glycemic treatment: standards of care in diabetes-2024. *Diabetes Care.* 2024;43(Suppl 1):S158-S178. PMID: 38078590

Davies MJ, Aroda VR, Collins BS, et al. Management of hyperglycemia in type 2 diabetes, 2022. A consensus report by the American Diabetes Association (ADA) and the European Association for the Study of Diabetes (EASD). *Diabetes Care.* 2022;45(11):2753-2786. PMID: 36148880

13 ANSWER: B) Once-daily basal insulin, plus correction insulin dose every 4 to 6 hours

Subcutaneous insulin is the recommended treatment for glycemic management in postoperative patients with type 2 diabetes who are in a noncritical care unit. If the patient were in the critical care setting, continuous intravenous insulin infusion (Answer A) would be the recommended method of glycemic management. However, if the patient is in a noncritical care setting, as in this case, a regimen of scheduled subcutaneous insulin injections is the best method for achieving glycemic targets.

Her glycemic status warrants basal insulin in addition to correction dose insulin. As she is not eating, meal insulin will not be provided. The dosing frequency of correction insulin depends on the type of insulin used. If a rapid-acting analogue is used, it may be given every 4 hours, and if regular insulin is used, it will be given every 6 hours (Answer B). These time intervals correspond to the known duration of action of each insulin and help avoid stacking of insulin and resulting hypoglycemia. Injections should align with meals and bedtime or every 4 to 6 hours if the patient is not consuming meals (thus, Answer C is incorrect).

Evidence clearly shows that sliding-scale insulin used alone (Answer E) is associated with increased rates of both hypoglycemia and hyperglycemia in patients with glucose concentrations greater than 180 mg/dL (>10.0 mmol/L), and its use is therefore not recommended. In addition, evidence from randomized controlled trials has demonstrated that a scheduled basal-plus-bolus treatment regimen results in better glycemic control and reduced hospital complications when compared with outcomes of sliding-scale insulin alone in general surgery patients with type 2 diabetes, further making the case for a basal-plus-bolus regimen. When this patient begins to eat, scheduled mealtime insulin will be added to her regimen.

Restarting home medications without insulin (Answer D) is incorrect, as the patient has nausea and also may be at risk for developing lactic acidosis.

EDUCATIONAL OBJECTIVE

Manage inpatient insulin treatment in the noncritical care setting.

REFERENCE(S)

American Diabetes Association Professional Practice Committee. 16. Diabetes care in the hospital: standards of care in diabetes-2024. *Diabetes Care.* 2024;47(Suppl 1):S295-S306. PMID: 38078585

Umpierrez GE, Smiley D, Jacobs S, et al. Randomized study of basal-bolus insulin therapy in the inpatient management of patients with type 2 diabetes undergoing general surgery (RABBIT 2 surgery). *Diabetes Care.* 2011;34(2):256-261. PMID: 21228246.

Migdal AL, Fortin-Leung C, Pasquel F, Wang H, Peng L, Umpierrez GE. Inpatient glycemic control with sliding scale insulin in noncritical patients with type 2 diabetes: who can slide? *J Hosp Med.* 2021;16(8):462-468. PMID: 34328842

14 ANSWER: E) Proteinuria

The turnover of serum proteins, mainly albumin, is more rapid than that of hemoglobin; thus, serum fructosamine values (glycated proteins, mostly albumin) reflect mean blood glucose values over a much shorter period (1 to 2 weeks). There is generally a good correlation between serum fructosamine and hemoglobin A_{1c} values. Fructosamine responds more rapidly to changes in blood glucose control than does hemoglobin A_{1c}. Falsely low fructosamine values in relation to mean blood glucose values occur with rapid albumin turnover, for example, in patients with protein-losing enteropathy or nephrotic syndrome (Answer E).

Biotin (Answer A), hemolysis (Answer B), and hypothyroidism (Answer C) do not falsely lower fructosamine.

Laboratory errors (Answer D) do rarely occur, but in this case, the heavy proteinuria explains the normal fructosamine value.

EDUCATIONAL OBJECTIVE

Diagnose nephrotic syndrome as a cause of falsely low fructosamine values.

REFERENCE(S)

Hassanein M, Shafi T. Assessment of glycemia in chronic kidney disease. *BMC Med.* 2022;20(1):117. PMID: 35414081

Copur S, Onal EM, Afsar B, et al. Diabetes mellitus in chronic kidney disease: biomarkers beyond HbA1c to estimate glycemic control and diabetes-dependent morbidity and mortality. *J Diabetes Complications.* 2020;34(11):107707. PMID: 32861562

Desouza CV, Rosenstock J, Kohzuma T, Fonseca VA. Glycated albumin correlates with time-in-range better than HbA1c or fructosamine. *J Clin Endocrinol Metab.* 2023;108(11):e1193-e1198. PMID: 37259605

15 ANSWER: A) Continue to control her glucose levels to achieve hemoglobin A_{1c} <7.0% (<53 mmol/mol)

Risk of nephropathy is associated with the hemoglobin A_{1c} level, starting with glycemic control at the time of diagnosis. Prolonged improvement in outcomes over time is known as the legacy effect. The best way to reduce this patient's risk is to focus on glycemic control with a hemoglobin A_{1c} target less than 7.0% (<53 mmol/mol) (Answer A). Risk of developin chronic kidney disease typically starts after a disease duration of 10 to 15 years.

The etiology of diabetic nephropathy is complex and multifactorial, but inherited risk factors are being identified. In fact, various genetic risk factors are associated with urinary albumin excretion, persistent proteinuria, and end-stage kidney disease in adults with diabetes. However, no specific genetic test is available at this time (thus, Answer B is incorrect).

Starting an ACE inhibitor or angiotensin receptor blocker is only recommended for individuals with diabetes and hypertension and/or an elevated albumin-to-creatinine ratio (thus, Answer D is incorrect).

In patients with a normal albumin-to-creatinine ratio, monitoring is not necessary more often than once annually (thus, Answer B is incorrect).

EDUCATIONAL OBJECTIVE

Discuss factors associated with the development of nephropathy in type 1 diabetes.

REFERENCE(S)

Zoccali C, Mallamaci F, Tripepi G, et al. The long-term benefits of early intensive therapy in chronic diseases-the legacy effect. *Clin Kidney J.* 2023;16(11):1917-1924. PMID: 37915902

DCCT/EDIC research group. Effect of intensive diabetes treatment on albuminuria in type 1 diabetes: long-term follow-up of the Diabetes Control and Complications Trial and Epidemiology of Diabetes Interventions and Complications study. *Lancet Diabetes Endocrinol.* 2014;2(10):793-800. PMID: 25043685

Jansson Sigfrids F, Groop PH. Progression and regression of kidney disease in type 1 diabetes. *Front Nephrol.* 2023;3:1282818. PMID: 38192517

Salem RM, Todd JN, Sandholm N, et al. Genome-wide association study of diabetic kidney disease highlights biology involved in glomerular basement membrane collagen. *J Am Soc Nephrol.* 2019;30(10):2000-2016. PMID: 31537649

16 ANSWER: C) Add an SGLT-2 inhibitor

Posttransplant diabetes (PTD) is important to diagnose and treat because it is a significant risk factor for complications after transplant. Over 5 years, the incidence of PTD is 10% to 20% for kidney transplant and 20% to 40% for liver, heart, and lung transplant. PTD is associated with worse outcomes, including infections, decreased organ survival, increased risk of cardiovascular disease and chronic kidney disease, and increased overall mortality. Risk factors for PTD are similar to those for diabetes in general (age, family history, ethnicity, obesity, etc), as well as the type of immunosuppression used. Hyperglycemia is very common in the early posttransplant period, although it generally resolves by the time of discharge. A formal diagnosis of PTD is made once the individual is stable on their posttransplant medications, usually at least 45 days after transplant. Diagnosing PTD is similar to diagnosing diabetes in general, although historically oral glucose tolerance testing performed 1 year after transplant was considered the gold standard. The use of fasting plasma glucose and hemoglobin A_{1c} measurement often supersedes the need for oral glucose tolerance testing.

The American Diabetes Association guidelines state that few randomized controlled studies have reported on the outcomes of short- and long-term use of antihyperglycemic agents in the setting of PTD. The guidelines recommend insulin therapy in an inpatient setting, which can also be considered after hospital discharge. However, given the lack of data on which agent to choose, the guidelines suggest selecting therapy based on the adverse effect profile of the medication, including possible interactions with immunosuppressive agents and the medication's potential kidney and cardiovascular benefits.

Although specific guidelines for treatment of PTD do not exist, following the overall guidelines for the management of type 2 diabetes is recommended, with the caveat of ensuring that the medications do not interfere with the patient's immunosuppressive therapy. The patient in this vignette has known cardiovascular disease, so the options would be use of an SGLT-2 inhibitor or a GLP-1 receptor agonist. Both have been assessed in smaller studies and have no effect on immunosuppression in most cases, although the delay in gastric emptying seen with GLP-1 receptor agonists is a concern. Starting an SGLT-2 inhibitor (Answer C) is reasonable, given the patient's clinical situation, mildly elevated hemoglobin A_{1c} value, and the absence of a compelling need to treat obesity.

Adding a sulfonylurea (Answer A) is incorrect, although it was previously recommended before the availability of newer agents to manage type 2 diabetes. Sulfonylureas can cause hypoglycemia and weight gain and are not recommended as first-line therapy for people with type 2 diabetes and cardiovascular disease.

Thiazolidinediones (Answer B) are not recommended as first-line therapy for people with type 2 diabetes and cardiovascular disease. However, they tend to be well tolerated after transplant and are considered potentially helpful for patients with metabolic dysfunction-associated steatotic liver disease. Thiazolidinediones are associated with weight gain and increased risk of heart failure.

Although insulin (Answer D) is recommended for use in hospitalized patients, it is not the first-line choice in the outpatient setting.

EDUCATIONAL OBJECTIVE

Identify new-onset diabetes after transplant and recommend appropriate treatment.

REFERENCE(S)

Ramakrishnan P, Garg N, Pabich S, Mandelbrot DA, Swanson KJ. Sodium-glucose cotransporter-2 inhibitor use in kidney transplant recipients. *World J Transplant.* 2023;13(5):239-249. PMID: 37746038

Chewcharat A, Prasitlumkum N, Thongprayoon C, et al. Efficacy and safety of SGLT-2 inhibitors for treatment of diabetes mellitus among kidney transplant patients: a systematic review and meta-analysis. *Med Sci (Basel).* 2020;8(4):47. PMID: 33213078

Munoz Pena JM, Cusi K. Posttransplant diabetes mellitus: recent developments in pharmacological management of hyperglycemia. *J Clin Endocrinol Metab.* 2023;109(1):e1-e11. PMID: 37410930

American Diabetes Association Professional Practice Committee. 2. Diagnosis and classification of diabetes: standards of care in diabetes-2024. *Diabetes Care.* 2024;47(Suppl 1):S20-S42. PMID: 38078585

17 ANSWER: C) Measure serum vitamin B_{12}

This patient has new neuropathic symptoms superimposed on a history and examination findings consistent with peripheral polyneuropathy. The symptoms and physical findings suggest posterior column and upper motor neuron disease, and in this setting, a positive Romberg sign and Babinski response would likely be present. Although this may represent progression of diabetic neuropathy, the latter findings are not typical of this alone. He has anemia, and the combination of neurologic and hematologic disturbance is compatible with vitamin B_{12} deficiency. Metformin has been associated with decreased plasma vitamin B_{12} levels in up to 30% of patients, and this medication doubles the risk of clinically significant B_{12} deficiency. While the mechanism is not entirely clear, most evidence points to interference with food-derived B_{12} absorption, primarily in the ileum. Replacement with oral or parenteral vitamin B_{12} is usually successful and precludes discontinuation of metformin. Numerous laboratory testing options are available to assess for the presence of B_{12} deficiency. Serum vitamin B_{12} measurement (Answer C) is most commonly used for initial assessment, while other tests, such as measurement of holotranscobalamin, methylmalonic acid, or homocysteine, are reserved for confirmatory testing.

Findings on electromyography and nerve conduction studies (Answer E) would most likely be abnormal in this man, but they are not specific for subacute combined degeneration (neuropathy due to vitamin B_{12} deficiency).

Vitamin B_6, pyridoxine, has a role in serotonin and norepinephrine metabolism and in the formation of myelin. Clinical symptoms of B_6 deficiency are bilateral, distal limb numbness (appears early) and distal limb burning paresthesia (replaces numbness later in the course). Distal limb weakness is rare. Thus, measuring vitamin B_6 (Answer B) is not the best next step.

This patient's presentation is not consistent with spinal or nerve root irritation from C-spine disease, which can manifest as pain in the neck and pain and numbness or weakness radiating down to the shoulder, arm, and hand. Thus, MRI of the cervical spine (Answer D) is incorrect.

γ-Glutamyltransferase (Answer A) would be elevated if he had alcohol-related neuropathy, but that is not suggested by his history.

EDUCATIONAL OBJECTIVE

Diagnose adverse effects of metformin, including vitamin B_{12} deficiency.

REFERENCE(S)

Pierce SA, Chung AH, Black KK. Evaluation of vitamin B12 monitoring in a veteran population on long-term, high-dose metformin therapy. *Ann Pharmacother.* 2012;46(11):1470-1476. PMID: 23115224

Bell DSH. Metformin-induced vitamin B12 deficiency can cause or worsen distal symmetrical, autonomic and cardiac neuropathy in the patient with diabetes. *Diabetes Obes Metab.* 2022;24(8):1423-1428. PMID: 35491956

Baig FA, Khan S, Rizwan A. Frequency of vitamin B12 deficiency in type 2 diabetic patients taking metformin. *Cureus.* 2022;14(3):e22924. PMID: 35399475

Ward PCJ. Modern approaches to the investigation of vitamin B12 deficiency. *Clin Lab Med.* 2002;22(2):435-445. PMID: 12134470

18 ANSWER: C) Pancreas transplant with or without a kidney transplant

Necrobiosis lipoidica is rare condition that occurs in 0.3% to 1.2% of patients with diabetes, more commonly in woman than in men, with an average age of onset of 45 years in people with diabetes. Among patients with necrobiosis lipoidica, 11% to 65% have diabetes. Necrobiosis lipoidica is an inflammatory granulomatous skin disorder in which microangiopathy appears to have a role in pathogenesis. The lesions are classically seen overlying the anterior shin, characterized by a shallow depression into the dermis that is erythematous, often with a slightly yellow hue (due to lipid deposition) and with telangiectasias. Lesion size varies considerably, ranging between 1 and several centimeters in diameter, and lesions can grow over time and are frequently bilateral. They may be subject to ulceration.

Evidence for any specific treatment is limited to case reports and small clinical trials, and there is no FDA-approved treatment. Pancreas transplant with or without a kidney transplant (Answer C) can resolve necrobiosis lipoidica, although not always. Kidney transplant alone (Answer B) does not.

Several studies have been published that examine the use of pentoxifylline (Answer D). Although it may lead to some improvement, it does not resolve the skin lesions.

Although JAK inhibitors (Answer A) are promising, they have been used too rarely to draw any conclusions. They are being studied in combination with topical calcineurin inhibitors (Answer E), and/or intralesional corticosteroids and compression therapy. Recent evidence has been published regarding the use of biologics, classic immunosuppressants, and topical therapies. Topical treatment with calcineurin inhibitors alone does not resolve the lesions, although in combination with glucocorticoids, they may lead to some improvement. Topical corticosteroids alone are beneficial in less than half of individuals treated.

Phototherapy is the most studied treatment. However, the most traditionally administered form of phototherapy, UVA1, has not shown significant overall benefit.

EDUCATIONAL OBJECTIVE

Explain the various treatments available for necrobiosis lipoidica.

REFERENCE(S)

Souza AD, El-Azhary RA, Gibson LE. Does pancreas transplant in diabetic patients affect the evolution of necrobiosis lipoidica? *Int J Dermatol.* 2009;48(9):964-970. PMID: 19702981

Mazur MJ, Lowney AC, Prigoff J, et al. Resolution of long-standing necrobiosis lipoidica diabeticorum (NLD) lesion after restoration of euglycemia following successful pancreas after kidney (PAK) transplantation: a case report. *Transplant Proc.* 2011;43(9):3296-3298. PMID: 22099781

Calzavara-Pinton P, Bettolini L, Tonon F, Rossi M, Venturini M. The realistic positioning of UVA1 phototherapy after 25 years of clinical experience and the availability of new biologics and small molecules: a retrospective clinical study. *Front Med (Lausanne).* 2023;10:1295145. PMID: 38076241

Nihal A, Caplan AS, Rosenbach M, Damsky W, Mangold AR, Shields BE. Treatment options for necrobiosis lipoidica: a systematic review. *Int J Dermatol.* 2023;62(12):1529-1537PMID: 37772666

Verheyden MJ, Rodrigo N, Gill AJ, Glastras SJ. A case series and literature review of necrobiosis lipoidica. *Endocrinol Diabetes Metab Case Rep.* 2022;2022:21-0185. PMID: 36001014

19 ANSWER: D) Now

Although the mainstay of diabetes prevention should always focus on lifestyle management, including diet and physical activity counseling, the screening guidelines vary. Current guidelines (American Diabetes Association, World Health Organization) suggest a BMI criterion of 23 kg/m^2 for type 2 diabetes screening in Asian Americans (decreased from 25 kg/m^2 in the general population) because data demonstrate that Asian Americans are at greater risk for diabetes at a lower BMI than non-Asian individuals. Therefore, this patient should be screened for type 2 diabetes now (Answer D). Delaying screening (Answers A and B) is not recommended. The general age for screening is now 35 years and older, regardless of BMI. Adults should be screened for diabetes regardless of symptoms (Answer C), as most people are asymptomatic at diagnosis.

In asymptomatic adults, diabetes screening should be considered in patients, regardless of age, who have overweight or obesity and 1 or more of the following risk factors: first-degree relative with diabetes, high-risk race/ethnicity, history of cardiovascular disease, hypertension, HDL-cholesterol concentration less than 35 mg/dL (<0.90 mmol/L) and/or triglyceride concentration greater than 250 mg/dL (>2.82 mmol/L), polycystic ovary syndrome (in women), and physical inactivity. Patients with prediabetes should have annual testing, and women diagnosed with gestational diabetes should have testing at least every 3 years.

According to the American Diabetes Association guidelines, screening for diabetes should begin at age 35 years regardless of other factors such as ethnicity, family history, BMI, blood pressure, and dyslipidemia.

EDUCATIONAL OBJECTIVE

Select the appropriate criteria for type 2 diabetes/prediabetes screening in patients of diverse racial/ethnic backgrounds.

REFERENCE(S)

American Diabetes Association Professional Practice Committee. 2. Diagnosis and classification of diabetes: standards of medical care in diabetes-2024. *Diabetes Care.* 2024;47(Suppl 1):S20-S42. PMID: 38078589

US Preventive Services Task Force, Davidson KW, Barry MJ, et al. Screening for prediabetes and type 2 diabetes. US Prevent Services Recommendation Statement. *JAMA.* 2021;326(8):736-743. PMID: 34427594

20 ANSWER: D) Restoration of hypoglycemia awareness

Following successful pancreas transplant alone, patients with diabetes are able to stop insulin therapy and have essentially normal β-cell function. A pancreas transplant provides normal counterregulatory hormone secretion and exocrine function. Therefore, hypoglycemia awareness is restored (Answer D).

After pancreas transplant alone, there is stabilization and, in some cases, improvement in peripheral and autonomic diabetic neuropathy. In addition, after successful pancreas transplant, the velocity of motor and sensory nerve conduction, as well as clinical neuropathy, stabilizes but does not regress (Answer A). Abnormalities of gastric motility do not improve (Answer B).

The effect of pancreas transplant on diabetic retinopathy is not clear. While some studies have found no benefit in terms of halting or reversing the progression of advanced retinopathy after pancreas transplant, other reports have noted stabilization or occasional regression of retinal lesions (Answer C) (but not at a proliferative stage as in this patient).

After pancreas transplant, serum triglyceride and LDL-cholesterol concentrations tend to fall, and serum HDL-cholesterol concentrations tend to rise. There are mixed data in terms of the effect on kidney function. This is due to a lack of comparator data, as well as a potential worsening of kidney function due to immunosuppressive therapy. Patients who do better regarding kidney function are those who have a pretransplant estimated glomerular filtration rate greater than 60 mL/min per 1.73 m^2.

EDUCATIONAL OBJECTIVE

Describe the potential benefits of pancreas transplant 5 years after successful transplant.

REFERENCE(S)

Fridell JA, Stratta RJ, Gruessner AC. Pancreas transplantation: current challenges, considerations, and controversies. *J Clin Endocrinol Metab.* 2023;108(3):614-623. PMID: 36377963

Boggi U, Baronti W, Amorese G, et al. Treating type 1 diabetes by pancreas transplant alone: a cohort study on actual long-term (10 years) efficacy and safety [Published correction appears in *Transplantation.* 2022;106(5):e286]. *Transplantation.* 2022;106(1):147-157. PMID: 33909390

21 ANSWER: D) Temporarily relax tight glucose targets

Up to 30% of patients with type 1 or longstanding type 2 diabetes have impaired or absent awareness of hypoglycemia. As plasma glucose levels fall, compromised physiologic counterregulatory defenses include failure of glucagon secretion to increase and attenuated epinephrine secretion. This, together with inability to reduce circulating insulin levels, results in the clinical syndrome of defective counterregulation, which markedly increases the risk of recurrent severe hypoglycemia. Hypoglycemia-attenuating defense against subsequent hypoglycemia is a concept referred to as hypoglycemia-associated autonomic failure. The treatment mainstay for this condition is the scrupulous avoidance of hypoglycemia. Patients with hypoglycemia unawareness and/or severe hypoglycemia and tight control should be advised to relax their glucose targets (Answer D) for a period to allow awareness to potentially return with adrenergic symptoms.

This patient should continue his usual dietary regimen (consistent carbohydrate or matching insulin to carbohydrates). Frequent small meals (Answer A) would not address the etiology of his problem.

Switching to insulin pump therapy (Answer C) would not address the underlying cause of the hypoglycemia unawareness (repetitive hypoglycemic episodes) or guarantee its avoidance. A pump with a closed-loop suspend or auto-suspend for hypoglycemia function might be considered in his long-term management plan. However, he has had tight glycemic control on a multiple daily injection regimen as evidenced by his hemoglobin A_{1c} value, and the urgent need here is to address the blunted glycemic awareness. There would also be a delay in initiating pump therapy and a learning curve regarding its use.

While a number of educational programs focusing on hypoglycemia detection and avoidance (Dose Adjustment for Normal Eating [DAFNE], Blood Glucose Awareness Training [BGAT], Hypoglycemia Awareness and Avoidance [HAAT]) have demonstrated effectiveness in reducing the occurrence of hypoglycemia, such an education program (Answer B) is not the most immediate fix for this patient, nor would it address the cause.

EDUCATIONAL OBJECTIVE

Recommend management for severe hypoglycemia and hypoglycemia unawareness in type 1 diabetes.

REFERENCE(S)

Cryer PE. Mechanisms of hypoglycemia-associated autonomic failure in diabetes. *N Engl J Med.* 2013;369(4):362-372. PMID: 23883381

American Diabetes Association Professional Practice Committee. 6. Glycemic goals and hypoglycemia: standards of care in diabetes-2024. *Diabetes Care.* 2024;47(Suppl 1);S111-S125. PMID: 38078586

Liakos A, Karagiannis T, Avgerinos I, Tsapas A, Bekiari E. Burden and coping strategies of hypoglycemia in people with diabetes. Curr *Diabetes Rev.* 2024;20(6):e201023222415. PMID: 37867276.

Yu X, Fan M, Zhao X, et al. Prevalence of impaired awareness of hypoglycaemia in people with diabetes mellitus: a systematic review and meta-analysis from 21 countries and regions. *Diabet Med.* 2023;40(9):e15129. PMID: 37143390

Takagi S, Miura J, Takita M, et al. Factors associated with hypoglycemia unawareness and severe hypoglycemia in type 1 diabetes mellitus patients. *J Diabetes Investig.* 2022;13(12):2018-2026. PMID: 35869856

22 ANSWER: D) Total iron-binding capacity and serum ferritin measurements

When diabetes is diagnosed, the possibility of secondary diabetes should be considered. Secondary diabetes occurs when a separate condition leads to hyperglycemia; this is considered distinct from routine type 1 or type 2 diabetes, although clinical features are often shared. Broad categories of secondary diabetes include medication-induced (eg, corticosteroids), other endocrinopathies (eg, acromegaly), pancreatic diseases (eg, pancreatitis), infections (eg, cytomegalovirus), and genetic conditions (eg, Rabson-Mendenhall syndrome).

One relatively common condition that should be considered is hemochromatosis, or iron overload. Primary hemochromatosis is a very common genetic disorder in the United States, affecting approximately 1 in every 200 to 300 Americans. It occurs more often in persons of Western European heritage. Hemochromatosis results from increased absorption of iron through the gastrointestinal tract, with excess iron deposition in many tissues (pancreas, liver, pituitary, etc). Traditional teaching has been that hyperglycemia results from iron deposition in the pancreas, leading to islet-cell dysfunction. However, recent data suggest that the pathogenesis involves primarily insulin resistance with secondary β-cell decompensation, as in routine cases of type 2 diabetes. Secondary hemochromatosis includes conditions characterized by increased red blood cell breakdown or a history of many blood transfusions (thalassemia, sideroblastic anemia, hemolytic anemia). The clues in this case include hypogonadism (due to hypogonadotropic hypogonadism from pituitary iron deposition) and hepatic dysfunction and enlargement. The initial approach to diagnosis is assessing markers of iron stores, which can be performed by measuring the total iron-binding capacity and serum ferritin (Answer D). These 2 tests are used to calculate the transferrin saturation, a more useful indication of iron stores than either measure alone.

Glutamic acid decarboxylase antibodies (Answer A) would be elevated if this patient had type 1 diabetes or latent autoimmune diabetes in adults, but these diagnoses seem unlikely.

Although liver ultrasonography (Answer B) could reveal fatty liver, it would not diagnose hemochromatosis.

Pituitary MRI (Answer C) is done after documenting secondary hypogonadism (after measuring free testosterone, LH, and FSH).

EDUCATIONAL OBJECTIVE

Diagnose hemochromatosis as a cause of secondary diabetes mellitus.

REFERENCE(S)

Hatunic M, Finucane FM, Brennan AM, Norris S, Pacini G, Nolan JJ. Effect of iron overload on glucose metabolism in patients with hereditary hemochromatosis. *Metabolism.* 2010;59(3):380-384. PMID: 19815242

Olynyk JK, Ramm GA. Hemochromatosis. *N Engl J Med.* 2022;387(23):2159-2170. PMID: 36477033

Savatt JM, Johns A, Schwartz MLB, et al. Testing and management of iron overload after genetic screening-identified hemochromatosis. *JAMA Netw Open.* 2023;6(10):e2338995. PMID: 37870835

23 ANSWER: A) Diabetes-related radiculopathy

Diabetic neuropathy is generally more common in patients with long disease duration and suboptimal glycemic control. Classification is subdivided into somatosensory, motor, and autonomic.

Diabetes-related radiculopathy (Answer A) manifests as acute sensory and/or motor neuropathy characterized by sudden pain and dysesthesias and/or muscle weakness in the distribution of 1 or more individual peripheral nerves or nerve roots. The patient in this vignette has right-sided facial pain and muscle weakness in the distribution of the facial (seventh cranial) nerve. This is an acute mononeuropathy or radiculitis. There is no specific therapy for this complication. The patient can be reassured that it typically resolves after 2 to 3 months. Neuropathy pain relief medications such as tricyclic antidepressants or selective serotonin and norepinephrine reuptake inhibitors may be given in the interim. The most common presentation of neuropathy with diabetes involves damage to sensory nerve fibers and typically affects the distal extremities in a "stocking-glove" distribution as this patient has on examination. Affected patients describe numbness, paresthesias, and occasionally sharp pains.

Autonomic dysfunction (Answer B) may affect 1 or several organ systems, including the vasculature (orthostatic hypotension), the heart (silent ischemia, abnormal cardiac rhythms), the gastrointestinal tract (gastroparesis, constipation, diarrhea from bacterial overgrowth), and the urinary bladder (atonic bladder, chronic urinary tract infections, overflow incontinence). It does not cause pain syndromes.

Herpes zoster (Answer C) can cause localized pain in a pattern similar to that described in this vignette, and pain can precede the typical rash, but the rash does not usually appear until about 1 week after the onset of pain.

Otitis media (Answer D) can spread to the facial nerve and inflame it, causing compression of the nerve in its canal; however, there is no evidence of otitis on this patient's examination.

Findings on his head CT do not suggest cerebrovascular accident (Answer E).

EDUCATIONAL OBJECTIVE

Diagnose less-common manifestations of diabetic neuropathy.

REFERENCE(S)

Bell DSH. Diabetic mononeuropathies and diabetic amyotrophy. *Diabetes Ther.* 2022;13(10):1715-1722. PMID: 35969368

Tesfaye S, Boulton AJ, Dyck PJ, et al; Toronto Diabetic Neuropathy Expert Group. Diabetic neuropathies: update on definitions, diagnostic criteria, estimation of severity, and treatments. *Diabetes Care.* 2010;33(10):2285-2293. PMID: 20876709

Casellini CM, Vinik AI. Clinical manifestations and current treatment options for diabetic neuropathies. *Endocr Pract.* 2007;13(5):550-566. PMID: 17872358

24 ANSWER: E) Zinc transporter 8 (ZnT8) antibody testing

In first-degree relatives of individuals with type 1 diabetes, screening before overt clinical symptoms develop, as occurred in this patient, can detect the disease in a clinically silent phase. Multiple positive antibodies are highly predictive of future disease development, while positivity for only 1 autoantibody may not indicate high risk. Several serum antibodies can be detected before the manifestation of autoimmune hyperglycemia, including islet-cell antibodies, insulin autoantibodies, glutamic acid decarboxylase antibodies, and antibodies to tyrosine phosphatase-like proteins. Analysis of zinc transporter 8 (ZnT8) antibodies (Answer E) increases the diagnostic sensitivity of islet autoantibodies for type 1 diabetes, as 26% of patients with antibody-negative type 1 diabetes (negative for insulin, glutamic acid decarboxylase, tyrosine phosphatase-like proteins, and islet-cell antibodies) have ZnT8 autoantibodies.

This patient's hemoglobin A_{1c} value is consistent with the high self-monitored blood glucose values. Measurement of fructosamine (Answer B) or 1,5-anhydroglucitol (Answer A) would not add any useful information. Both values would be high, similar to her hemoglobin A_{1c}.

This patient is much more likely to have type 1 diabetes than maturity-onset diabetes of the young (MODY), both statistically and because of her family history, and testing for pathogenic variants in the *GCK* gene (Answer C) or the *HNF1A* gene (Answer D) would only be indicated if the ZnT8 antibody measurement is negative.

EDUCATIONAL OBJECTIVE

Select the best test to confirm the diagnosis of type 1 diabetes.

REFERENCE(S)

Rochmah N, Faizi M, Windarti SW. Zinc transporter 8 autoantibody in the diagnosis of type 1 diabetes in children. *Clin Exp Pediatr.* 2020;63(10):402-405. PMID: 33050689

Williams CL, Long AE. What has zinc transporter 8 autoimmunity taught us about type 1 diabetes? *Diabetologia.* 2019;62(11):1969-1976. PMID: 31444530

Mrena S, Virtanen SM, Laippala P, et al. Models for predicting type 1 diabetes in siblings of affected children. *Diabetes Care.* 2006;29(3):662-667. PMID: 16505523

Andersson C, Vaziri-Sani F, Delli A, et al; BDD Study Group. Triple specificity of ZnT8 autoantibodies in relation to HLA and other islet autoantibodies in childhood and adolescent type 1 diabetes. *Pediatr Diabetes.* 2013;14(2):97-105. PMID: 22957668

Gorus FK, Balti EV, Vermeulen I, et al. Screening for insulinoma antigen 2 and zinc transporter 8 autoantibodies: a cost-effective and age-dependent strategy to identify rapid progressors to clinical onset among relatives of type 1 diabetic patients. *Clin Exp Immunol.* 2013;171(1):82-90. PMID: 23199327

25 ANSWER: C) Lifestyle intervention

For this patient, lifestyle intervention (Answer C) would be preferred over metformin (Answer D) based on findings from available studies, mainly the landmark Diabetes Prevention Program. In the Diabetes Prevention Program, 3234 patients with obesity (average BMI, 34 kg/m^2) aged 25 to 85 years (average age, 51 years) at high risk for diabetes (based on BMI ≥24 kg/m^2 and fasting and 2-hour plasma glucose concentrations of 96 to 125 mg/dL [5.3-6.9 mmol/L] and 140 to 199 mg/dL [7.8-11.1 mmol/L], respectively) were randomly assigned to one of the following groups:

- Intensive lifestyle changes with the aim of reducing weight by 7% through a behavioral modification program aimed at a low-fat diet and exercise for 150 minutes per week
- Treatment with metformin (850 mg twice daily) plus information on diet and exercise
- Placebo plus information on diet and exercise

After an average follow-up of 3 years, fewer patients in the intensive lifestyle group developed diabetes, as diagnosed by fasting plasma glucose and 2-hour postload glucose concentrations (14% vs 22% and 29% in the metformin and placebo groups, respectively). The intensive lifestyle and metformin interventions reduced the cumulative incidence of diabetes by 58% and 31%, respectively. Lifestyle intervention was effective in men and women in all age groups and in all ethnic groups.

In a follow-up observational study (the Diabetes Prevention Program Outcomes Study), the benefit of lifestyle intervention was shown to persist more than 10 years. In this study, 85% of patients originally enrolled in the Diabetes Prevention Program joined the long-term follow-up and were offered group-implemented lifestyle intervention. Patients originally assigned to metformin continued receiving it (unblinded). During a cumulative 10 years of follow-up, the incidence of diabetes in the lifestyle and metformin groups was significantly reduced by 34% and 18%, respectively, compared with placebo. In older individuals (≥60 years of age at baseline), lifestyle intervention was particularly effective (72% reduction in diabetes compared with reduction in placebo group), while metformin was relatively less effective. Conversely, metformin was particularly effective in individuals who were younger (<60 years), had a higher BMI (>35 kg/m^2), and were at highest risk of developing diabetes.

The Actos Now for Prevention of Diabetes study assessed the ability of pioglitazone (Answer E) (30 to 45 mg daily) to reduce the risk of developing diabetes in 600 patients with impaired glucose tolerance and 1 or more components of the metabolic syndrome. After a median follow-up period of 2.4 years, fewer patients randomly assigned to pioglitazone developed diabetes (5.0% vs 16.7% with placebo; hazard ratio, 0.28 [95% CI, 0.16-0.49]). Weight gain was significantly greater with pioglitazone (3.9 vs 0.77 kg), and edema was more common (12.9% vs 6.4%). Pioglitazone should not be used for diabetes prevention in this patient because of potential adverse effects (fluid retention, weight gain, heart failure), especially since she already has 2+ edema on examination.

There are no studies on empagliflozin (Answer B) or dulaglutide (Answer A) with respect to diabetes prevention, although in cardiovascular outcome trials, individuals with prediabetes treated with an SGLT-2 inhibitor or incretin therapy showed a decrease in progression to diabetes that lasts as long as the medications are continued.

EDUCATIONAL OBJECTIVE

Identify prediabetes (impaired fasting glucose and impaired glucose tolerance) and recommend the best way to prevent progression to diabetes.

REFERENCE(S)

Dunkley AJ, Bodicoat DH, Greaves CJ, et al. Diabetes prevention in the real world: effectiveness of pragmatic lifestyle interventions for the prevention of type 2 diabetes and of the impact of adherence to guideline recommendations: a systematic review and meta-analysis. *Diabetes Care.* 2014;37(4):922-933. PMID: 24652723

Knowler WC, Barrett-Connor E, Fowler SE, et al; Diabetes Prevention Program Research Group. Reduction in the incidence of type 2 diabetes with lifestyle intervention or metformin. *N Engl J Med.* 2002;346(6):393-403. PMID: 11832527

Diabetes Prevention Program Research Group, Knowler WC, Fowler SE, et al. 10-year follow-up of diabetes incidence and weight loss in the Diabetes Prevention Program Outcomes Study [published correction appears in *Lancet.* 2009;374(9707):2054]. *Lancet.* 2009;374(9702):1677-1686. PMID: 19878986

DeFronzo RA, Tripathy D, Schwenke DC, et al; ACT NOW Study. Pioglitazone for diabetes prevention in impaired glucose tolerance [published corrections appear in *N Engl J Med.* 2011;365(2):189 and *N Engl J Med.* 2011;365(9):869]. *N Engl J Med.* 2011;364(12):1104-1115. PMID: 21428766

Diabetes Prevention Program Research Group. Long-term effects of lifestyle intervention or metformin on diabetes development and microvascular complications over 15-year follow-up: the Diabetes Prevention Program Outcomes Study. *Lancet Diabetes Endocrinol.* 2015;3(11):866-875. PMID: 26377054

26 ANSWER: C) 500-1000 mL/h of 0.9% NaCl; no insulin bolus, start 10 units/h

The recommended fluid replacement is 500 to 1000 mL/h of 0.9% NaCl for the first 2 to 4 hours, watching for any issues with fluid overload. An insulin bolus is not recommended, and the starting dose of intravenous insulin should be 0.1 unit/kg per h, which is 10 units/h for this patient (Answer C).

He meets the criteria for the hyperosmolar hyperglycemic state. The diagnostic criteria are a plasma glucose concentration greater than 600 mg/dL (>33.3 mmol/L), effective serum

	2a. DKA Diagnostic Criteria	
DKA	**D**iabetes/hyperglycemia	Glucose ≥200 mg/dL (11.1 mmol/L) *OR* prior history of diabetes
	Ketosis	β-hydroxybutyrate concentration ≥3.0 mmol/L *OR* urine ketone strip 2+ or greater
	Metabolic **A**cidosis	pH <7.3 and/or bicarbonate concentration <18 mmol/L
	2b. HHS Diagnostic Criteria	
HHS	**H**yperglycemia	Plasma glucose ≥600 mg/dL (33.3 mmol/L)
	Hyperosmolarity	Calculated effective serum osmolality >300 osm/kg (calculated as [2xNa⁺ (mmol/L) + glucose (mmol/L)]), *OR* total serum osmolality >320 osm/kg [(2xNa⁺ (mmol/L) + glucose (mmol/L) + urea (mmol/L)]
	Ab**S**ence of significant ketonemia	β-hydroxybutyrate concentration <3.0 mmol/L *OR* urine ketone strip less than 2+
	Absence of acidosis	pH ≥7.3 and bicarbonate concentration ≥15 mmol/L

Reprinted from "Hyperglycemic Crises in Adults with Diabetes: A Consensus Report," Guillermo E. Umpierrez et al. *Diabetes Care*, June 22, 2024. © by The American Diabetes Association and the European Association.

osmolality greater than 300 mOsm/kg (>300 mmol/kg), arterial pH greater than 7.3, serum bicarbonate concentration greater than 15 mEq/L (>15 mmol/L), and β-hydroxybutyrate concentration less than 3.1 mg/dL (<300 μmol/L).

The most common precipitating factors for hyperosmolar hyperglycemic state are infection (often pneumonia or urinary tract infection) and discontinuation of or inadequate insulin therapy. Compromised water intake due to underlying medical conditions, particularly in older patients, can promote the development of severe dehydration and the hyperosmolar hyperglycemic state. Other conditions and factors associated with the hyperosmolar hyperglycemic state include acute major illnesses such as myocardial infarction, cerebrovascular accident, sepsis, or pancreatitis, etc.

The hyperosmolar hyperglycemic state is treated with fluids and insulin. Because of severe dehydration, isotonic 0.9% NaCl is initiated at a rate of 500 to 1000 mL/h over the first 2 to 4 hours (thus, Answers D and E are incorrect).

After restoration of intravascular volume, the subsequent choice for fluid replacement depends on the patient's state of hydration. The goal is to correct the estimated deficits within the first 24 to 48 hours, with caution in older adults and those with comorbid conditions who could be negatively affected by rapid fluid replacement.

The decline in glucose should not exceed 90 to 120 mg/dL per h, the decline in serum sodium should not exceed 10 mEq/L in 24 hours, and the decline in osmolality should be no greater than 3.0 to 8.0 mOsm/kg per h. The administration of 0.45% sodium chloride is only indicated if osmolality is not decreasing despite adequate positive fluid balance and insulin administration.

A decision is then made as to whether to continue the 0.9% NaCl or switch to 0.45% NaCl depending on volume status and corrected serum sodium. In fact, in this patient, the corrected serum sodium was 145 mEq/L (145 mmol/L) (serum sodium may be corrected by adding 1.6 mg/dL to the measured serum sodium for each 100 mg/dL of glucose above 100 mg/dL [>5.6 mmol/L]).

For treatment of the hyperosmolar hyperglycemic state, intravenous insulin should be initiated with an intravenous drip of fixed-rate regular insulin at 0.1 units/kg body weight. In this patient, who weighs approximately 100 kg, this calculates to be 10 units/h. An initial bolus of insulin is not recommended for most people with hyperosmolar hyperglycemic state (thus, Answers A and B are incorrect).

EDUCATIONAL OBJECTIVE

Manage the hyperosmolar hyperglycemic state.

REFERENCE(S)

Umpierrez GE, Davis GM, ElSayed NA, et al. Hyperglycaemic crises in adults with diabetes: a consensus report. *Diabetologia*. 2024 [Online ahead of print]

Diabetes Mellitus, Section 2 Board Review

Marie McDonnell, MD

27 **ANSWER: E) Semaglutide**

Metabolic dysfunction-associated steatotic liver disease (MASLD) is the term used to identify a spectrum of conditions ranging from macrovesicular hepatic steatosis only (or with mild inflammation) to steatohepatitis (metabolic steatohepatitis [MASH]) to cirrhosis in the absence of ongoing or recent consumption of significant amounts of alcohol (defined as ingestion of >21 standard drinks per week in men and >14 standard drinks per week in women over a 2-year period preceding evaluation) or the presence of other secondary causes of fatty liver disease. Recent studies in adults estimate that MASLD is present in more than 70% of people with type 2 diabetes, half of whom have MASH. MASH also adds significantly to the already increased cancer risk among those with diabetes and/or obesity.

Many studies have illustrated that relying on transaminitis as a MASLD indicator is not sensitive, yet abdominal imaging alone is not sufficient. The Fibrosis 4 (FIB-4) tool was therefore appropriately used in this vignette as the most cost-effective first discriminatory test to determine the risk of advanced MASLD. The patient's value was found to be in the indeterminant range. FIB-4 estimates the risk of hepatic cirrhosis and is calculated from the computation of age, plasma aminotransferase concentrations (AST and ALT), and platelet count. A value less than 1.3 is considered lower risk (fibrosis stage 0 or 1), while a value greater than 2.67 indicates a high probability of advanced fibrosis (fibrosis stage 4). An indeterminate value should lead, as in this case, to a second noninvasive test such as elastography to measure liver stiffness.

In this patient, elastography showed a low likelihood of advanced cirrhosis. Thus, a therapeutic approach should be selected that reduces or resolves MASH, with the goal of preventing advanced liver disease. Current first-line treatment in these patients is lifestyle intervention to achieve weight loss and improve cardiometabolic comorbidities, but there is no approved MASH-specific pharmacotherapeutic treatment. In a phase 3 randomized controlled trial, 320 individuals with and without type 2 diabetes and/or obesity were assigned to either low-dosage semaglutide (Answer E) (0.1 to 0.4 mg) or placebo. MASH resolution was achieved with no worsening of fibrosis stage in 40% to 59% of individuals in the semaglutide group in a dosage-dependent manner vs 17% in the placebo group. This may have been mediated mainly by weight loss, which was 13% in the semaglutide arm and 1% in the placebo arm. Importantly, this benefit was not apparent in a population of patients with MASH and established cirrhosis (fibrosis stage 4) in a recently published randomized controlled trial.

Pioglitazone (Answer D) would be the most appropriate choice for a patient with MASLD and established fibrosis (fibrosis stages 1-3) after weight loss is achieved by lifestyle and/or medical therapies. Pioglitazone should be avoided in those exhibiting signs of volume overload on examination, as in this patient who has pedal edema.

Phentermine (Answer C) could induce beneficial weight loss, but it has not been shown to improve MASH and is not the best choice in the setting of suboptimally controlled blood pressure.

Icosapent ethyl (Answer A) would likely reduce triglyceride levels, which is an important clinical goal in MASLD-oriented management, but it has not been shown to improve MASH in humans.

Resuming metformin (Answer B) is a good choice for adjunctive diabetes therapy, and could be resumed safely, but it is unknown whether it directly improves MASH.

EDUCATIONAL OBJECTIVE

Select the best therapies to treat patients with diabetes and metabolic steatohepatitis.

REFERENCE(S)

Newsome PN, Buchholtz K, Cusi K, et al; NN9931-4296 Investigators. A placebo-controlled trial of subcutaneous semaglutide in nonalcoholic steatohepatitis. *N Engl J Med.* 2021;384(12):1113-1124. PMID: 33185364

Kanwal F, Shubrook JH, Younossi Z, et al. Preparing for the NASH epidemic: a call to action. *Obesity (Silver Spring).* 2021;29(9):1401-1412. PMID: 34365735

American Diabetes Association Professional Practice Committee. 4. Comprehensive medical evaluation and assessment of comorbidities: standards of care in diabetes-2024. *Diabetes Care.* 2024;47(Suppl 1):S52-S76. PMID: 38078591

28 ANSWER: B) BMI >30 kg/m^2

Medical transplant committees are designed to determine an individual's transplant candidacy by thoughtfully and carefully weighing the 2 sides of the medical decision-making equation; namely, risk and benefit. While selection criteria for pancreas transplant vary by center, general criteria include age younger than 65 years, insulin-requiring diabetes, labile blood glucose (usually with hypoglycemia), fasting C-peptide concentration less than 10 ng/mL (<3.3 nmol/L), and BMI less than 30 kg/m^2 (thus, Answer B is correct). The maximum allowable BMI for pancreas transplant varies among centers, but it is often lower than that for kidney transplant because pancreas transplant requires intra-abdominal surgery. As a result, postoperative wound healing and complications are thought to be affected to a greater extent by elevated BMI. Moreover, in some studies, increasing recipient BMI is an independent risk factor for pancreas graft loss in both the short and long term. While her BMI would not disqualify her from pancreas transplant in many programs in the United States, any potential benefits of transplant must be balanced by this increased risk. Most centers therefore use a BMI threshold of 30 kg/m^2. Some centers consider performing simultaneous pancreas-kidney transplant in selected patients with a BMI in the range of 30 to 35 kg/m^2, whereas very few pancreas transplants are performed in patients with a BMI greater than 35 kg/m^2.

Another consideration is that some have reported improved endogenous insulin production over time after starting targeted therapy for cystic fibrosis. Therefore, in this case, the committee voiced questions about the long-term benefit of pancreas transplant, especially in light of the risk, and decided to reevaluate the patient in 6 months to determine the potential benefit and her ability to lose weight.

Time since last transplant is not a consideration (thus, Answer A is incorrect). Overall health and kidney graft function have a role in determining the best approach. This patient's kidney function is acceptable for pancreas transplant, and, in fact, a diminished estimated glomerular filtration rate would generally expedite being listed for pancreas transplant to benefit long-term kidney graft function (thus, Answer D is incorrect).

Although pancreas transplant is overall less common in people with advanced cystic fibrosis–related diabetes than in people with type 1 and type 2 diabetes, patients who meet the above criteria should be considered for pancreas transplant (thus, Answer C is incorrect).

Having a hemoglobin A_{1c} value less than 8.0% (<64 mmol/mol) is generally not a major criterion to determine benefit of pancreas transplant (thus, Answer E is incorrect).

Importantly, evidence of diminished quality of life or diabetes-related distress is also an important consideration in weighing risk and benefit. In many centers, diabetes-related distress is measured or similar tools are used, such as the Type 1 Diabetes Distress scale. Based on what this patient reported to the clinical team, she would likely have a score greater than 3, indicating severe distress. This adds substantially to the benefit side of the equation for pancreas-after-kidney transplant.

EDUCATIONAL OBJECTIVE

Determine selection considerations for pancreas transplant.

REFERENCE(S)

Nordheim E, Lindahl JP, Carlsen RK, et al. Patient selection for islet or solid organ pancreas transplantation: experiences from a multidisciplinary outpatient-clinic approach. *Endocr Connect.* 2021;10(2):230-239. PMID: 33544090

Bédat B, Niclauss N, Jannot AS, Andres A, Toso C, Morel P, Berney T. Impact of recipient body mass index on short-term and long-term survival of pancreatic grafts. *Transplantation.* 2015;99(1):94-9. PMID: 24914570

Hessler DM, Fisher L, Polonsky WH, et al. Diabetes distress is linked with worsening diabetes management over time in adults with type 1 diabetes. *Diabet Med.* 2017;34(9):1228-1234. PMID: 28498610

Fridell JA, Bozic MA, Ulrich BJ, Lutz AJ, Powelson JA. Pancreas transplantation for cystic fibrosis: a frequently missed opportunity. *Clin Transplant.* 2021;35(9):e14371. PMID: 34032335

Taelman V, Declercq D, Van Biervliet S, Weygaerde YV, Lapauw B, Van Braeckel E. Effect of 18 months elexacaftor-tezacaftor-ivacaftor on body mass index and glycemic control in adults with cystic fibrosis. *Clin Nutr ESPEN.* 2023;58:73-78. PMID: 38057039

29 ANSWER: D) Order echocardiography

This patient has a high risk of cardiovascular disease given her history of longstanding suboptimal control of major risk factors, and she now presents with overall decompensation after a period of good glycemic control. Her concern of general fatigue led to an appropriately focused but comprehensive evaluation, including thyroid function tests, vitamin B_{12} measurement (given long-term metformin use), and natriuretic peptide measurement (to screen for heart failure). Adults with diabetes are at increased risk for the development of asymptomatic cardiac structural or functional abnormalities (stage B heart failure) or symptomatic (stage C) heart failure. Both the American Diabetes Association and the American Heart Association now recommend that measurement of natriuretic peptide (B-type natriuretic peptide [BNP] or N-terminal pro-BNP [NT-proBNP]) be considered when screening for asymptomatic heart failure in people with diabetes to facilitate the prevention of, or progression to, symptomatic stages of heart failure. This is based on observational data from large studies, showing, for example, that a baseline NT-proBNP concentration of 125 pg/mL or higher predicts heart failure hospitalization and all-cause mortality. In people with diabetes and an abnormal natriuretic peptide value, echocardiography (Answer D) is recommended as the next step to screen for structural heart disease, and echocardiographic Doppler indices should be used to identify evidence of diastolic dysfunction and increased filling pressure.

When ordering measurement of natriuretic peptides, one must remember that both peptides can be elevated in the setting of suboptimal glycemic control, and they improve once glucose is lowered. Other conditions can cause elevations, such as kidney insufficiency (which could be a factor in this case), pulmonary disease (eg, pulmonary hypertension and chronic obstructive lung disease), obstructive sleep apnea, ischemic and hemorrhagic stroke, and anemia. There is also an inverse relationship between NT-proBNP levels and BMI, which is not a concern in the absence of obesity, as in this case.

Adding carvedilol (Answer A) or increasing the losartan dosage (Answer B) may be appropriate steps following a diagnosis of heart failure, but neither is the best next step since that diagnosis has not been made.

Currently, the dual SGLT-1/2 inhibitor sotagliflozin (Answer E) is recommended for people with diabetes and established heart failure to reduce risk of worsening heart failure and cardiovascular death. However, it has not yet been compared head-to-head with SGLT-2 inhibitors for this or other indications. In this case, since the diagnosis of heart failure has not been established and empagliflozin has similar cardiovascular benefits, there is no reason to consider switching from empagliflozin.

Determining the ankle-brachial index (Answer C) is recommended given that she is older than 50 years and has microvascular disease. However, because she does not have a specific symptom or finding on examination suggestive of severe peripheral arterial disease, evaluation of elevated natriuretic peptide should be prioritized.

EDUCATIONAL OBJECTIVE

Guide screening for heart failure by measuring natriuretic peptides in individuals with type 2 diabetes who are at high risk.

REFERENCE(S)

American Diabetes Association Professional Practice Committee. 10. Cardiovascular Disease and Risk Management: Standards of Care in Diabetes—2024. *Diabetes Care.* 2024;47(Suppl 1):S179-S218). PMID: 38078592

Dal K, Ata N, Yavuz B, et al. The relationship between glycemic control and BNP levels in diabetic patients. *Cardiol J.* 2014;21(3):252-256. PMID: 23990181

Pandey A, Vaduganathan M, Patel KV, et al. Biomarker-based risk prediction of incident heart failure in pre-diabetes and diabetes. *JACC Heart Fail.* 2021;9(3):215-223. PMID: 33422434

Bhatt DL, Szarek M, Steg PG, et al; SOLOIST-WHF Trial Investigators. Sotagliflozin in patients with diabetes and recent worsening heart failure. *N Engl J Med.* 2021;384(2):117-128. PMID: 33200892

30 ANSWER: D) Pioglitazone

Pioglitazone (Answer D) is the third thiazolidinedione to be marketed and is the most widely used drug from this class of antihyperglycemic medications. Following FDA approval of the first agent in 1997, thiazolidinediones were initially celebrated as potent glucose-lowering agents that directly target the fundamental problem of insulin resistance in classic type 2 diabetes. Pioglitazone was also the first diabetes drug in this class shown to lower the risk of cardiovascular events in people with type 2 diabetes who are at high cardiovascular risk. Pioglitazone also lowers hemoglobin A_{1c} and triglyceride levels. However, postmarketing studies, published cases, and eventually prospective trials indicated several serious potential adverse effects, including volume overload in individuals with congestive heart failure, new-onset clinical congestive heart failure, peripheral edema, weight gain, and bone fractures. There were also concerns about a potential link between thiazolidinediones and bladder cancer, which has resulted in the warning on the package insert to avoid use in those with a family or personal history of bladder cancer. Several studies have shown that these adverse effects are dosage related.

In treatment guidelines, pioglitazone is recommended in selected individuals after balancing potential risks and benefits. There are several reasons why benefits likely outweigh risks for the patient in this clinical vignette. First, he does not have any contraindications to the medication, and his N-terminal pro-B-type natriuretic peptide concentration is reassuringly in the normal range, making the risk of new-onset clinical heart failure low. Second, his glycemic control is suboptimal. Because he is in good overall health with some nephropathy, a hemoglobin A_{1c} target near 7.0% (53 mmol/mol) is most appropriate. Pioglitazone is as potent as metformin for glucose lowering, achieving 0.5% to 1% lowering of hemoglobin A_{1c}. Third, 2 large randomized controlled clinical trials document the cardiovascular safety and potential benefit of pioglitazone. In the IRIS trial (Pioglitazone after Ischemic Stroke or Transient Ischemic Attack), more than 3000 individuals with insulin resistance and a history of stroke or transient ischemic attack were randomly assigned to either pioglitazone or placebo. Over an average follow-up of 4.8 years, patients assigned to pioglitazone experienced a 24% relative risk reduction in fatal and nonfatal stroke or myocardial infarction (hazard ratio, 0.76 [95% CI, 0.62-0.93]; $P = .007$; absolute risk reduction, 2.8%). While the IRIS trial did not include people with overt diabetes, it is plausible that this benefit could be extended to individuals with type 2 diabetes since the benefit was seen in trial participants who had prediabetes. In the PROspective pioglitAzone Clinical Trial In macroVascular Events (PROactive) study, 5000 patients with type 2 diabetes and a history of macrovascular disease were randomized assigned to pioglitazone or placebo and were followed for up to 3 years. While the study failed to show a significant reduction in the primary composite outcome, there was a consistent reduction in most of the individual components of the primary end point. The risk of mortality, nonfatal myocardial infarction, silent myocardial infarction, stroke, major leg amputation, and acute coronary syndromes was lower with pioglitazone relative to risk in the placebo group. In addition, for the main secondary end point, which included all-cause mortality, nonfatal myocardial infarction and stroke, pioglitazone was associated with a 16% relative risk reduction ($P = .02$), demonstrating the number needed to treat of 48 patients for 3 years to avoid 1 first major cardiovascular event.

Linagliptin (Answer B) is not likely to achieve hemoglobin A_{1c} lowering of more than 0.4%, and it therefore lacks sufficient potency.

Glyburide (Answer A), a sulfonylurea, is not preferred in older adults due to concerns regarding hypoglycemia. Moreover, glyburide is the least-preferred sulfonylurea agent, particularly in those with cardiovascular disease, because safety data from prospective trials are lacking.

Oral semaglutide (Answer C) is a GLP-1 receptor agonist, and the patient has already declined being rechallenged with this drug class. At this time, there are no proven cardiovascular benefits of the oral form of semaglutide.

The premeal secretogogue repaglinide (Answer E) is a reasonable option, but it is not ideal in this case because it requires more than once-daily dosing to achieve the desired degree of glycemic control, and the patient has indicated this would not be feasible for him.

EDUCATIONAL OBJECTIVE

Select patients who would benefit from thiazolidinedione therapy.

REFERENCE(S)

Dormandy JA, Charbonnel B, Eckland DJA, et al; PROactive Investigators. Secondary prevention of macrovascular events in patients with type 2 diabetes in the PROactive Study (PROspective pioglitAzone Clinical Trial In macroVascular Events): a randomised controlled trial. *Lancet.* 2005;366(9493):1279-1289. PMID: 16214598

Kernan WN Viscoli CM, Furie K, et al; IRIS Trial Investigators. Pioglitazone after ischemic stroke or transient ischemic attack. *N Engl J Med.* 2016;374(14):1321-1231. PMID: 26886418

Pavo I, Jermendy G, Varkonyi TT, et al. Effect of pioglitazone compared with metformin on glycemic control and indicators of insulin sensitivity in recently diagnosed patients with type 2 diabetes. *J Clin Endocrinol Metab.* 2003;88(4):1637-1645. PMID: 12679450

31 ANSWER: D) Discontinue tramadol

Post–gastric bypass hypoglycemia is defined as recurrent episodes of postmeal glucose values less than 70 mg/dL (<3.9 mmol/L) with classic symptoms relieved by the ingestion of glucose. This patient has had stable post–gastric bypass hypoglycemia for some time while following a low-carbohydrate diet and taking acarbose before meals. A posthospital exacerbation of a previously controlled chronic condition should always prompt a careful medication review. In this case, moderate- to high-dosage tramadol use is the most likely explanation for renewed difficulty in managing her postmeal hypoglycemia. Based on numerous case reports, reported episodes to the FDA, and analyses of public data from clinical trials, hypoglycemia is considered an adverse drug reaction of tramadol, which can be observed in people with or without diabetes. Tramadol should therefore be discontinued in this patient (Answer D).

Given the results of inpatient glucose monitoring and the hemoglobin A_{1c} value, she still has some degree of glucose dysregulation after Roux-en-Y gastric bypass, so metformin is likely to be of continued benefit and should not be discontinued (Answer C). She takes it at bedtime, and she was tolerating it before her recent hospitalization.

While acetaminophen can lead to falsely low readings on some continuous glucose monitoring devices, this is not the case with hospital-approved, point-of-care blood glucose monitors, so acetaminophen does not need to be stopped (Answer B).

Acarbose is an effective treatment for most cases of post–gastric bypass hypoglycemia, and reinitiating it would not be expected to increase the frequency or severity of episodes. Thus, it does not need to be discontinued (Answer A).

Likewise, a balanced diet that relies on proteins, fats, and undigestible fiber (and less on carbohydrates) is the general nutritional strategy for post–gastric bypass hypoglycemia. In this case, diet is not likely a key factor contributing to her worsening hypoglycemia, given her previous success, and a reduction in dietary fat (Answer E) is not needed.

EDUCATIONAL OBJECTIVE

Identify medications that increase the risk of clinically significant hypoglycemia.

REFERENCE(S)

Juba KM, van Manen RP, Fellows SE. A review of the Food and Drug Administration Adverse Event Reporting System for tramadol-related hypoglycemia. *Ann Pharmacother.* 2020;54(3):247-253. PMID: 31648533

De Canecaude C, Rousseau V, Sommet A, Montastruc JL. Tramadol-induced hypoglycemia: a pharmacovigilance study. *Fundam Clin Pharmacol.* 2021;35(5):933-936. PMID: 33511683

Salehi M, Vella A, McLaughlin T, Patti ME. Hypoglycemia after gastric bypass surgery: current concepts and controversies. *J Clin Endocrinol Metab.* 2018;103(8):2815-2826. PMID: 30101281

Patience N, Sheehan A, Cummings C, Patti ME. Medical nutrition therapy and other approaches to management of post-bariatric hypoglycemia: a team-based approach. *Curr Obes Rep.* 2022;11(4):277-286. PMID: 36074258

32 ANSWER: A) Add eplerenone, 25 mg daily

The most important factor to address in this case is uncontrolled hypertension in the face of recurrent stroke risk. People with diabetes and confirmed resistant hypertension should be evaluated for secondary causes of hypertension, including primary hyperaldosteronism, renal artery stenosis, diabetic kidney disease, and obstructive sleep apnea. In general, barriers to taking medication (such as cost and adverse effects) should be identified and addressed. In patients whose hypertension is uncontrolled while taking medications from each of the 3 main antihypertensive drug classes (ACE/ARB, calcium channel blocker, and diuretic), the next therapeutic step is to add a mineralocorticoid receptor antagonist with good blood pressure–lowering effect such as eplerenone (Answer A) or spironolactone. This guidance is in recognition of the fact that excess mineralocorticoid activity has a role in most cases of resistant hypertension.

Evaluating for secondary causes or risk factors is critical in resistant hypertension. Since her aldosterone concentration is normal without a suppressed or low renin value and her metanephrine concentration is normal, neither primary aldosteronism nor pheochromocytoma (which would benefit from surgical intervention) is a likely diagnosis. Thus, imaging the adrenal glands (Answer D) is not necessary.

She has no symptoms of sleep apnea, as she feels refreshed in morning and does not require a nap during the day. A sleep study (Answer E) might be considered in the future, but it is not the best next step.

While labetalol (Answer B) is often used as a fourth-line agent for hypertension management, in most people with diabetes, this is not preferred over mineralocorticoid antagonism.

In 2023, the US FDA approved sotagliflozin (Answer C), a dual inhibitor of SGLT 1 and 2, for people with either heart failure or type 2 diabetes to reduce the risk of death from cardiovascular causes, hospitalization for heart failure, and urgent heart failure visits. These indications are based on the design and results of the phase 3 clinical trials

SOLIST-WHF and SCORED. Although sotagliflozin has a modest blood pressure–lowering effect, it is not indicated to treat hypertension, and it is less effective than eplerenone. Compared with outcomes with placebo, mean lowering of systolic blood pressure is approximately 3.85 mm Hg with sotagliflozin vs 9.21 mm Hg with eplerenone.

EDUCATIONAL OBJECTIVE

Treat resistant hypertension in people with diabetes.

REFERENCE(S)

American Diabetes Association Professional Practice Committee. 4. Comprehensive medical evaluation and assessment of comorbidities: standards of care in diabetes-2024. *Diabetes Care.* 2024;47(Suppl 1):S52-S76. PMID: 38078591

Williams B, MacDonald TM, Morant S, et al; British Hypertension Society's PATHWAY Studies Group. Spironolactone versus placebo, bisoprolol, and doxazosin to determine the optimal treatment for drug-resistant hypertension (PATHWAY-2): a randomised, double-blind, crossover trial. *Lancet.* 2015;386(2059-2068. PMID: 26414968

Bakris GL, Agarwal R, Chan JC, et al; Mineralocorticoid Receptor Antagonist Tolerability Study–Diabetic Nephropathy (ARTS-DN) Study Group. Effect of finerenone on albuminuria in patients with diabetic nephropathy: a randomized clinical trial. *JAMA.* 2015;314(9):884-894PMID: 26325557

Wu J, Zhao X, Chen H, Zhu S. Metabolic effects of the dual SGLT 1/2 inhibitor sotagliflozin on blood pressure and body weight reduction in people with diabetes: an updated meta-analysis of randomized controlled trials. *J Diabetes Complications.* 2022;36(12):108352. PMID: 36370667

Tam TS, Wu MH, Masson SC, et al. Eplerenone for hypertension. *Cochrane Database Syst Rev.* 2017;2(2):CD008996. PMID: 28245343

33 **ANSWER: C) 3 years**

The US Preventive Task Force recommends screening for prediabetes and type 2 diabetes in adults aged 35 to 70 years who have overweight or obesity. In recognition of the lack of sensitivity of BMI as a predictor of type 2 diabetes in some ethnic groups, the American Diabetes Association recommends a more aggressive screening approach, suggesting that screening should begin at age 35 years regardless of other factors such as ethnicity, family history, BMI, blood pressure, and dyslipidemia. Moreover, per the American Diabetes Association, in asymptomatic adults younger than 35 years, diabetes screening should be considered in patients who have overweight or obesity and have 1 or more of the following risk factors: first-degree relative with diabetes, high-risk race/ethnicity, history of cardiovascular disease, hypertension, HDL-cholesterol concentration less than 35 mg/dL (<0.91 mmol/L) and/or triglyceride concentration greater than 250 mg/dL (>2.83 mmol/L), polycystic ovary syndrome (in women), and physical inactivity. Recent additions to this risk factor list are people who are prescribed medications that could increase the risk of developing diabetes, including second-generation antipsychotic medications, glucocorticoids, statins, thiazide diuretics, and HIV medications, emphasizing the importance of screening before any of these agents are initiated.

Repeat testing over the lifespan depends on the result of the initial screening test and the presence of other risk factors, but in most adults, screening should be repeated at least every 3 years. While adults with a prediabetes-range hemoglobin A_{1c} value should have annual testing, women diagnosed with gestational diabetes should have lifelong testing at least every 3 years (Answer C). As this patient does not have prediabetes, annual screening (Answer B) is not indicated, although this could be considered if her overall risk increases (eg, in the setting of weight gain), newly identified hypertension, or starting one of the aforementioned medications).

Screening every 5 years (Answer D) or every 10 years (Answer E) is too infrequent for most at-risk adults. This is particularly true for this woman because the risk of developing diabetes following gestational diabetes is estimated to be 50% within the first 5 years postpartum, and it continues to increase by approximately 10% every year thereafter.

EDUCATIONAL OBJECTIVE

Guide diabetes screening in adults at high risk based on standard recommendations.

REFERENCE(S)

American Diabetes Association Professional Practice Committee. 2. Diagnosis and classification of diabetes: standards of care in diabetes-2024. *Diabetes Care.* 2024;47(Suppl 1):S20-S42. PMID: 38078589

US Preventive Services Task Force. Prediabetes and Type 2 Diabetes: Screening. 2021. https://www.uspreventiveservicestaskforce.org/uspstf/recommendation/screening-for-prediabetes-and-type-2-diabetes

34 ANSWER: B) Increase glucose target to 130 mg/dL (7.2 mmol/L) for 4 hours after a run and take carbohydrate as needed every 30 minutes

Continuous glucose monitoring allows for a patient-tailored approach to reduce hypoglycemia due to exercise in people with diabetes, as addressed in detail in a multisociety expert consensus statement. According to this statement, this patient has a moderate risk of hypoglycemia based on the time-below-range between 4% and 8%, with heightened concern given the time-very-below-range (<54 mg/dL [<3.0 mmol/L]) of 2%. Although he reports awareness of and lack of fear about hypoglycemia, he has at least a moderate baseline risk of severe episodes.

The guidance highlights the risk of delayed postexercise hypoglycemia in certain individuals. During the first 90 minutes following exercise, an interstitial glucose range of 80 to 180 mg/dL (4.4-10.0 mmol/L) might be targeted in most people with type 1 diabetes who are at a low risk of hypoglycemia, but people with an elevated risk of hypoglycemia are recommended to increase the lower limit of sensor glucose to 90 mg/dL (5.0 mmol/L) or 100 mg/dL (5.6 mmol/L) during the postexercise period and to potentially extend the period with the higher target. The most efficient way to avoid glucose concentrations lower than this suggested limit is to raise the programmed target glucose in his pump. Given that his risk period extends for as long as 4 hours, it is reasonable to increase his usual target from 100 to 130 mg/dL (5.6 to 7.2 mmol/L) for 4 hours after a run (Answer B). He could also opt to extend the "exercise activity" (target of 150 mg/dL [8.3 mmol/L] on his automated insulin delivery pump) for up to 4 hours as well, but this is likely to cause hyperglycemia and was not presented as an option.

If the lower limit is reached, consumption of simple carbohydrates every 30 minutes depends on the direction that the continuous glucose monitor's arrow recommends. For example, 10 g of carbohydrates is recommended if the trend arrow is horizontal; 15 g of carbohydrates if the trend arrow is slight downward; and 30 g or more if the trend arrow is rapidly falling downward. Treatment should be repeated if sensor glucose does not rise within 30 minutes as reflected by trend arrows.

Unnecessary hyperglycemia should be avoided before, during, and after exercise, as this can reduce efficiency and relative insulin deficiency and/or cause sluggishness and subsequent hypoglycemia from overcorrection, as seen in this case. For this reason, ingesting a gel oral supplement with 30 g of carbohydrate every 15 minutes of exercise as long as glucose is between 126 and 180 mg/dL (7.0-10.0 mmol/L) (Answer D) and ingesting a meal with 60 g of carbohydrate without an insulin bolus before a run (Answer C) are incorrect because they would likely produce significant hyperglycemia.

Glucagon (Answer E) is an important therapy for severe hypoglycemia, but it should not be relied on after exercise, which is a state of glycogen depletion.

If the sensor glucose is rapidly increasing in the postexercise phase (detected by continuous glucose monitoring when using the rate-of-change alert), then an insulin correction can be considered, but this should be 50% of the typical correction dose. A correction factor of 1:20 (Answer A) is more aggressive than 1:40, so this would be incorrect.

EDUCATIONAL OBJECTIVE

Manage delayed postexercise hypoglycemia in patients with diabetes.

REFERENCE(S)

Moser O, Riddell MC, Eckstein ML, et al. Glucose management for exercise using continuous glucose monitoring (CGM) and intermittently scanned CGM (isCGM) systems in type 1 diabetes: position statement of the European Association for the Study of Diabetes (EASD) and of the International Society for Pediatric and Adolescent Diabetes (ISPAD) endorsed by JDRF and supported by the American Diabetes Association (ADA). *Diabetologia.* 2020;63(12):2501-2520. PMID: 33047169

35 ANSWER: E) Repeat hemoglobin A_{1c} measurement

This scenario addresses the consensus recommendation to perform a second confirmatory test in most patients for the purpose of diagnosing diabetes (thus, Answer A is incorrect). According to the American Diabetes Association, in the absence of a clear clinical diagnosis (eg, classic symptoms of hyperglycemia and a random plasma glucose ≥200 mg/dL [11.1 mmol/L]), diagnosis requires 2 abnormal screening test results, measured either at the same time or at 2 different time points (with as little time between tests as possible). Two different tests (eg, hemoglobin A_{1c} and fasting plasma glucose measurement) with results above the diagnostic threshold when collected at the same time or at 2 different time points would also confirm the diagnosis. However, if an individual has discordant results from 2 different tests, then the test result that is above the diagnostic threshold is the one that should be repeated. Exceptions to this include conditions that render the hemoglobin A_{1c} value potentially unreliable, for example, in the setting of anemia. The diagnosis is then made based on the confirmatory screening test.

The most important goal of screening individuals at high risk is to avoid a missed diagnosis due to using an insensitive test. In this case, the patient's hemoglobin A_{1c} value is above the currently standard diagnostic threshold for diabetes. Thus, there is no compelling reason to use glucose measurement (Answer D) for confirmation. Some organizations do support performing a 2-hour oral glucose tolerance test (with measurement of fasting and 2-hour glucose) for all women with polycystic ovary syndrome at initial diagnosis to prevent a delayed diagnosis. If this is not feasible, fasting glucose should be measured together with hemoglobin A_{1c}. The rationale for an oral glucose tolerance test is that a standard fasting glucose measurement and hemoglobin A_{1c} measurement lack the sensitivity to detect impaired glucose tolerance or early type 2 diabetes that could be identified by oral glucose tolerance testing in a substantial number of women with polycystic ovary syndrome. However, in this vignette, the patient's hemoglobin A_{1c} is already elevated, and the best next step is to repeat hemoglobin A_{1c} measurement for confirmation (Answer E).

Additionally, fasting and carbohydrate restriction can falsely elevate glucose with an oral glucose challenge. The general recommendation is that patients should consume a mixed diet with at least 150 g of carbohydrates in the 3 days before the glucose tolerance test (thus, Answer B is incorrect).

There is currently insufficient evidence to support the use of continuous glucose monitoring (Answer C) to screen for or diagnose diabetes.

EDUCATIONAL OBJECTIVE

Guide screening for prediabetes and type 2 diabetes in women with polycystic ovary syndrome.

REFERENCE(S)

American Diabetes Association Professional Practice Committee. 2. Diagnosis and classification of diabetes: standards of medical care in diabetes-2024. *Diabetes Care.* 2024;47(Suppl 1):S20-S42. PMID: 38078589

Velling Magnussen L, Mumm H, Andersen M, Glintborg D. Hemoglobin A1c as a tool for the diagnosis of type 2 diabetes in 208 premenopausal women with polycystic ovary syndrome. *Fertil Steril.* 2011;96(5):1275-1280. PMID: 21982282

36 ANSWER: A) Assessment for ketones

In people with type 1 diabetes, ketone testing (Answer A) should be performed in the home environment if the blood glucose concentration is above 300 mg/dL (>16.7 mmol/L) for unexplained reasons, especially if the person feels unwell at the time. Testing for ketones (usually by urine, but home blood testing kits are also currently approved for use; breath analyzers are not yet FDA approved) should also be performed during periods of illness or stress or if there are symptoms compatible with ketoacidosis such as nausea, vomiting, and abdominal pain. If ketones are elevated in the setting of hyperglycemia, diabetic ketoacidosis should be suspected, and additional confirmatory tests are usually necessary (measurement of serum ketones, electrolytes, bicarbonate, pH, etc). In the case of moderate to severe ketoacidosis, patients should be referred to the hospital environment for standard therapy with intravenous fluids and an evidence-based insulin protocol.

Importantly, patients commonly lack awareness of the signs and symptoms of ketosis. In a study conducted in 6 Swiss and 3 German endocrine outpatient clinics specialized in the treatment of diabetes, participants rated their own knowledge of diabetic ketoacidosis significantly lower than that of their physicians ($P < .0001$). Of all the participants, 46% were unable to name a symptom of diabetic ketoacidosis, 45% were unaware of its potential causes, and 64% reported never testing for ketones.

While basal rate testing (Answer B), diabetes education (Answer C), and a continuous glucose sensor (Answer D) are all needed to help this patient achieve a lower hemoglobin A_{1c}, none of these options is the best immediate step to take now. These steps can be done over weeks to months.

Therapy for stress management (Answer E) is appropriate if she is willing to explore it, but again, this is not immediately necessary.

EDUCATIONAL OBJECTIVE

Determine when urine ketones should be measured in a patient with type 1 diabetes.

REFERENCE(S)

Huang J, Yeung AM, Bergenstal RM, et al. Update on measuring ketones. *J Diabetes Sci Technol.* 2023;18(3):714-726. PMID: 36794812.

Hepprich M, Roser P, Stiebitz S, et al. Awareness and knowledge of diabetic ketoacidosis in people with type 1 diabetes: a cross-sectional, multicenter survey. *BMJ Open Diabetes Res Care.* 2023;11(6):e003662. PMID: 37949471

Albanese-O'Neill A, Wu M, Miller KM, et al; T1D Exchange Clinic Network. *Diabetes Care.* 2017;40(4):e38-e39. PMID: 28100607

Marks BE, Wolfsdorf JI. Monitoring of pediatric type 1 diabetes. *Front Endocrinol (Lausanne).* 2020;11:128. PMID: 32256447

Weber C, Kocher S, Neeser K, Joshi SR. Prevention of diabetic ketoacidosis and self-monitoring of ketone bodies: an overview. *Curr Med Res Opin.* 2009;25(5):1197-1207. PMID: 19327102

37 ANSWER: B) Reduce glargine to 20 units, reduce lispro to 4 units, and start linagliptin

Patients with suboptimally controlled type 2 diabetes may be prescribed multiple daily insulin injections. It is increasingly recognized that this can impose a self-care burden, particularly among older patients. Measuring blood glucose and injecting insulin multiple times daily and, where appropriate, problem solving to adjust insulin doses and/or take correction doses require complex self-care decision-making skills. The use of rapid- or short-acting insulin also increases hypoglycemia risk, which is of concern in older patients, such as the one in this vignette.

Hypoglycemia in elderly patients with diabetes increases the risk of cardiovascular and cerebrovascular events, progression of dementia, injurious falls, emergency department visits, and hospitalization. Hypoglycemic episodes are often difficult to diagnose in this population and are easily missed by intermittent fingerstick blood glucose measurements, as has been shown using continuous glucose monitoring.

In addition, large studies have shown lack of benefit and higher risk of morbidity and mortality with tight glycemic control. Both the Endocrine Society and the American Diabetes Association, as well as several other organizations, recommend relaxing glycemic control for older adults, with a goal of 7.0% to 7.5% (53-58 mmol/mol) in otherwise healthy older adults with few coexisting chronic conditions and intact cognitive and functional status. Among those with multiple coexisting conditions, cognitive impairment or functional dependence goals that are less stringent (eg, <8.0% [<64 mmol/mol] or <8.5% [<69 mmol/mol]), would be considered appropriate.

This patient's basal insulin dose should be reduced, as she becomes hypoglycemic when lunch is late. Her erratic morning blood glucose values suggest that she is also having nocturnal hypoglycemia. Her multiple daily insulin injection regimen requires problem solving, as she must determine when and how to take correction insulin doses. Her C-peptide concentration indicates that she is still making insulin, and she is taking fewer than 10 units of rapid-acting analogue before meals, so it is reasonable to reduce her mealtime insulin and add an oral agent that does not independently cause hypoglycemia, such as linagliptin (Answer B). Ideally, insulin lispro would be discontinued as soon as stable control is achieved.

Referring her to a diabetes educator (Answer C) is a reasonable adjunctive measure, but it would not lower her risk for hypoglycemia without a concurrent adjustment in her antihyperglycemic medication regimen.

Reducing her insulin doses and continuing the multiple daily injection regimen (Answer A) may reduce the frequency of hypoglycemia, but this would still require her to problem solve, which seems to be challenging for her.

Stopping both of her insulins (Answer D) is likely to result in hyperglycemia, as her total daily dose is currently 52 units. Repaglinide with meals might be a reasonable oral agent for this patient, as we know she is still able to secrete C-peptide. However, repaglinide would need to be taken 3 times daily and it could cause hypoglycemia. Thus, a once-daily agent such as a DPP-4 inhibitor is a preferred next step.

EDUCATIONAL OBJECTIVE

Simplify the antihyperglycemic regimen to prevent hypoglycemia in older adults with type 2 diabetes.

REFERENCE(S)

LeRoith D, Biessels GJ, Braithwaite SS, et al. Treatment of diabetes in older adults: an Endocrine Society clinical practice guideline. *J Clin Endocrinol Metab.* 2019;104(5):1520-1574. PMID: 30903688

Munshi MN, Slyne C, Segal AR, Saul N, Lyons C, Weinger K. Simplification of insulin regimen in older adults and risk of hypoglycemia. *JAMA Intern Med.* 2016;176(7):1023-1025. PMID: 27273335

Kirkman MS, Briscoe VJ, Clark N, et al. Diabetes in older adults. *Diabetes Care.* 2012;35(12):2650-2664. PMID: 23100048

38 ANSWER: D) Panretinal laser photocoagulation

This photograph reveals proliferative retinopathy with florid neovascularization (*blue arrow*) arising from the disc and retinal vessels (*red arrow*), as well as intraretinal hemorrhages (*see image*).

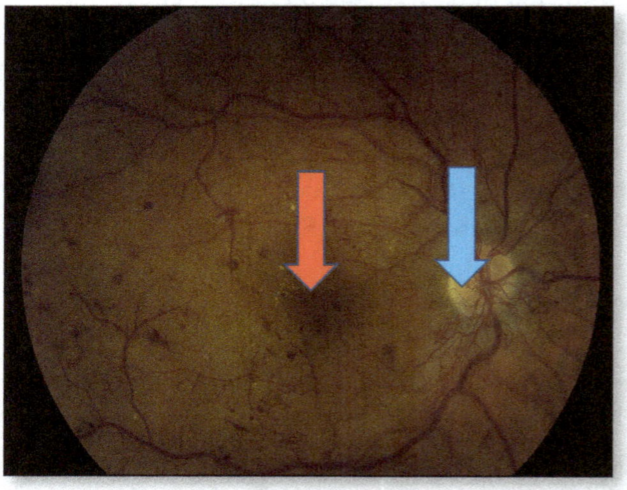

Diabetic retinopathy is divided into 2 major forms: nonproliferative and proliferative, named for the absence or presence of abnormal new blood vessels emanating from the retina. Nonproliferative diabetic retinopathy consists of a variable display of nerve-fiber layer infarcts (cotton wool spots), intraretinal hemorrhages, and hard exudates and microvascular abnormalities (including microaneurysms, occluded vessels, and dilated or tortuous vessels), primarily in the macula and posterior retina. Vision loss in nonproliferative diabetic retinopathy is mainly due to the development of macular edema. Proliferative diabetic retinopathy is marked by the presence of neovascularization arising from the disc and/or retinal vessels and the consequences of this neovascularization, including preretinal and vitreous hemorrhage, subsequent fibrosis, and traction retinal detachment. The severity of proliferative diabetic retinopathy can be classified as early, high risk, and severe. In early proliferative diabetic retinopathy, new vessels are present as fine loops or networks, but they do not meet the criteria for the high-risk category. There is a 75% 5-year risk of progression from early- to high-risk stages. Untreated high-risk proliferative diabetic retinopathy results in a 60% risk of severe vision loss at 5 years. Macular edema can be present with any degree of proliferative diabetic retinopathy and should be addressed as part of the overall treatment strategy.

Treatment for proliferative retinopathy must be quickly initiated to prevent progression and vision loss. Both panretinal photocoagulation and anti-VEGF agents (intravitreal once-a-month injection) have been shown to be effective in preventing progression of proliferative diabetic retinopathy and subsequent vision loss. Five-year data comparing initial treatment of proliferative diabetic retinopathy with ranibizumab vs panretinal photocoagulation show equivalent visual acuity outcomes. Although anti-VEGF agents are more effective in the short term, delays in treatment (missed appointments) can lead to significant disease progression, whereas panretinal photocoagulation is a more durable treatment than anti-VEGF inhibitors to prevent severe vision loss. Therefore, in this patient who is not adherent to her treatment regimen and will most likely miss appointments, panretinal laser photocoagulation (Answer D) is the better option.

Anti-VEGF agents (Answer A) would be incorrect because there is a significant risk of proliferative diabetic retinopathy recurrence and/or progression with loss to follow-up after treatment with these agents.

Focal laser photocoagulation (Answer B) is an established treatment for macular edema alone, not for proliferative retinopathy.

Vitrectomy (Answer E) is a technique used in cases of proliferative retinopathy that progress to vitreous hemorrhage that is nonclearing (or prevents photocoagulation) or traction retinal detachment (not the case with this patient).

Intravitreal glucocorticoid monotherapy (Answer C) may have some benefit in patients with refractory macular edema, but not proliferative retinopathy. However, these benefits are counterbalanced by an often transient response and an increased risk of adverse effects, including glaucoma and cataract.

EDUCATIONAL OBJECTIVE

Diagnose and manage proliferative diabetic retinopathy.

REFERENCE(S)

Douglas VP, Douglas KAA, Vavvas DG, Miller JW, Miller JB. Short- and long-term visual outcomes in patients receiving intravitreal injections: the impact of the coronavirus 2019 disease (COVID-19)-related lockdown. *J Clin Med.* 2022;11(8):2097. PMID: 35456189

Sabanayagam C, Banu R, Chee ML, et al. Incidence and progression of diabetic retinopathy: a systematic review. *Lancet Diabetes Endocrinol.* 2019;7(2):140-149. PMID: 30005958

Wubben TJ, Johnson MW; Anti-VEGF Treatment Interruption Study Group. Anti-vascular endothelial growth factor therapy for diabetic retinopathy: consequences of inadvertent treatment interruptions. *Am J Ophthalmol.* 2019;204:13-18. PMID: 30878488

Gross JG, Glassman AR, Liu D, et al; Diabetic Retinopathy Clinical Research Network. Five-year outcomes of panretinal photocoagulation vs intravitreous ranibizumab for proliferative diabetic retinopathy: a randomized clinical trial. *JAMA Ophthalmol.* 2018;136(10):1138-1148. PMID: 30043039

39 ANSWER: E) Pramlintide

Pramlintide (Answer E), an analogue of the naturally occurring hormone amylin, increases satiety, decreases body weight, slows gastric emptying, and suppresses glucagon secretion in conjunction with insulin in both type 1 and type 2 diabetes. It is associated with a modest degree of weight loss in most individuals. None of the other listed drugs are approved by the US FDA for use in type 1 diabetes, although they are frequently used off label.

Metformin (Answer D) is generally considered weight neutral or is associated with a mild degree of weight loss. It has been shown in some studies to reduce the amount of insulin required, but it has no significant effect on hemoglobin A_{1c} levels or cardiovascular outcomes. Metformin is also not approved by the US FDA for use in type 1 diabetes because of a relative concern regarding risk of lactic acidosis.

α-Glucosidase inhibitors (Answer A) have been tested in type 1 diabetes and have some effect on postprandial glucose levels and body weight, but they do not significantly reduce hemoglobin A_{1c} values in individuals with type 1 diabetes.

There is some evidence that GLP-1 receptor agonists (Answer B) have beneficial effects on β-cell function, but this is mainly derived from small observational studies. However, research is ongoing to investigate this potential beneficial effect in humans, particularly in the settings of recent-onset type 1 diabetes and islet-cell transplant.

Although SGLT-2 inhibitors (Answer C) may improve glycemic control and cause weight loss, they have not been adequately studied in persons with type 1 diabetes, nor are they recommended or approved for use in this setting. Also, SGLT-2 inhibitors may increase the risk of diabetic ketoacidosis. Some GLP-1 receptor agonists and SGLT-2 inhibitors may be selected based on their cardio-renal benefits if the patient has chronic kidney disease or congestive heart failure, etc. However, none of these situations is present in this vignette.

EDUCATIONAL OBJECTIVE

Recommend adjunctive treatments to manage type 1 diabetes.

REFERENCE(S)

Lane K, Freeby M. Adjunctive therapies in type 1 diabetes mellitus. *Curr Opin Endocrinol Diabetes Obes.* 2021;28(1):8-13. PMID: 33332928

Garg SK, Kaur G, Haider Z, Rodriquez E, Beatson C, Snell-Bergeon J. Efficacy of semaglutide in overweight and obese patients with type 1 diabetes. *Diabetes Technol Ther.* 2024;26(3):184-189. PMID: 38444317

Taylor SI, Blau JE, Rother KI, Beitelshees AL. SGLT2 inhibitors as adjunctive therapy for type 1 diabetes: balancing benefits and risks. *Lancet Diabetes Endocrinol.* 2019;7(12):949-958. PMID: 31585721

40 ANSWER: A) Dapagliflozin

This individual with obesity, type 2 diabetes, heart failure with reduced ejection fraction (HFrEF), and chronic kidney disease is at high risk for both cardiovascular mortality and kidney disease progression. In this case, overall *disease control* includes designing a therapeutic approach that addresses each of these conditions both individually and ideally concurrently, since control of one of these conditions can have a major impact on the others. Because dapagliflozin (Answer A) has been shown to both reduce progression of chronic kidney disease in those with an estimated glomerular filtration rate of 25 mL/min per 1.73 m^2 or higher, as well as reduce important outcomes due to HFrEF in those with an estimated glomerular filtration rate of 30 mL/min per 1.73 m^2 or higher, it should be prioritized above the other options in this case.

Importantly, based on a hemoglobin A_{1c} value that is below usual targets for diabetes control, this patient does not require more robust glucose management and would likely benefit from simplifying his regimen by eliminating the rapid-acting insulin. This is especially the case because he reports rarely taking it. Dapagliflozin is not FDA approved for the purpose of improving glycemic control in people with diabetes who have an estimated glomerular filtration rate less than 45 mL/min per 1.73 m^2, mainly due to reduced overall volume of urine and hence less glucose excretion. Thus, while it may provide a small degree of glucose lowering, it should not be considered for that purpose in this case.

Glimepiride (Answer C) increases the risk of hypoglycemia when prescribed in combination with insulin therapy, especially in the setting of chronic kidney disease stage 3b. Additionally, as noted, there is no need to enhance glucose lowering at this time. Similarly, pramlintide (Answer E) is an analogue of the amylin peptide approved for use in combination with insulin therapy in people with diabetes. Pramlintide also typically produces beneficial weight loss. However, it is prescribed as 3 doses per day, which the patient has found difficult, and it also increases the risk of hypoglycemia.

While linagliptin (Answer D) is beneficial in controlling glucose during hospitalization in certain patients in the hospital setting, and it is safe in the setting of advanced chronic kidney disease, it would not have any expected long-term benefits regarding overall disease control as described above.

Obesity management is another important consideration in this case, and dulaglutide (Answer B) is established as a weight-lowering medication for the treatment of type 2 diabetes. However, the potential benefit of dulaglutide in heart failure and/or chronic kidney disease has been derived only from post hoc analyses of cardiovascular outcome trials. Moreover, the heart failure post hoc analysis did not show reduced events. In contrast, another GLP-1 receptor agonist, semaglutide (not given as an answer option), has been shown in targeted outcome trials to be effective not only in reducing weight and improving glycemic control, but also in reducing morbidity from heart failure and progression of kidney disease (the STEP-≥ DM trial and FLOW trials, respectively). However, current published data support the benefit of a GLP-1 receptor agonist on heart failure with preserved, not reduced, ejection fraction in the setting of obesity (the STEP-HFpEF DM trial).

EDUCATIONAL OBJECTIVE

Explain the relative risks and benefits of antihyperglycemic agents for type 2 diabetes management in the setting of chronic kidney disease and heart failure.

REFERENCE(S)

Dapagliflozin [package insert]. Wilmington, DE: AstraZeneca Pharmaceuticals LP; 2024.

McMurray JJV, Solomon SD, Inzucchi SE, et al; DAPA-HF Trial Committees and Investigators. Dapagliflozin in patients with heart failure and reduced ejection fraction. *N Engl J Med.* 2019;381(21):1995-2008. PMID: 31535829

Heerspink HJL, Stefánsson BV, Correa-Rotter R, et al; DAPA-CKD Trial Committees and Investigators. Dapagliflozin in patients with chronic kidney disease. *N Engl J Med.* 2020;383(15):1436-1446. PMID: 32970396

Branch KRH, Dagenais GR, Avezum A, et al. Dulaglutide and cardiovascular and heart failure outcomes in patients with and without heart failure: a post-hoc analysis from the REWIND randomized trial. *Eur J Heart Fail.* 2022;24(10):1805-1812. PMID: 36073143

Kosiborod MN, Petrie MC, Borlaug BA, et al; STEP-HFpEF DM Trial Committees and Investigators. Semaglutide in patients with obesity-related heart failure and type 2 diabetes. *N Engl J Med.* 2024;390(15):1394-1407. PMID: 38587233

Perkovic V, Tuttle KR, Rossing P, et al; FLOW Trial Committees and Investigators. Effects of semaglutide on chronic kidney disease in patients with type 2 diabetes. *N Engl J Med.* 2024 [online ahead of print] PMID: 38785209

41 ANSWER: D) Leptin measurement

This patient has acquired generalized lipodystrophy. The lipodystrophy syndromes are a heterogeneous group of rare disorders that have in common selective deficiency of adipose tissue in the absence of nutritional deprivation or catabolic state.

Lipodystrophies are categorized based on etiology (genetic or acquired) and distribution of lost adipose tissue affecting the entire body (generalized) or only regions (partial). This yields 4 major categories:

- Congenital generalized lipodystrophy
- Familial partial lipodystrophy
- Acquired generalized lipodystrophy
- Acquired partial lipodystrophy

Acquired generalized lipodystrophy, also known as Lawrence syndrome, is very rare. Generalized fat loss is not present at birth but develops later in life.

It occurs over a variable period, ranging from a few weeks to years. Although the pathogenesis of acquired generalized lipodystrophy is unknown, it is hypothesized to be linked to autoimmune destruction of adipocytes. Some patients with acquired generalized lipodystrophy initially present with an autoimmune disease that includes dermatomyositis, Sjogren syndrome, rheumatoid arthritis, systemic sclerosis, and systemic lupus erythematosus. It has also been described after exposure to immune checkpoint inhibitor cancer drugs. Fat loss occurs within a few weeks to years after the onset of the autoimmune condition.

In people with acquired generalized lipodystrophy, metabolic abnormalities associated with severe insulin resistance (eg, hypertriglyceridemia, diabetes, hepatic steatosis, acanthosis nigricans, menstrual irregularities, and polycystic ovary syndrome) may develop soon after the recognition of fat loss. Affected patients have suppressed leptin levels and adiponectin. Thus, leptin measurement (Answer D) is the best next step. Currently, metreleptin (recombinant human methionyl leptin) is the only drug approved specifically for lipodystrophy. It is approved in the United States as an adjunct to diet for treatment of metabolic complications in patients with generalized lipodystrophy, and it appears to have a substantial disease-modifying effect.

Glutamic acid decarboxylase antibodies (Answer A) would be assessed to evaluate for type 1 diabetes, which is inconsistent with the patient's severe insulin resistance.

HNF1A gene testing (Answer B) is done to diagnose maturity-onset diabetes of the young (MODY), which is not the diagnosis in this case given the patient's lack of response to a sulfonylurea (most forms of MODY respond to this treatment) and the presence of severe insulin resistance.

Pathogenic variants in the insulin receptor gene (Answer C) cause type A insulin resistance; affected patients do not have loss of subcutaneous fat as is observed in acquired generalized lipodystrophy.

While Cushing syndrome is a form of acquired lipodystrophy due to chronically elevated circulating cortisol, this patient does not exhibit the classic phenotype of truncal obesity (including the anterior and posterior cervical area) with loss of fat in the limbs. Additionally, she has no other classic signs of hypercortisolemia such as bruising or hypertension. Thus, measuring urinary free cortisol excretion (Answer E) is incorrect.

EDUCATIONAL OBJECTIVE

Diagnose lipodystrophic syndromes.

REFERENCE(S)

Araújo-Vilar D, Santini F. Diagnosis and treatment of lipodystrophy: a step-by-step approach. *J Endocrinol Invest.* 2019;42(1):61-73. PMID: 29704234

Cook K, Ali O, Akinci B, et al. Effect of leptin therapy on survival in generalized and partial lipodystrophy: a matched cohort analysis. *J Clin Endocrinol Metab.* 2021;106(8):e2953-e2967. PMID: 33822100

Brown RJ, Oral EA, Cochran E, et al. Long-term effectiveness and safety of metreleptin in the treatment of patients with generalized lipodystrophy. *Endocrine.* 2018;60(3):479-489. PMID: 29644599

42 ANSWER: B) Exercise 150 minutes per week plus follow a reduced-calorie diet

This individual has hypogonadism based on a low testosterone concentration and a normal SHBG concentration accompanied by symptoms of reduced libido and depressed mood. Some observational data have indicated that treating low testosterone (Answer E) may be protective against diabetes, but until recently, this had not been prospectively studied in a clinical trial. A prespecified subgroup analysis of the Testosterone Replacement Therapy for Assessment of Long-Term Vascular Events and Efficacy Response in Hypogonadal Men (TRAVERSE) study attempted to answer the question of whether treatment of hypogonadism in men with prediabetes prevented the incidence of overt type 2 diabetes. Of the 5204 randomized participants, 1175 had prediabetes, with a mean age of 64 years. The study found that risk of progression to diabetes did not differ significantly between testosterone and placebo groups over the course of 48 months. The investigators concluded that in men with hypogonadism and prediabetes, the incidence of progression from prediabetes to diabetes did not differ significantly between testosterone- and placebo-treated men, suggesting that testosterone replacement should not be used as the primary therapeutic intervention to prevent diabetes in men with hypogonadism. As an additional note, before testosterone replacement is considered, this patient requires an evaluation of the gonadal axis to determine the correct diagnosis.

Behavioral lifestyle intervention that includes exercise and reduced caloric intake (Answer B) is preferred over metformin (Answer D) on the basis of findings from available studies, mainly the landmark Diabetes Prevention Program study. In this study, 3234 patients with obesity (average BMI = 34 kg/m^2) aged 25 to 85 years (average age = 51 years) at high risk for diabetes (based on fasting and 2-hour plasma glucose concentrations of 96 to 125 mg/dL [5.3-6.9 mmol/L] and 140 to 199 mg/dL [7.8-11.1 mmol/L], respectively) were randomly assigned to one of the following groups:

- Intensive lifestyle changes with the aim of reducing weight by 7% through a behavioral modification program focused on a low-fat diet and exercise for 150 minutes per week
- Treatment with metformin (850 mg twice daily) plus information on diet and exercise
- Placebo plus information on diet and exercise

After an average follow-up of 3 years, fewer patients in the intensive lifestyle group developed diabetes, as diagnosed by fasting plasma glucose and 2-hour postload glucose concentrations (14% vs 22% and 29% in the metformin and placebo groups, respectively). The intensive lifestyle and metformin interventions reduced the cumulative incidence of diabetes by 58% and 31%, respectively. Lifestyle intervention was effective in men and women in all age groups and in all ethnic groups. In a follow-up observational study (the Diabetes Prevention Program Outcomes Study), the benefit of the lifestyle intervention was shown to persist more than 10 years, particularly in older individuals (≥60 years of age at baseline).

Treatment with 3-hydroxy-3-methylglutaryl-coenzyme A reductase (HMGCR) inhibitors, or statins, has been associated with increased incidence of type 2 diabetes. However, stopping the statin (Answer A) for the purpose of avoiding transition from prediabetes to overt diabetes is problematic for 2 reasons: (1) there are no data to support that stopping a statin can delay the onset of type 2 diabetes, and (2) stopping a statin would significantly reduce the cardiopreventive effect of his medication regimen, which is overall counterproductive since the goal of preventing diabetes is, in essence, to prevent cardiovascular disease.

There are no studies on empagliflozin (Answer C) with respect to diabetes prevention.

EDUCATIONAL OBJECTIVE

Identify prediabetes (impaired fasting glucose and impaired glucose tolerance) and recommend the best approach to prevent progression to diabetes.

REFERENCE(S)

Knowler WC, Barrett-Connor E, Fowler SE, et al; Diabetes Prevention Program Research Group. Reduction in the incidence of type 2 diabetes with lifestyle intervention or metformin. *N Engl J Med.* 2002;346(6):393-403. PMID: 11832527

Bhasin S, Lincoff AM, Nissen SE, et al. Effect of Testosterone on Progression From Prediabetes to Diabetes in Men With Hypogonadism: a substudy of the TRAVERSE randomized clinical trial. *JAMA Intern Med.* 2024;184(4):353-362. PMID: 38315466

Mansi I, Frei CR, Wang CP, Mortensen EM. Statins and new-onset diabetes mellitus and diabetic complications: a retrospective cohort study of US healthy adults. *J Gen Intern Med.* 2015;30(11):1599-1610. PMID: 25917657

43 ANSWER: D) Perform polysomnography

In both men and women, the strongest risk factor for obstructive sleep apnea (OSA) is obesity. The prevalence of OSA progressively increases as BMI and associated markers increase (eg, neck circumference, waist-to-hip ratio). In a prospective study of nearly 700 adults with 4-year longitudinal follow-up, a 10% increase in weight was associated with a 6-fold increase in the risk of incident OSA. In a population-based study of more than 1000 adults who underwent polysomnography, moderate-to-severe obstructive sleep apnea (apnea-hypopnea index ≥15 events/h) was present in 11% of patients who were normal weight, 21% of those who were overweight (BMI, 25-30 kg/m^2), and 63% of those with obesity (BMI >30 kg/m^2).

Conversely, the presence of OSA impacts overall metabolic control. The results of a 2016 meta-analysis of different cohort studies including more than 60,000 patients with OSA indicated that the presence of OSA has a comparable impact on developing type 2 diabetes as traditional risk factors such as excess body weight, family predisposition, and physical inactivity. Moreover, the diagnosis of OSA in people with diabetes and obesity is important because treatment with continuous positive airway pressure appears to positively affect glycemic control.

Most patients with OSA first come to the attention of a clinician because of fatigue, daytime sleepiness, or report by the patient's bed partner of loud snoring, gasping, snorting, or interruptions in breathing while sleeping. Diagnostic testing for OSA should be performed in any patient with unexplained excessive daytime sleepiness, which is the clinically relevant symptom of OSA that is most responsive to treatment. In the absence of excessive daytime sleepiness, diagnostic testing is pursued if the patient snores and either works in a mission-critical profession (eg, airline pilots, bus drivers, and truck drivers) or has 2 or more additional clinical features of OSA.

Full-night, attended, in-laboratory polysomnography (Answer D) is considered the gold-standard diagnostic test for OSA. It involves monitoring the patient during a full night's sleep. Patients in whom OSA is diagnosed and who choose positive airway pressure therapy are subsequently brought back for another study, during which their positive airway pressure device is titrated. Split-night, attended, in-laboratory polysomnography is similar, except the diagnostic portion of the study is performed during the first part of the night only. Those patients in whom OSA is diagnosed during the first part of the night and who choose positive airway pressure therapy can have their positive airway pressure device titrated during the second part of the night.

There is no role for a cosyntropin-stimulation test (Answer B) in this case. The patient has no other symptoms suggestive of adrenal insufficiency, and he has a normal morning cortisol concentration, blood pressure, and electrolytes.

Total testosterone can be lower than normal because of obesity. Obesity decreases the serum concentration of SHBG, thereby decreasing the serum total testosterone concentration, usually without lowering the free testosterone concentration. The binding abnormality is proportional to the degree of obesity and is corrected by weight loss. Therefore, before diagnosing or treating hypogonadism (Answer E), serum free testosterone should be measured by equilibrium dialysis. If the value is normal, pituitary MRI (Answer C) would not be indicated. This patient also has normal libido, which is consistent with a normal gonadal axis; erectile dysfunction is most likely due to diabetes and other comorbidities.

While aspirin therapy is no longer recommended for primary prevention of cardiovascular events, it is not contributing to his symptom of fatigue and therefore discontinuing it (Answer A) is incorrect.

EDUCATIONAL OBJECTIVE

Diagnose obstructive sleep apnea in patients with obesity and type 2 diabetes.

REFERENCE(S)

Kapur VK, Auckley DH, Chowdhuri S, Kuhlmann DC, Mehra R, Ramar K, Harrod CG. Clinical practice guideline for diagnostic testing for adult obstructive sleep apnea: an American Academy of Sleep Medicine clinical practice guideline. *J Clin Sleep Med.* 2017;13(3):479-504. PMID: 28162150

Anothaisintawee T, Reutrakul S, Van Cauter E, Thakkinstian A. Sleep disturbances compared to traditional risk factors for diabetes development: systematic review and meta-analysis. *Sleep Med Rev.* 2016;30:11-24. PMID: 26687279

Herth J, Sievi NA, Schmidt F, Kohler M. Effects of continuous positive airway pressure therapy on glucose metabolism in patients with obstructive sleep apnoea and type 2 diabetes: a systematic review and meta-analysis. *Eur Respir Rev.* 2023;32(169):230083. PMID: 37673425

Peppard PE, Young T, Barnet JH, Palta M, Hagen EW, Hla KM. Increased prevalence of sleep-disordered breathing in adults. *Am J Epidemiol.* 2013;177(9):1006-1014. PMID: 23589584

44 ANSWER: D) Tissue transglutaminase antibodies

About 5% of patients with type 1 diabetes develop celiac disease (gluten-sensitive enteropathy diagnosed by a positive small-bowel biopsy sample), and 7% to 10% have detectable tissue transglutaminase antibodies (Answer D). The 2022 American Diabetes Association guidelines state that adults with type 1 diabetes should be screened for celiac disease in the presence of gastrointestinal symptoms, signs, or laboratory manifestations suggestive of celiac disease. However, for children and adolescents (defined by the World Health Organization to include individuals aged 10 to 19 years), the recommendation is to screen with antibodies soon after diagnosis given the higher prevalence of celiac disease in persons with youth-onset type 1 diabetes.

Although 15% to 30% of patients with type 1 diabetes have positive antithyroid antibodies (TPO and/or thyroglobulin antibodies) (Answer E), the preferred screening test for hypothyroidism in adults and adolescents is measurement of TSH rather than TPO antibodies. This is, in part, due to the fact that studies have shown a TPO-antibody positivity rate between 12% and 15% in the general healthy euthyroid population, and even higher rates in older women. An abnormal TSH value is also required for diagnosis and treatment of hypothyroidism.

Measurement of antinuclear antibodies (Answer B) is done to identify rheumatologic conditions such as systemic lupus erythematosus in patients presenting with consistent symptoms, and it should not be used as a general screening test.

Less than 1% to 2% of children and adolescents with type 1 diabetes have autoimmune adrenalitis with circulating antibodies to steroid 21-hydroxylase (Answer A). Overall, the prevalence of Addison disease is relatively low. Testing should be driven by signs and symptoms of a low cortisol state, and antibodies should only be measured after a confirmed diagnosis of primary adrenal insufficiency.

Screening for risk of pernicious anemia with antiparietal cell antibodies (Answer C) in people with type 1 diabetes is not recommended for 2 reasons. First, pernicious anemia occurs in only 2.5% to 4.0% of individuals with type 1 diabetes, and second, it is more reliable to periodically measure B_{12} levels and complete blood cell count in this setting.

EDUCATIONAL OBJECTIVE

Recommend appropriate screening for autoimmune conditions in persons with type 1 diabetes.

REFERENCE(S)

American Diabetes Association Professional Practice Committee. 14. Children and adolescents: standards of care in diabetes-2024. *Diabetes Care.* 2024;47(Suppl 1):S258-S281. PMID: 38078582

Kahaly GJ, Hansen MP. Type 1 diabetes associated autoimmunity. *Autoimmun Rev.* 2016;15(7):644-648. PMID: 26903475

Janovsky CCPS, Bittencourt MS, Goulart AC, et al. Prevalence of antithyroperoxidase antibodies in a multiethnic Brazilian population: the ELSA-Brasil Study. *Arch Endocrinol Metab.* 2019;63(4):351-357. PMID: 31038589

Amouzegar A, Gharibzadeh S, Kazemian E, Mehran L, Tohidi M, Azizi F. The prevalence, incidence and natural course of positive antithyroperoxidase antibodies in a population-based study: Tehran Thyroid Study. *PLoS One.* 2017;12(1):e0169283. PMID: 28052092

45 ANSWER: C) Myocardial infarction (decreased), stroke (decreased), cardiovascular death (decreased)

Published in 1993, the Diabetes Control and Complications Trial (DCCT) was a landmark study that compared the effects of intensive vs conventional control on the onset and progression of diabetes-related complications over 6.5 years in more than 1400 patients with type 1 diabetes. The DCCT demonstrated a substantial benefit of intensive insulin therapy in the primary prevention of diabetic retinopathy: at 9 years (mean 6.5 years), the incidence of new-onset retinopathy was 12% in the intensive therapy group vs 54% in the conventional therapy group. In addition to its efficacy in primary prevention, intensive insulin therapy also slows the rate of progression of mild to moderate retinopathy. At follow-up of up to 9 years (mean 6.5 years), intensive therapy led to a significant reduction in the incidence of new-onset microalbuminuria (16.4% vs 23.9%; adjusted risk reduction 39%). There was also a significant reduction in new-onset macroalbuminuria in the entire study population (3.2% vs 7.2%; adjusted risk reduction 51%). The incidence of confirmed clinical neuropathy (defined as findings from the history and physical examination that were confirmed by neurologic testing) was reduced by 64% with intensive insulin therapy. The DCCT documented a nonsignificant trend toward fewer cardiovascular events with intensive therapy (3.2% vs 5.4%; $P = .08$). The incidence of death was not reduced.

Following completion of the DCCT in 1993, the conventional treatment group was offered intensive treatment, and 93% of DCCT participants (n = 1394) agreed to participate in the observational Epidemiology of Diabetes Interventions and Complications (EDIC) study. Differences in glycated hemoglobin levels between the intensive and conventional treatment groups at the end of the DCCT trial (7.4% and 9.1%, respectively) narrowed at the end of the 11-year follow-up EDIC study (7.9% and 7.8%, respectively). Cardiovascular outcomes for the EDIC study were defined as the occurrence of nonfatal myocardial infarction, stroke, cardiovascular death, documented angina, or coronary revascularization. The analysis of cardiovascular events according to original DCCT treatment assignment was predetermined to conclude when 50 patients in the original conventional treatment group had experienced a cardiovascular event. During the entire follow-up period (mean 17 years), 46 events had occurred in 31 patients from the DCCT intensive therapy group, compared with 98 events in 52 patients from the conventional therapy group (0.38 vs 0.80 events per 100 patient-years). This represented a 42% decrease in any cardiovascular event (95% CI, 9%-63%); there was also a 57% reduction in a serious cardiovascular event (nonfatal myocardial infarction, stroke, or death of cardiovascular disease [95% CI, 12%-79%]) in the original DCCT intensive therapy group compared with the DCCT conventional treatment group (thus, Answer C is correct and Answers A, B, and D are incorrect).

EDUCATIONAL OBJECTIVE

Recall the findings of the Epidemiology of Diabetes Interventions and Complications study regarding myocardial infarction, stroke, and death.

REFERENCE(S)

Diabetes Control and Complications Trial Research Group. The effect of intensive treatment of diabetes on the development and progression of long-term complications in insulin-dependent diabetes mellitus. *N Engl J Med.* 1993;329(14):977-986. PMID: 8366922

Diabetes Control and Complications Trial Research Group. Progression of retinopathy with intensive versus conventional treatment in the Diabetes Control and Complications Trial. *Ophthalmology.* 1995;102(4):647-661. PMID: 7724182

Nathan DM, Clearly PA, Backlund JY, et al; Diabetes Control and Complications Trial/Epidemiology of Diabetes Interventions and Complications (DCCT/EDIC) Study Research Group. Intensive diabetes treatment and cardiovascular disease in patients with type 1 diabetes. *N Engl J Med.* 2005;353(25):2643-2653. PMID: 16371630

46 ANSWER: A) Insulin degludec; take it at his convenience once daily

The duration of action of insulin degludec (Answer A) is longer than 42 hours; the half-life is approximately 25 hours, and it reaches steady state in 2 to 3 days. It may be given safely and effectively with a minimum of 8 hours and maximum of 40 hours between doses. This makes it well suited to being used during travel, as long as the patient generally takes it once daily. Here, degludec would be the alternative to the more commonly prescribed U100 insulin glargine (Answer C), which is incorrect because it would require careful attention to timing of dosing to ensure administration at least, but not more often than, every 24 hours to optimize control and minimize hypoglycemia.

NPH insulin at bedtime, given at the same time when traveling (Answer B), is an impractical regimen as it is difficult to give it at the same time when crossing multiple time zones.

The half-life of U300 insulin glargine (Answer D) is about 23 hours. It reaches a steady state in 4 days, and the duration of action is less than or equal to 36 hours. Data regarding U300 insulin support its safety and efficacy up to a ± 3-hour window for administration, so this also may not be ideal for dosing when traveling.

EDUCATIONAL OBJECTIVE

Optimize basal insulin therapy for travel across time zones.

REFERENCE(S)

Ritzel R, Rouseel R, Bolli GB, et al. Patient-level meta-analysis of the EDITION 1, 2 and 3 studies: glycemic control and hypoglycaemia with new insulin glargine 300 U/ml versus glargine 100 U/mL in people with type 2 diabetes. *Diabetes Obes Metab.* 2015;17(9):859-867. PMID: 25929311

Matheiu C, Hollander P, Miranda-Palma B, et al. Efficacy and safety of insulin degludec in a flexible dosing regimen vs insulin glargine in patients with type 1 diabetes (BEGIN: Flex T1): a 26-week randomized, treat-to-target trial with a 26-week extension. *J Clin Endocrinol Metab.* 2013;98(3):1154-1162. PMID: 23393185

47 ANSWER: A) β-Hydroxybutyrate measurement

This patient has a year-long history consistent with progressive hypoglycemia that has reached a worrisome level of severity. Although her symptoms only occur during the day with an apparent relationship to meals, she has adopted protective behaviors such as eating a snack containing a balanced amount of carbohydrate and fat before bed. She presents with a fasting glucose concentration below 55 mg/dL (<3.1 mmol/L), and both her insulin and C-peptide concentrations are inappropriately elevated for her degree of hypoglycemia. Moreover, she presented with a neuroadrenergic symptom that resolved with sugar intake. On the basis of the available laboratory values and her history, the clinical picture raises the possibility of insulinoma.

While a supervised 72-hour fast is often required to accurately and safely assess clinical hypoglycemia, episodes can occasionally be "captured" in usual care settings as in this case. In addition to direct measurement of endogenous insulin production with C-peptide and insulin, and in the absence of indicators for other causes, it is most helpful to measure other physiologic markers of excess insulin secretion to confirm an insulin-mediated cause. Specifically, the ketone body β-hydroxybutyrate (Answer A) is low or low-normal in the context of insulin-mediated hypoglycemia, but it is high-normal or elevated in the context of non–insulin-mediated causes.

Heavy alcohol use is associated with hypoglycemia and would yield an elevated β-hydroxybutyrate concentration. However, there is no indication of alcoholism relapse, and she does not appear to be intoxicated. Thus, measuring blood alcohol (Answer B) is incorrect.

IGF-2–secreting tumors should be suspected in individuals who appear unwell, as these are typically large tumors that grow quickly. Because she is otherwise well, measuring IGF-2 (Answer C) is not necessary.

Insulin antibodies (Answer D) should be measured in cases where the insulin concentration is very elevated, as it may indicate the presence of high-affinity insulin antibodies causing intermittent severe hypoglycemia due to erratic release of bound insulin in the blood stream. Since her insulin concentration is not substantially elevated, this is unlikely to be helpful.

Screening for hypoglycemic agents such as sulfonylureas (Answer E) is typically done in cases of suspected insulin-mediated hypoglycemia, but in this case, one would expect a higher insulin concentration, typically greater than 20 µIU/mL (>138.9 pmol/L).

EDUCATIONAL OBJECTIVE

Appropriately evaluate hypoglycemia.

REFERENCE(S)

De León DD, Stanley CA. Determination of insulin for the diagnosis of hyperinsulinemic hypoglycemia. *Best Pract Res Clin Endocrinol Metab.* 2013;27(6):763-769. PMID: 24275188

48 ANSWER: A) Measure hemoglobin A_{1c} now; if normal, perform a 75-g oral glucose tolerance test at 24 to 28 weeks' gestation

Given the increased risk of type 2 diabetes in women with a history of gestational diabetes, current American Diabetes Association guidelines recommend screening for undiagnosed type 2 diabetes at the time that pregnancy is established (thus, Answer C is incorrect). Hemoglobin A_{1c} measurement, fasting plasma glucose measurement, and the 75-g oral glucose tolerance test may all be used as screening tests for type 2 diabetes; however, oral glucose tolerance testing is the most sensitive modality. Importantly, hemoglobin A_{1c} measurement is not accurate beyond the first trimester because of altered red blood cell turnover (thus, Answer D is incorrect).

The recurrence rate of gestational diabetes is high; at least 50% of future pregnancies will be affected. If type 2 diabetes is not present, oral glucose tolerance testing should be repeated at the standard time of 24 to 28 weeks' gestation to screen for gestational diabetes. This could consist of a 2-step process (50-g oral glucose tolerance test and then, depending on threshold criteria, the 100-g oral glucose tolerance test) or a 1-step process (75-g oral glucose tolerance test). Neither Answer B nor Answer C includes the required steps to be paired with the recommendations. The 1-step process has significantly increased the number of women identified with gestational diabetes because it requires only 1 abnormal value rather than 2. However, because this increased identification has not clearly translated into improved maternal or neonatal outcomes, the 2-step approach to diagnosing gestational diabetes is still supported by several organizations, including the American College of Obstetrics and Gynecology.

EDUCATIONAL OBJECTIVE

Recommend a screening protocol for gestational diabetes.

REFERENCE(S)

American Diabetes Association Professional Practice Committee. 15. Management of diabetes in pregnancy: *standards of care in diabetes-2024. Diabetes Care.* 2024;47(Suppl 1):S282-S294. PMID: 38078583

Sarker MR, Ramos GA. Routine screening for gestational diabetes: a review. *Curr Opin Obstet Gynecol.* 2024;36(2):97-103. PMID: 38259247

49 ANSWER: A) Initiate continuous glucose monitoring

Men with type 1 diabetes are approximately 2 to 3 times more likely to have erectile dysfunction than men who do not have diabetes, and the prevalence increases with longer duration of diabetes. In a study published in 1980 of 541 men aged 20 to 59 years who had type 1 diabetes, the best predictors of erectile dysfunction were age, presence of peripheral or autonomic neuropathy, retinopathy, long duration of disease, and suboptimal glycemic control. Erectile dysfunction is considered a microvascular complication, the risk of which has been shown to be modifiable by improving glycemic control in the DCCT trial (Diabetes Control and Complications Trial), In fact, this is an opportune time to encourage glycemic control for the direct indication of preventing erectile dysfunction along with other microvascular dysfunction. Of the available answers, the only option that has been demonstrated to lower hemoglobin A_{1c} is the initiation of continuous glucose monitoring (thus, Answer A is correct and Answer D is incorrect). Additionally, testosterone measurement at regular intervals (Answer C) is not recommended as a screening approach for hypogonadism, but rather as a confirmatory test in the presence of consistent symptoms.

Many drugs are associated with erectile dysfunction, including β-adrenergic blockers and thiazides, but not ACE inhibitors. Thus, there is no need to stop lisinopril (Answer E).

Saw palmetto (Answer B) has not been shown to prevent erectile dysfunction.

EDUCATIONAL OBJECTIVE

Counsel a man with type 1 diabetes about the risk of developing erectile dysfunction.

REFERENCE(S)

McCulloch DK, Campbell IW, Wu FC, Prescott RJ, Clarke BF. Prevalence of diabetic impotence. *Diabetologia.* 1980;18(4):279-283. PMID: 7418954

Diabetes Control and Complications Trial Research Group; Nathan DM, Genuth S, Lachin J, et al. The effect of intensive treatment of diabetes on the development and progression of long-term complications in insulin-dependent diabetes mellitus. *N Engl J Med.* 1993;329(14):977-986. PMID: 8366922

Akturk HK, Rompicherla S, Rioles N, et al. Factors associated with improved A1C among adults with type 1 diabetes in the United States. *Clin Diabetes.* 2023;41(1):76-80. PMID: 36714244

50 ANSWER: C) Lowers the renal threshold for glucose excretion to less than 100 mg/dL

SGLTs cotransport sodium and glucose into cells using the sodium gradient produced by sodium-potassium ATPase pumps at the basolateral cell membranes. SGLT-2 is expressed in segments S1 and S2 of the proximal convoluted tubules and is responsible for renal reabsorption of glucose. Renal tubular reabsorption is known to undergo adaptations in the setting of uncontrolled diabetes. Particularly relevant in this context is the up-regulation of renal SGLT-2, which is an important adaptation in diabetes to maintain renal tubular glucose reabsorption. SGLT-2 is not present in the S3 segment (thus, Answer E is incorrect) or in the distal tubule (thus, Answers A and B are incorrect).

SGLT-2 inhibitors reduce filtered glucose reabsorption by epithelial cells of the kidney proximal tubule. The renal threshold for glucose reabsorption in patients with type 2 diabetes was reported to be between 200 and 250 mg/dL, which is higher than that of persons without type 2 diabetes (170-200 mg/dL). SGLT-2 inhibitors, by blocking SGLT-2, lower the threshold from around 220 to 240 mg/dL to less than 100 mg/dL (thus, Answer C is correct and Answer D is incorrect).

EDUCATIONAL OBJECTIVE

Explain the mechanism of action of SGLT-2 inhibitors at the kidney level.

REFERENCE(S)

Nair S, Wilding JP. Sodium glucose cotransporter 2 inhibitors as a new treatment for diabetes mellitus. *J Clin Endocrinol Metab.* 2010;95(1):34-42. PMID: 19892839

Osaki A, Okada S, Saito T, et al. Renal threshold for glucose reabsorption predicts diabetes improvement by sodium glucose cotransporter 2 inhibitor therapy. *J Diabetes Investig.* 2016;7(5):751-754. PMID: 27181936

51 ANSWER: B) Does not sufficiently decrease blood glucose levels

SGLT-2 inhibitors act by reducing the renal threshold for glucose excretion, thereby lowering blood glucose by increasing renal glucose clearance. These drugs do cause weight loss, as monotherapy and in combination, although the mechanism is not fully understood. In clinical trials, weight loss persists for at least 6 to 12 months and often longer (thus, Answer A is incorrect).

Although SGLT-2 inhibitors can transiently worsen the estimated glomerular filtration rate, in the longer term they provide kidney protection (thus, Answer D is incorrect).

No adverse effects on blood pressure or hepatic function have been described (thus, Answers C and E are incorrect).

The glucose-lowering effects of SGLT-2 inhibitors are dependent on the estimated glomerular filtration rate, and hemoglobin A_{1c} lowering decreases to approximately 0.4% at rates below 60 mL/min per 1.73 m^2. In this woman with an estimated glomerular filtration rate of 42 mL/min per 1.73 m^2, the addition of empagliflozin is unlikely to help achieve her hemoglobin A_{1c} goal (thus, Answer B is correct).

EDUCATIONAL OBJECTIVE

Determine when an SGLT-2 inhibitor is appropriate in the treatment of type 2 diabetes.

REFERENCE(S)

Tsapas A, Avgerinos I, Karagiannis T, et al. Comparative effectiveness of glucose-lowering drugs for type 2 diabetes: a systematic review and network meta-analysis. *Ann Intern Med.* 2020;173(4):278-286. PMID: 32598218

52 ANSWER: E) Repeat measurement of the urinary albumin-to-creatinine ratio

A normal urinary albumin-to-creatinine ratio is less than 30 mg/g of creat; persistently elevated values between 30 and 300 mg/g creat are characterized as moderately increased albuminuria (the new terminology for what was formerly called "microalbuminuria"). A ratio above 300 mg/g creat is considered to represent severely increased albuminuria (the new terminology for what was formerly called "macroalbuminuria," overt albuminuria, or dipstick-positive albuminuria).

However, the urinary albumin-to-creatinine ratio is a continuous measurement, and differences within the normal and abnormal ranges are associated with kidney and cardiovascular outcomes. Furthermore, because of high biologic variability of more than 20% between measurements in urinary albumin excretion, 2 of 3 specimens collected within a 3- to 6-month period should be abnormal before considering a patient to have increased albuminuria. In addition, exercise within 24 hours, infection, fever, congestive heart failure, marked hyperglycemia, menstruation, and marked hypertension can elevate the urinary albumin-to-creatinine ratio independently of kidney damage.

This patient with excellent glycemic control (hemoglobin A_{1c} <7.0% [<53 mmol/mol]) suddenly has a urinary albumin-to-creatinine ratio greater than 300 mg/g creat, while 3 months ago, it was normal. This is suspicious for menstruation causing a high ratio. Therefore, the urinary albumin-to-creatinine ratio measurement must be repeated (Answer E), and the patient should be given instructions not to provide a urine sample during her menses.

Lowering the patient's hemoglobin A_{1c} level to less than 6.5% (Answer D) is incorrect because the increase in her hemoglobin A_{1c} from 6.4% to 6.9% (46 to 52 mmol/mol) would not increase the urinary albumin-to-creatinine ratio to greater than 300 mg/g creat. At a hemoglobin A_{1c} value of 6.9%, she is still at goal and there is no need to intensify her insulin regimen.

Treatment with an ACE inhibitor (Answer C) or angiotensin receptor blocker (Answer B) should not be initiated based on a single abnormal urinary albumin-to-creatinine ratio measurement.

Adding canagliflozin (Answer A) is incorrect because it is not indicated for type 1 diabetes. Canagliflozin has a kidney indication only in patients with type 2 diabetes when the urinary albumin-to-creatinine ratio is greater than 300 mg/g creat.

EDUCATIONAL OBJECTIVE

Interpret the urinary albumin-to-creatinine ratio in a patient with diabetes.

REFERENCE(S)

American Diabetes Association Professional Practice Committee; 11. Chronic kidney disease and risk management: *standards of care in diabetes-2024. Diabetes Care.* 2024;47(Suppl 1):S219-S230. PMID: 38078574

Kidney Disease: Improving Global Outcomes (KDIGO) Diabetes Work Group. KDIGO 2022 clinical practice guideline for diabetes management in chronic kidney disease. *Kidney Int.* 2022;102(5S):S1-S127. PMID: 36272764

Tankeu AT, Kaze FF, Noubiap JJ, Chelo D, Dehayem MY, Sobngwi E. Exercise-induced albuminuria and circadian blood pressure abnormalities in type 2 diabetes. *World J Nephrol.* 2017;6(4):209-216. PMID: 28729969

Female Reproduction Board Review

Margaret Flynn Lippincott, MD

1 ANSWER: B) Serum 17-hydroxyprogesterone measurement

The diagnosis of polycystic ovary syndrome (PCOS) requires 2 of the following 3 criteria: (1) ovulatory dysfunction; (2) biochemical and/or clinical hyperandrogenism; (3) polycystic ovarian morphology on ultrasonography. The new 2023 International Guidelines also allow for an elevated antimullerian hormone value to substitute for polycystic ovarian morphology on ultrasonography.

The vignette describes symptoms consistent with lifelong ovulatory dysfunction: more than 3 years between breast development and the start of menses and menstrual cycles less than 21 days when the patient is more than 3 years past menarche. The vignette also provides the information needed to deduce that the patient has clinical hyperandrogenism (her race and her modified Ferriman-Gallwey) as cutoffs for hirsutism vary by race. Given that she has ovulatory dysfunction and clinical hyperandrogenism, she does not require any additional testing to assess for polycystic ovaries such as serum free testosterone measurement (Answer C), calculated free testosterone value (which requires measurement of SHBG [Answer D]), or transvaginal ultrasonography (Answer E).

Since PCOS is a diagnosis of exclusion, she does require a 17-hydroxyprogesterone measurement to rule out late-onset congenital adrenal hyperplasia (thus, Answer B is correct, and Answer A is incorrect). She has the type of clinical hyperandrogenism most specific for PCOS—hirsutism. However, she has no signs of virilization to suggest an adrenal tumor, and her total testosterone concentration is normal. Her hirsutism is mild and not associated with any glucose dysregulation, suggesting she does not have premenopausal ovarian hyperthecosis. Her primary care physician has already ruled out thyroid dysfunction, hyperprolactinemia, and early ovarian aging.

EDUCATIONAL OBJECTIVE

Diagnose polycystic ovary syndrome.

REFERENCE(S)

Teede HJ, Tay CT, Laven JJE, et al. Recommendations from the 2023 international evidence-based guideline for the assessment and management of polycystic ovary syndrome. *J Clin Endocrinol Metab.* 2023;108(10):2447-2469. PMID: 37580314

Legro RS, Arslanian SA, Ehrmann DA, et al; Endocrine Society. Diagnosis and treatment of polycystic ovary syndrome: an Endocrine Society clinical practice guideline. *J Clin Endocrinol Metab.* 2013;98(12):4565-4592. PMID: 24151290

ACOG committee opinion No. 651: menstruation in girls and adolescents: using the menstrual cycle as a vital sign. *Obstet Gynecol.* 2015;126(6):e143-e146. PMID: 26595586

2 ANSWER: C) Mammography and PSA measurement

Cancer screening in transgender individuals is recommended to commence at the same time as in their cis-gender counterparts. For Black cis-gendered men, discussion about prostate cancer screening should begin at age 45 years. While some population level studies suggest that transwomen are at a decreased risk for prostate cancer, case reports in the literature have described metastatic prostate cancer in transwomen. Transwomen who start GnRH agonist therapy at an older age may be at increased risk for prostate cancer compared with those who start earlier. While uncertainty remains, this patient is older than 45 years and is Black; thus, it is recommended that she have a conversation with her provider about screening for prostate cancer with PSA measurement, taking into account her preferences. As the patient in this vignette indicated that she would like to be up to date on cancer screening, PSA measurement would be recommended (thus, Answer E is incorrect). In transwomen, a PSA threshold of 1.0 ng/mL (1.0 µg/L) is recommended to prompt additional workup. In transwomen who have had vaginoplasty, the prostate can typically be felt during a vaginal exam rather than a digital rectal exam.

There is some controversy about the optimal age at which to initiate screening for breast cancer. This 48-year-old patient is of the age where both the US Preventive Services Task Force (age 40) and the American Cancer Society (age 45) recommend screening, although evidence suggests that transwomen who have been exposed to less than 30 years of estrogen therapy are likely at low risk for breast cancer. Thus, combined screening with both PSA and mammography is indicated (thus, Answer C is correct and Answers B and D are incorrect).

Her blood pressure is at her therapeutic goal according to the 2018 American Heart Association and 2023 European Society of Hypertension guidelines, so there is no indication to increase her lisinopril dosage (Answer A).

EDUCATIONAL OBJECTIVE

Explain cancer screening recommendations for transwomen.

REFERENCE(S)

Hembree WC, Cohen-Kettenis PT, Gooren L, et al. Endocrine treatment of gender-dysphoric/gender-incongruent persons: an Endocrine Society clinical practice guideline. *J Clin Endocrinol Metab.* 2017;102(11):3869-3903. PMID: 28945902

Crowley F, Mihalopoulos M, Gaglani S, et al. Prostate cancer in transgender women: considerations for screening, diagnosis and management. *Br J Cancer.* 2023;128(2):177-189. PMID: 36261584

Whelton PK, Carey RM, Aronow WS, et al. 2017 ACC/AHA/AAPA/ABC/ACPM/AGS/APha/ASH/ASPC/NMA/PCNA guideline for the prevention, detection, evaluation, and management of high blood pressure in adults: a report of the American College of Cardiology/American Heart Association Task Force on Clinical Practice Guidelines. *J Am Coll Cardiol.* 2018;71:e127-e248. PMID: 29146535

Mancia G, Kreutz R, Brunström M, et al. 2023 ESH guidelines for the management of arterial hypertension the Task Force for the management of arterial hypertension of the European Society of Hypertension: endorsed by the International Society of Hypertension (ISH) and the European Renal Association (ERA). *J Hypertens.* 2023;41(12):1874-2071. PMID: 37345492

3 ANSWER: D) Levonorgestrel-releasing intrauterine device

In addition to contraception, this patient requires endometrial protection for her irregular periods. Thus, a copper intrauterine device (Answer A) would not be a good choice.

Carbamazepine decreases the efficacy of combined oral contraceptives, especially low-dose formulations, and progestin-only contraceptive pills (Answers B and E).

Her blood pressure is a relative contraindication to any estrogen-containing contraceptive pill or ring (Answers B and C).

The only option with no relative or absolute contraindications that provides both endometrial protection and contraception is a levonorgestrel-releasing intrauterine device (Answer D).

EDUCATIONAL OBJECTIVE

Select the best birth control for women with complex medical histories.

REFERENCE(S)

Curtis KM, Tepper NK, Jatlaoui TC, et al. U.S. medical eligibility criteria for contraceptive use, 2016. *MMWR Recomm Rep.* 2016;65(No. RR-3):1-104. PMID: 27467196

4 ANSWER: B) Prescribe fezolinetant, 45 mg daily

This patient has a 10-year risk of atherosclerotic cardiovascular disease of 21%, and the primary factor increasing her risk from intermediate to high is her race (Black women have a higher risk for cardiovascular disease compared with risk in White women). Therefore, she has a contraindication to estrogen therapy (Answer C) for vasomotor symptoms.

Fezolinetant (Answer B) is a neurokinin B receptor antagonist that is FDA approved for the treatment of menopausal vasomotor symptoms. The most common adverse effect is headache. It is recommended that patients taking fezolinetant have liver enzymes monitored at baseline and at 3, 6, and 9 months.

In an evidence-based literature review by the North American Menopause Society, clonidine (Answer A) is not recommended because of limited efficacy and significant adverse effects.

Mindfulness-based interventions and cooling techniques (Answers D and E) require more research before they can be recommended.

EDUCATIONAL OBJECTIVE

Recommend options for nonhormonal treatment of vasomotor symptoms of menopause.

REFERENCE(S)

The 2023 Nonhormone Therapy Position Statement of The North American Menopause Society Advisory Panel. The 2023 nonhormone therapy position statement of The North American Menopause Society. *Menopause.* 2023;30(6):573-590. PMID: 37252752

Stuenkel CA, Davis SR, Gompel A, et al. Treatment of symptoms of the menopause: an Endocrine Society Clinical Practice Guideline. *J Clin Endocrinol Metab.* 2015;100(11):3975-4011. PMID: 26444994

5 ANSWER: E) Selective serotonin reuptake inhibitor

This patient has premenstrual dysphoric disorder (PMDD). Women with PMDD experience a wide variety of cyclic and recurrent physical, emotional, behavioral, and cognitive symptoms that start in the luteal phase and stop after the onset of menses. Major symptoms include affective symptoms such as depression, angry outbursts, irritability, and anxiety, and somatic symptoms such as breast pain, bloating, swelling, and headache. For PMDD to be diagnosed, the patient's symptoms must interfere with her daily life.

The first-line treatment is a selective serotonin reuptake inhibitor (Answer E). Selective serotonin reuptake inhibitors can be given continuously or cyclically limited to the luteal phase of the cycle. Given that this patient has polycystic ovary syndrome, a continuous serotonin reuptake inhibitor is recommended because of her irregular ovulation.

Because progestins can worsen PMDD, there is no indication for a progestin-only pill (Answer D).

A cyclic low-dosage oral contraceptive pill (Answer A) is the first-line therapy for polycystic ovary syndrome to address menstrual cycle regulation and patient-important hirsutism, but it is not first-line therapy for PMDD. She is not bothered by hirsutism and does not need endometrial protection. A continuous low-dosage oral contraceptive pill, specifically one containing drospirenone, or a contraceptive patch (Answer C) is a second-line treatment for mild to moderate PMDD and could be considered if the patient desires contraception.

GnRH agonists, such as leuprolide (Answer B), can be used to suppress ovulation in treatment-resistant, moderately severe cases of PMDD. However, she would require hormone add-back therapy, including progesterone, which could trigger PMDD.

EDUCATIONAL OBJECTIVE

Recommend treatment options for women with premenstrual dysphoric disorder.

REFERENCE(S)

Ismaili E, Walsh S, O'Brien PMS, et al; Consensus Group of the International Society for Premenstrual Disorders. Fourth consensus of the International Society for Premenstrual Disorders (ISPMD): auditable standards for diagnosis and management of premenstrual disorder. *Arch Womens Ment Health.* 2016;19(6):953-958. PMID: 27378473

Marjoribanks J, Brown J, O'Brien PMS, Wyatt K. Selective serotonin reuptake inhibitors for premenstrual syndrome. *Cochrane Database Syst Rev.* 2013;2013(6):CD001396. PMID: 23744611

Carlini SV, Lanza di Scalea T, McNally ST, Lester J, Deligiannidis KM. Management of premenstrual dysphoric disorder: a scoping review. *Int J Womens Health.* 2022;14:1783-1801. PMID: 36575726

Management of premenstrual disorders: ACOG Clinical Practice Guideline No. 7. *Obstet Gynecol.* 2023;142(6):1516-1533. PMID: 37973069

6 ANSWER: A) No treatment

No treatment is necessary for this patient now (Answer A) because it appears that she is recovering from functional hypothalamic amenorrhea. Her laboratory values are consistent with recent ovulation (likely in the luteal phase and will have a period soon). The serum progesterone concentration of 3.5 ng/mL (11.1 nmol/L) confirms that she has ovulated. While progesterone levels are also high in pregnancy, but they are considerably higher than 3.5 ng/mL (>11.1 nmol/L) and her pregnancy test was negative. Serum LH and FSH vary across the cycle but are relatively low in the late luteal phase (just before the important small rise in serum FSH that is responsible for the recruitment of the cohort of follicles for the subsequent menstrual cycle). Serum estradiol concentrations peak just before the midcycle surge, but there is also a secondary rise in the luteal phase that corresponds with the rise in serum progesterone (both hormones secreted by the corpus luteum). The best option is to reassure her that she is recovering and will likely have a period.

If there were no evidence of recovery, the next step would be to start a physiologic dose of estrogen (Answer E), rather than an oral contraceptive (Answer D), which contains a pharmacologic dose.

Bisphosphonates (Answer C) should not be given in this setting.

Isoflavone supplements (Answer B) are unlikely to change the course of her recovery.

EDUCATIONAL OBJECTIVE

Identify a postovulatory pattern of gonadotropin and gonadal steroid levels.

REFERENCE(S)

Perkins RB, Hall JE, Martin KA. Aetiology, previous menstrual function, and patterns of neuro-endocrine disturbance as prognostic indicators in hypothalamic amenorrhoea. *Hum Reprod.* 2001;16(10):2198-2205. PMID: 11574516

Filicori M, Santoro N, Merriam GR, Crowley WF Jr. Characterization of the physiological pattern of episodic gonadotropin secretion throughout the human menstrual cycle. *J Clin Endocrinol Metab.* 1986;62(6):1136-1144. PMID: 3084534

Gordon CM, Ackerman KE, Berga SL, et al. Functional hypothalamic amenorrhea: an Endocrine Society clinical practice guideline. *J Clin Endocrinol Metab.* 2017;102(5):1413-1439. PMID: 28368518

7 ANSWER: C) Estradiol and prolactin

Functional hypothalamic amenorrhea is a diagnosis of exclusion. Excessive stress, exercise, low weight, and eating disorders may alter the GnRH pulse generator, thereby affecting the necessary switch of pulse frequency and amplitude across the menstrual cycle to induce ovulation and ensure regular periods. Hyperprolactinemia due to mild thyroid dysfunction, medications, or prolactin-secreting pituitary tumors can turn off the GnRH pulse generator and present as hypothalamic amenorrhea. Furthermore, premature ovarian insufficiency can present with shortening and then missed menstrual cycles. FSH would be normal or low in the setting of hypothalamic amenorrhea or hyperprolactinemia, but high in premature ovarian insufficiency. Estrogen is low in the settings of hypothalamic amenorrhea and hyperprolactinemia, but it would be high if the patient were pregnant. In addition to FSH, the best laboratory analytes to measure next are estradiol and prolactin (Answer C).

Androgens (Answer E) should be measured in a patient who has acne and hirsutism.

A stimulated 17-hydroxyprogesterone measurement (Answer A) is the best test to diagnose congenital adrenal hyperplasia, but there is no reason to suspect that diagnosis in this vignette because the patient did not describe hyperandrogenic symptoms or early development of pubic hair.

Progesterone (Answer B) is measured to assess ovulation and luteal-phase function in women attempting fertility.

Cushing syndrome may result in amenorrhea due to inhibition of gonadotropin secretion by excess cortisol. However, an evaluation for hypercortisolism (Answer D) is not indicated in this case.

EDUCATIONAL OBJECTIVE

Recommend appropriate hormone testing based on the history, examination findings, and presentation in amenorrheic women.

REFERENCE(S)

Gordon CM, Ackerman KE, Berga SL, et al. Functional hypothalamic amenorrhea: an Endocrine Society clinical practice guideline. *J Clin Endocrinol Metab.* 2017;102(5):1413-1439. PMID: 28368518

Christin-Maitre S, Givony M, Albarel F, et al. Position statement on the diagnosis and management of premature/primary ovarian insufficiency (except Turner Syndrome). *Ann Endocrinol (Paris).* 2021;82(6):555-571. PMID: 34508691

Caronia LM, Martin C, Welt CK, et al. A genetic basis for functional hypothalamic amenorrhea. *N Engl J Med.* 2011;364(3):215-225. PMID: 21247312

Melmed S, Casanueva FF, Hoffman AR, et al; Endocrine Society. Diagnosis and treatment of hyperprolactinemia: an Endocrine Society clinical practice guideline. *J Clin Endocrinol Metab.* 2011;96(2):273-288. PMID: 21296991

8 ANSWER: D) Letrozole

Women with polycystic ovary syndrome can have intermittent ovulation or anovulation, hyperandrogenism, and insulin resistance. Before planning for fertility, lifestyle should be optimized with diet and exercise. A relatively small amount of weight loss sometimes restores ovulatory cycles. The addition of metformin as an insulin sensitizer can help regulate cycles and suppress androgens, and it may make lifestyle intervention more effective.

Historically, if fertility was desired, clomiphene citrate (Answer A) (50 mg on cycle days 5 through 9) was prescribed to induce ovulation. Clomiphene citrate is more effective than metformin therapy (Answer B) to achieve live births. Although clomiphene citrate is a potential approach to induce ovulation, the Reproductive Network Trial comparing the second-generation aromatase inhibitor letrozole (Answer D) with clomiphene citrate demonstrated a convincingly higher rate of ovulation induction and live births with letrozole, particularly in women with obesity and polycystic ovary syndrome.

Progesterone suppositories (Answer E) are sometimes prescribed for women with hypothalamic amenorrhea—not for women with polycystic ovary syndrome. They improve menstrual cyclicity, but they have not been shown to increase rates of ovulation induction.

Gonadotropin therapy with recombinant FSH (Answer C) is not used as first-line therapy for ovulation induction in women with polycystic ovary syndrome, as it has a greater risk of multiple gestation and ovarian hyperstimulation syndrome. It is typically used in women who have not responded to letrozole and clomiphene.

EDUCATIONAL OBJECTIVE

Compare the treatment effectiveness of clomiphene citrate with that of aromatase inhibitors for ovulation induction in women with polycystic ovary syndrome who would like to become pregnant.

REFERENCE(S)

Palomba S. Aromatase inhibitors for ovulation induction. *J Clin Endocrinol Metab.* 2015;100(5):1742-1747. PMID: 25710566

Legro RS, Brzyski RG, Diamond MP, et al; NICHD Reproductive Medicine Network. Letrozole versus clomiphene for infertility in the polycystic ovary syndrome [published correction appears in *N Engl J Med.* 2014;317(15):1465]. *N Engl J Med.* 2014;371(2):119-129. PMID: 25006718

Franik S, Kremer JA, Nelen WL, Farquhar C, Marjoribanks J. Aromatase inhibitors for subfertile women with polycystic ovary syndrome: summary of a Cochrane review. *Fertil Steril.* 2015;103(2):353-355. PMID: 25455536

Legro RS, Arslanian SA, Ehrmann DA, et al; Endocrine Society. Diagnosis and treatment of polycystic ovary syndrome: An Endocrine Society clinical practice guideline. *J Clin Endocriol Metab.* 2013;98(12):4565-4592. PMID: 24151290

9 **ANSWER: B) 21-Hydroxylase antibodies**

This patient has spontaneous primary ovarian insufficiency (POI). Additional evaluation is needed once this condition is diagnosed. Although the etiology of POI remains unknown in most cases, several tests should be ordered after the diagnosis of POI is established. These investigations include karyotype analysis (primarily to diagnose Turner syndrome) and genetic testing for the fragile X premutation (approximately 6% of POI cases are associated with premutations in the *FMR1* gene, the gene responsible for fragile X syndrome and fragile X–associated tremor/ataxia syndrome). Women with a premutation often have POI, but the main concern is expansion to a full mutation in male offspring, causing intellectual disability.

Approximately 3% of women with spontaneous POI have asymptomatic autoimmune adrenal insufficiency—the diagnosis of POI typically precedes that of adrenal insufficiency by several years. As a screen for the presence of asymptomatic autoimmune adrenal insufficiency, serum 21-hydroxylase antibodies (Answer B) should be measured in all women with a 46,XX karyotype at the time spontaneous POI is diagnosed. Women with adrenal autoimmunity detected by the presence of autoantibodies have a 50% chance of developing adrenal insufficiency. These women should then be evaluated by measuring 8 AM serum cortisol and plasma ACTH. Testing for 21-hydroxylase antibodies may serve the dual purpose of screening for autoimmune adrenal insufficiency and diagnosing autoimmune oophoritis. Autoimmune oophoritis is characterized by theca-cell destruction; granulosa cells are preserved.

Inhibin B levels (Answer D) are normal in women with autoimmune POI but are low in women with other types of POI. Therefore, affected women present with serum LH concentrations that are higher than FSH concentrations.

Measurement of serum ovarian antibodies (Answer E) (with an indirect immunofluorescence assay using cynomolgus monkey ovary) has poor predictive value for autoimmune POI. The prevalence of ovarian antibodies is similar (30%-50%) in women with normal cycles and in women with spontaneous POI.

IGF-1 measurement (Answer C) would not provide useful clinical information about POI.

GAD-65 antibodies (Answer A) would provide insight into her potential risk for type 1 diabetes, but the most important first step is evaluation for adrenal insufficiency and autoimmune oophoritis.

EDUCATIONAL OBJECTIVE

Determine the etiology of primary ovarian insufficiency.

REFERENCE(S)

Bakalov VK, Anasti JN, Calis KA, et al. Autoimmune oophoritis as a mechanism of follicular dysfunction in women with 46,XX spontaneous premature ovarian failure. *Fertil Steril.* 2005;84(4):958-965. PMID: 16213850

Welt CK, Hally JE, Adams JM, Taylor AE. Relationship of estradiol and inhibin to the follicle-stimulating hormone variability in hypergonadotropic hypogonadism or premature ovarian failure. *J Clin Endocrinol Metab.* 2005;90(2):826-830. PMID: 15562017

Novosad JA, Kalantaridou SN, Tong ZB, Nelson LM. Ovarian antibodies as detected by indirect immunofluorescence are unreliable in the diagnosis of autoimmune premature ovarian failure: a controlled evaluation. *BMC Womens Health.* 2003;3(1):2. PMID: 12694633

10 ANSWER: D) Unscheduled bleeding (breakthrough bleeding)

Unscheduled bleeding (also referred to as breakthrough bleeding) (Answer D) is the most common early adverse effect that women experience with combined estrogen-progestin oral contraceptives (COCs), and the most common reason for COC discontinuation. Unscheduled bleeding is more common with lower-dosage estrogen COCs (10 mcg, 20 mcg ethinyl estradiol) and with continuous administration of COCs. The bleeding typically decreases and resolves over subsequent months. If pills have not been missed, the patient can be reassured that unscheduled bleeding does not indicate a lack of contraceptive efficacy. The cause of the bleeding is progressive endometrial atrophy, as low-dosage COCs and continuous regimens are progestin-dominant formulations.

Although many women have concerns that COCs are associated with weight gain (Answer E), most evidence now suggests that the lower-dosage COCs currently used (20 to 35 mcg ethinyl estradiol) are weight neutral.

Sexual dysfunction (decline in libido) (Answer C) is another common concern, given that COCs suppress ovarian androgen secretion. However, available evidence has not shown a consistent negative impact of COCs on sexual function.

Data on the risk of developing depression (Answer A) while taking COCs are mixed. In a large observational study, the absolute rates of first antidepressant use on COCs was 2.2 per 100 woman-years in hormonal contraceptive users compared with 1.7 per 100 woman-years in nonusers (difference of 0.5 per 100 women-years). Although COCs may cause a slight increase in systolic blood pressure in some women, they have not been associated with new-onset hypertension (Answer B).

EDUCATIONAL OBJECTIVE

Describe the early adverse effects of combined estrogen-progestin oral contraceptives.

REFERENCE(S)

Gallo MF, Nanda K, Grimes DA, Schulz KF. 20 mcg versus >20 mcg estrogen combined oral contraceptives for contraception. *Cochrane Database Syst Rev.* 2005;(2):CD003989. PMID: 15846690

Skovlund CW, Mørch LS, Kessing LV, Lidegaard Ø. Association of hormonal contraception with depression. *JAMA Psychiatry.* 2016;73(11):1154-1162. PMID: 27680324

Hickey M, Agarwal S. Unscheduled bleeding in combined oral contraceptive users: focus on extended-cycle and continuous-use regimens. *J Fam Plann Reprod Health Care.* 2009;35(4):245-248. PMID: 19849921

Hee L, Kettner LO, Vejtorp M. Continuous use of oral contraceptives: an overview of effects and side-effects. *Acta Obstet Gynecol Scand.* 2013;92(2):125-136. PMID: 23083413

Boozalis A, Tutlam NT, Chrisman Robbins C, Peipert JF. Sexual desire and hormonal contraception. *Obstet Gynecol.* 2016;127(3):563-572. PMID: 26855094

11 ANSWER: B) Luteomas of pregnancy

This patient has gestational hyperandrogenism, with bilateral solid ovarian masses, which makes luteomas of pregnancy (Answer B) the most likely diagnosis. Luteomas are unilateral or bilateral nonneoplastic ovarian masses associated with pregnancy that regress in the postpartum period. Serum androgens rise during normal pregnancy (serum total testosterone increases up to about 120 ng/dL), but it is uncommon for women to experience worsening or new hyperandrogenic symptoms and very rare for them to become virilized. This is because they are protected by both the pregnancy-associated rise in SHBG and by placental aromatase, the enzyme that converts androgen precursors to estrogens. Luteomas are usually asymptomatic. However, in approximately 30% to 35% of cases, affected women have extremely high androgen concentrations and present with virilizing signs. However, serum androgen concentrations are not a reliable predictor of virilization. If the mother becomes virilized, there is an 80% chance that a female fetus will also be virilized. If the mother is not virilized, then the fetus will not virilize. Fetal virilization was not observed in this case.

Theca lutein cysts (Answer E) are benign cysts without solid components, which distinguishes them from luteomas or malignancy. Ovaries that contain theca lutein cysts can cause pressure symptoms, as they can be as large as 10 to 15 cm. Approximately 30% of pregnant women with theca lutein cysts develop hirsutism or become virilized; however, female fetuses do not virilize.

Women with polycystic ovary syndrome (Answer D) may experience higher serum androgens than women without polycystic ovary syndrome during pregnancy, but they do not have levels high enough to cause virilization.

Dietary supplements (Answer A) would not cause this clinical picture unless they contained significant doses of androgens.

Nonclassic congenital adrenal hyperplasia (Answer C) has not been associated with gestational hyperandrogenism.

EDUCATIONAL OBJECTIVE

Determine the most likely cause of virilization in a pregnant woman.

REFERENCE(S)

Wang YC, Su HY, Liu JY, Chang FW, Chen CH. Maternal and female fetal virilization caused by pregnancy luteomas. *Fertil Steril.* 2005;84(2):509. PMID: 16086574

Wadzinski TL, Altowaireb Y, Gupta R, Conroy R, Shoukri K. Luteoma of pregnancy associated with nearly complete virilization of genetically female twins. *Endocr Pract.* 2014;20(2):e18-e23. PMID: 24126228

Kuijper EA, Ket JC, Caanen MR, Lambalk CB. Reproductive hormone concentrations in pregnancy and neonates: a systematic review. *Reprod Biomed Online.* 2013;27(1):33-63. PMID: 23669015

12 ANSWER: E) Transvaginal ultrasonography

Postmenopausal hirsutism or virilization of recent onset with a serum testosterone concentration greater than 150 ng/dL (>5.2 nmol/L) or a serum DHEA-S concentration greater than 700 to 800 μg/dL (18.97 to 21.68 μmol/L) suggests a neoplastic source of hyperandrogenism. Signs of virilization include deepening of the voice, increased muscle mass, and clitoromegaly. Clitoromegaly is defined by a clitoral length greater than 10 mm or a clitoral index (length × width) greater than 35 mm^2. Virilization is only seen with more severe hyperandrogenemia (serum testosterone >150 ng/dL [>5.2 nmol/L]). Postmenopausal women with polycystic ovary syndrome do not have serum testosterone levels in this range, nor are they virilized.

Women with ovarian hyperthecosis typically develop symptoms gradually, but some with severe hyperthecosis have a more rapid course with severe hyperandrogenemia that mimics androgen-secreting tumors. Women with androgen-secreting adrenal tumors often present with symptoms of Cushing syndrome in addition to virilization. Unlike ovarian tumors, adrenal androgen-secreting tumors often, but not always, cause elevation in serum DHEA-S. However, DHEA-S can be normal in androgen-secreting adrenal tumors. Androgen-secreting ovarian tumors include Sertoli-Leydig–cell tumors, arrhenoblastomas, or hilus-cell tumors.

The first step in the evaluation of severe hyperandrogenism in postmenopausal women is transvaginal ultrasonography (Answer E) to look for a tumor or asymmetry of the ovaries (as the tumors are typically very small). If findings on ultrasonography are normal, adrenal CT (Answer A) should be performed, because there are occasional cases of adrenal tumors that secrete only testosterone. However, adrenal CT would not be the preferred initial imaging. In addition, ultrasonography is a better imaging choice than abdominal CT for visualizing the ovaries.

Dexamethasone-suppression testing (Answer B) is used in the workup of Cushing syndrome and might be indicated if an adrenal mass were detected. With adrenal Cushing syndrome, the presentation would be different from this patient's and the testosterone level would not be as high as it is in this vignette.

Serum inhibin (Answer D) is a marker for some ovarian tumors, including granulosa-cell tumors and sex-cord stromal tumors, but ultrasonography is the more important next step.

Serum 17-hydroxyprogesterone (Answer C) would be measured when there are concerns for nonclassic congenital adrenal hyperplasia due to 21-hydroxylase deficiency (which is associated with hirsutism, but not virilization).

EDUCATIONAL OBJECTIVE

Evaluate postmenopausal hyperandrogenism.

REFERENCE(S)

Alpañés M, González-Casbas JM, Sánchez J, Pián H, Escobar-Morreale HF. Management of postmenopausal virilization. *J Clin Endocrinol Metab.* 2012;97(8):2584-2588. PMID: 22669303

Meczekalski B, Szeliga A, Maciejewska-Jeske M, et al. Hyperthecosis: an underestimated nontumorous cause of hyperandrogenism. *Gynecol Endocrinol.* 2021;37(8):677-682. PMID: 33759685

Pugeat M, Déchaud H, Raverot V, Denuzière A, Cohen R, Boudou P; French Endocrine Society. Recommendations for investigation of hyperandrogenism. *Ann Endocrinol (Paris).* 2010;71(1):2-7. PMID: 20096825

Carmina E, Dewailly D, Escobar-Morreale HF, et al. Non-classic congenital adrenal hyperplasia due to 21-hydroxylase deficiency revisited: an update with a special focus on adolescent and adult women. *Hum Reprod Update.* 2017;23(5):580-599. PMID: 28582566

13 ANSWER: D) Oral 17β-estradiol, 2 mg daily

This patient is an excellent candidate for estrogen. The results of the Women's Health Initiative are not relevant to her, as the mean patient age was 63 years, and she is only 42. She should be approached like any woman with primary ovarian insufficiency and be treated with estrogen until the average age of menopause (50/51 years). She has severe symptoms that are interfering with her quality of life and her ability to function, so estrogen is indicated. Women with primary ovarian insufficiency are prescribed higher dosages of estrogen than other women; therefore, a progesterone-only option (Answer C) is incorrect. The best answer is oral 17β-estradiol, 2 mg daily (Answer D). She could also use unopposed transdermal estrogen, but it is not necessary (and was not offered as an option).

A combination estrogen-progestin option is listed (Answer A), which she does not need. Progestin therapy is not indicated in a patient after a hysterectomy, as its only role is to prevent endometrial hyperplasia.

Venlafaxine (Answer E) and gabapentin (Answer B) are nonhormonal alternatives—these are options for some patients with breast cancer who cannot take estrogen.

EDUCATIONAL OBJECTIVE

Recommend the optimal approach to managing severe hot flashes in a premenopausal woman after total hysterectomy and bilateral salpingo-oophorectomy.

REFERENCE(S)

Stuenkel CA, Davis SR, Gompel A, et al. Treatment of symptoms of the menopause: an Endocrine Society clinical practice guideline. *J Clin Endocrinol Metab.* 2015;100(11):3975-4011. PMID: 26444994

The NAMS 2017 Hormone Therapy Position Statement Advisory Panel. The 2017 hormone therapy position statement of The North American Menopause Society. *Menopause.* 2017;24(7):728-753. PMID: 28650869

Committee on Gynecologic Practice. Committee opinion No. 698: hormone therapy in primary ovarian insufficiency. *Obstet Gynecol.* 2017;129(5):e134-e141. PMID: 28426619

14 ANSWER: A) Daily prospective symptom diary for 2 cycles

This patient appears to have premenstrual dysphoric disorder. However, it is necessary to have prospective documentation of the timing of her symptoms to confirm the diagnosis (Answer A). Unlike other mood disorders, premenstrual dysphoric disorder symptoms should resolve in the follicular phase.

In some cases, perimenopause must be ruled out with a cycle day 3 measurement of serum FSH (Answer B) and serum antimullerian hormone (Answer D), as there can be some overlap in clinical mood symptoms.

Patients with thyroid disease may also have similar mood changes, but their symptoms would not be cyclic. Thus, TSH measurement (Answer E) is not the best next step.

Unipolar depression that worsens before menses is not considered to be premenstrual dysphoric disorder. Therefore, depression screening (Answer C) is not the best next step.

EDUCATIONAL OBJECTIVE

Identify the symptoms of premenstrual dysphoric disorder and diagnose this condition.

REFERENCE(S)

Cohen LS, Soares CN, Otto MW, Sweeney BH, Liberman RF, Harlow BL. Prevalence and predictors of premenstrual dysphoric disorder (PMDD) in older premenopausal women. The Harvard Study of Moods and Cycles. *J Affect Disord.* 2002;70(2):125-132. PMID: 12117624

Freeman EW, Halberstadt SM, Rickels K, Legler JM, Lin H, Sammel MD. Core symptoms that discriminate premenstrual syndrome. *J Womens Health (Larchmt).* 2011;20(1):29-35. PMID: 21128818

Endicott J, Nee J, Harrison W. Daily record of severity of problems (DRSP): reliability and validity. *Arch Womens Ment Health.* 2006;9(1):41-49. PMID: 16172836

15 ANSWER: B) 46,XX

This patient most likely has mullerian agenesis. Mullerian agenesis or hypoplasia leads to variable uterine development and congenital absence of the vagina, termed the Mayer-Rokitansky-Kuster-Hauser syndrome. The uterus may be underdeveloped or absent. Affected persons have a normal female phenotype at birth, functioning ovaries, normal external genitalia, and a 46, XX karyotype (Answer B). These individuals are raised as girls. Breast development and pubic hair growth are also normal.

Patients with complete androgen insensitivity who are diagnosed during their teenage years present with primary amenorrhea, absence of axillary or pubic hair, serum testosterone within or above the normal range for boys and men, high LH, and normal FSH. Mullerian structures are absent (blind vaginal pouch and absent uterus and cervix), and the karyotype is 46,XY (Answer C). This disorder is due to a defect in the androgen receptor that results in complete resistance to androgens.

Women with Turner syndrome have short stature, primary hypogonadism, a high rate of cardiovascular anomalies, a number of comorbidities, and a 45,X karyotype (Answer A). Women with Turner syndrome mosaicism often have a 45,X/46,XX karyotype (Answer D).

A 47,XXY karyotype (Answer E) is the etiology of Klinefelter syndrome, and affected individuals have a male phenotype.

EDUCATIONAL OBJECTIVE

Distinguish between complete androgen insensitivity syndrome and mullerian agenesis in young women who present with primary amenorrhea.

REFERENCE(S)

Doehnert U, Bertelloni S, Werner R, Dati E, Hiort O. Characteristic features of reproductive hormone profiles in late adolescent and adult females with complete androgen insensitivity syndrome. *Sex Dev.* 2015;9(2):69-74. PMID: 25613104

Grimbizis GF, Gordts S, Di Spiezio Sardo A, et al. The ESHRE/ESGE consensus on the classification of female genital tract congenital anomalies. *Hum Reprod.* 2013;28(8):2032-2044. PMID: 23771171

16 ANSWER: B) Leuprolide, 3.75 mg intramuscularly, plus estradiol, 50 mcg by transdermal patch

As is the case in postmenopausal women, the use of estrogen in transgender patients is associated with an increased risk of venous thromboembolism. In the case described, the patient is already at increased risk of venous thromboembolism by having an inherited thrombophilia. Therefore, when selecting the most appropriate hormone regimen, the priority is to identify the one with the lowest thrombogenic potential.

The risk of venous thromboembolism conferred by estrogen depends on the dosage, formulation, and route of administration.

Incorporating a GnRH agonist into the hormone regimen for a transgender female patient has the advantage of causing profound suppression of endogenous testosterone, so that only physiologic doses of estrogen need to be administered. Of the 2 hormone regimens that include a GnRH agonist, the option with the estrogen patch (Answer B) is correct, as transdermal estrogen is associated with a lower clotting risk than oral formulations (Answer A) because it bypasses the liver and therefore leads to less of an increase in clotting factors.

Unlike GnRH analogues, antiandrogens such as spironolactone cause more modest suppression of testosterone, so higher estrogen dosages are needed to achieve the desired degree of testosterone suppression. Therefore, a regimen consisting of spironolactone without estrogen would not be potent enough to suppress testosterone even if combined with a 5α-reductase inhibitor such as finasteride (Answer D). Spironolactone, 200 mg, plus estradiol, 1 mg orally, (Answer E) is also incorrect because it adds oral estradiol to the regimen of a patient with an inherited thrombophilia.

Of the different types of estrogen available, risk of venous thromboembolism is highest with ethinyl estradiol (Answer C), which should therefore be avoided.

EDUCATIONAL OBJECTIVE

Guide the initiation of hormone therapy in a transgender woman at increased risk of venous thromboembolism.

REFERENCE(S)

Hembree WC, Cohen-Kettenis PT, Gooren L, et al. Endocrine treatment of gender dysphoric/gender incongruent persons: an Endocrine Society clinical practice guideline. *J Clin Endocrinol Metab.* 2017;102(11):3869-3903. PMID: 28945902

T'Sjoen G, Arcelus J, Gooren L, Klink DT, Tangpricha V. Endocrinology of transgender medicine. *Endocr Rev.* 2019;40(1):97-117. PMID: 30307546

Safer JD, Tangpricha V. Care of transgender persons. *N Engl J Med.* 2019;381(25):2451-2460. PMID: 31851801

Male Reproduction Board Review

Stephanie Page, MD, PhD

1 ANSWER: D) Repeat morning fasting total and free testosterone measurement with concomitant LH and FSH in 1 month
The diagnosis of late-onset male hypogonadism requires both symptomatic and biochemical evidence of hypogonadism. This patient has fatigue, a nonspecific sign of hypogonadism, as well as decreased libido. Decreases in libido and sexual function, while not diagnostic of hypogonadism, are the most specific signs associated with male hypogonadism. He has had 2 low serum testosterone measurements; however, one of these was performed in the context of acute illness. Acute illness suppresses the hypothalamic-pituitary-gonadal axis, an effect that can take 2 to 3 months to recover from, and it has been documented in the setting of COVID-19 infection. Moreover, the timing of his initial referring blood draw is not known, and his hypothalamic-pituitary-testicular axis appears to be recovering with an increase in serum testosterone over the last 2 months. The diagnosis of male hypogonadism requires 2 measurements documenting low fasting morning (7-10 AM) serum total testosterone or free testosterone concentrations while in stable health. Thus, before prescribing testosterone replacement (Answers A and B), this patient should have another testosterone measurement, as well as an evaluation of primary vs secondary hypogonadism, which requires LH and FSH measurement (Answer D). A trial of testosterone replacement is indicated only in men who have an established diagnosis of male hypogonadism.

Although weight loss and lifestyle changes (Answer C) can raise serum testosterone concentrations, this patient should have complete evaluation for hypogonadism, including investigation of the etiology.

Similarly, while depression (Answer E) and late-onset hypogonadism have some symptom overlap, evaluation for hypogonadism should be completed given his presenting symptoms and low testosterone on his first sample.

EDUCATIONAL OBJECTIVE
Guide the diagnostic evaluation of male hypogonadism in older men, particularly in the setting of acute illness.

REFERENCE(S)

Bhasin S, Brito JP, Cunningham GR, et al. Testosterone therapy in men with hypogonadism: an Endocrine Society clinical practice guideline. *J Clin Endocrinol Metab.* 2018;103(5):1715-1744. PMID: 29562364

Cinislioglu AE, Cinislioglu N, Demirdogen SO, et al. The relationship of serum testosterone levels with the clinical course and prognosis of COVID-19 disease in male patients: a prospective study. *Andrology.* 2022;10(1):24-33. PMID: 34288536

2 ANSWER: A) Improve his anemia
The double-blinded, randomized controlled Testosterone Trials (T-Trials) provide the most definitive data to date regarding the benefits of testosterone therapy in older men with low testosterone and at least 1 symptom of hypogonadism. The study population was symptomatic men older than 65 years old who had a total testosterone concentration less than 275 ng/dL (<9.5 mmol/L). Participants randomly assigned to testosterone therapy had increases in total testosterone and experienced (1) improvements in sexual activity and libido; (2) mild improvements in mood and reduced severity of depressive symptoms; and (3) improvements in

physical function as assessed by a 6-minute walk test. Importantly, in those participants with unexplained anemia, those receiving testosterone had a clinically significant increase in hemoglobin (Answer A).

While testosterone therapy increases bone mineral density and may increase bone strength (effects observed in the T-Trials and other studies), no randomized controlled trials of testosterone therapy have been powered to address fracture risk, and recent reports from the TRAVERSE study have not supported a benefit of testosterone therapy in preventing fracture (thus, Answer D is incorrect).

Testosterone therapy does not reproducibly improve mental cognition in men, an effect that was also not observed in the "Vitality" substudy nested within the T-Trials (thus, Answer B is incorrect).

While the T-Trials were not powered to assess cardiovascular risk with testosterone therapy, no increase in events was seen compared with placebo, and the recent TRAVERSE study, a noninferiority trial in men at high risk for cardiovascular disease, demonstrated no increase in cardiovascular disease events with testosterone therapy compared with placebo (thus, Answer C is incorrect).

Finally, while oral testosterone therapy reduces serum HDL cholesterol, testosterone therapy does not significantly lower LDL cholesterol (thus, Answer E is incorrect).

EDUCATIONAL OBJECTIVE

Explain the current evidence regarding the risks and benefits of testosterone therapy in older men with symptomatic, late-onset hypogonadism.

REFERENCE(S)

Lincoff AM, Bhasin S, Flevaris P, et al; TRAVERSE Study Investigators. Cardiovascular safety of testosterone-replacement therapy. *N Engl J Med.* 2023;389(3):107-117. PMID: 37326322

Roy CN, Snyder PJ, Stephens-Shields AJ, et al. Association of testosterone levels with anemia in older men: a controlled clinical trial. *JAMA Intern Med.* 2017;177(4):480-490. PMID: 28241237

Snyder PJ, Bhasin S, Cunningham GR, et al; Testosterone Trials Investigators. Effects of testosterone treatment in older men. *N Engl J Med.* 2016;374(7):611-624. PMID: 26886521

3 ANSWER: C) Ensure that he is up to date with mammography

The Endocrine Society Guidelines for transgender care recommend continued health maintenance screening as per the biological gender. Thus, for this patient, who is in his fifties and has a first-degree relative with breast cancer and is thus at increased risk himself, ongoing breast cancer screening (Answer C) is warranted. There is currently no indication for oophorectomy (Answer E). Given his family history, he could be referred at some point to medical genetics for consideration of *BRCA* or other genetic screening, but oophorectomy for transgender men older than 50 years in the absence of further indication is currently not recommended.

When monitoring the effectiveness of gender-affirming hormone therapy, hormone concentrations also help guide therapy and should target the physiologic reference range for the transgender. When delivering hormone therapy via intramuscular injections, hormone concentrations may be assessed at the mid-dose or trough dose time intervals. This patient has normal testosterone concentrations midweek through the dosing interval and thus does not need a dose adjustment (Answers A and B).

Testosterone administration, particularly intramuscular injections, stimulates erythrocytosis, and polycythemia can be dose-limiting. However, this patient's hematocrit value is normal. Prostate cancer is not a concern in transgender men, as there is no prostate tissue. Thus, PSA measurement (Answer D) is not recommended.

EDUCATIONAL OBJECTIVE

Guide monitoring and health care maintenance for transgender men taking gender-affirming hormone therapy.

REFERENCE(S)

Hembree WC, Cohen-Kettenis PT, Gooren L, et al. Endocrine treatment of gender-dysphoric/gender-incongruent persons: an Endocrine Society clinical practice guideline. *J Clin Endocrinol Metab.* 2017;102(11):3869-3903. PMID: 28945902

Gorton RN, Erickson-Schroth L. Hormonal and surgical treatment options for transgender men (female-to-male). *Psychiatr Clin North Am.* 2017;40(1):79-97. PMID: 28159147

4 ANSWER: A) Perform pituitary MRI

This otherwise healthy patient presents with adult-onset secondary, symptomatic hypogonadism (low testosterone with low serum gonadotropins) that requires further evaluation before initiation of therapy. While the yield for pituitary imaging is low in older men with late-onset hypogonadism, this 44-year-old man has acute symptoms and very low serum testosterone on 2 morning measurements and no suggestion of hemochromatosis. Despite normal thyroid function and prolactin concentrations, he may harbor a pituitary adenoma suppressing his gonadotropin production without affecting other pituitary hormones. Thus, pituitary imaging (Answer A) is indicated.

Initiation of hypogonadism treatment (Answers C and D) may address his symptoms, but it would not establish the cause of secondary hypogonadism.

Similarly, treatment of erectile dysfunction (Answer B) may improve his sexual health, but it would not improve his low testosterone.

While chronic narcotics can suppress gonadotropin production, resulting in secondary hypogonadism, this degree of testosterone and gonadotropin deficiency is not attributable to occasional use of low-potency narcotics (Answer E) and is not an appropriate strategy for delaying his evaluation.

EDUCATIONAL OBJECTIVE

Determine when pituitary imaging is indicated in the evaluation of male hypogonadism.

REFERENCE(S)

Bhasin S, Brito JP, Cunningham GR, et al. Testosterone therapy in men with hypogonadism: an Endocrine Society clinical practice guideline. *J Clin Endocrinol Metab.* 2018;103(5):1715-1744. PMID: 2956236

Dalvi M, Walker BR, Strachan MWJ, Zammitt NN, Gibb FW. The prevalence of structural pituitary abnormalities by MRI scanning in men presenting with isolated hypogonadotrophichypogonadism. *Clin Endocrinol (Oxf).* 2016;84(6):858–861. PMID: 26733239

5 ANSWER: C) Start a phosphodiesterase inhibitor

Phosphodiesterase inhibitors (Answer C) have been shown to consistently improve erectile function in clinical trials, and they are the mainstay of treating erectile dysfunction in otherwise healthy men without contraindications.

While this patient's testosterone concentration is at the lower end of the reference range, he does not have biochemical hypogonadism. Thus, there is no indication for hCG therapy (Answers D and E). Furthermore, the co-administration of testosterone and sildenafil has been studied in men with low testosterone, and the addition of testosterone has not been shown to provide additional benefit. In a double-blind, randomized, placebo-controlled trial, middle-aged men (40-70 years) who had erectile dysfunction with low total testosterone (<330 ng/dL [<11.5 nmol/L] or free testosterone <5.0 ng/dL [<0.2 nmol/L]) were treated with sildenafil and then randomly assigned to an additional 14 weeks of sildenafil alone or sildenafil plus testosterone therapy (testosterone gel). No difference in erectile function was observed between the groups, and the investigators concluded that the addition of testosterone treatment to sildenafil did not improve erectile function. A second blinded, randomized controlled trial in middle-aged and older men (45-80 years) with mild hypogonadism found no difference in erectile function between men for whom phosphodiesterase treatment failed and were then randomly assigned to testosterone gel plus tadalafil compared with tadalafil alone. The investigators did observe some benefit from the addition of testosterone therapy to tadalafil in men with total testosterone concentrations less than 300 ng/dL (<10.4 nmol/L). On the basis of these recent trial findings, the addition of testosterone replacement to phosphodiesterase inhibitor therapy is unlikely to improve erectile function in this patient with a low-normal serum testosterone concentration.

This patient has normal gonadotropins, serum testosterone, and thyroid function; thus, pituitary imaging (Answer A) is not indicated.

With normal seminal fluid analysis, history of fertility, and infrequent intercourse complicated by erectile dysfunction, referral for assisted reproductive services (Answer B) is premature.

EDUCATIONAL OBJECTIVE

Evaluate and treat erectile dysfunction and describe the limited role of exogenous testosterone in the treatment of erectile dysfunction.

REFERENCE(S)

McVary KT. Clinical practice. Erectile dysfunction. *N Engl J Med.* 2007;357(24):2472-2481. PMID: 18077811

Bhasin S, Brito JP, Cunningham GR, et al. Testosterone therapy in men with hypogonadism: an Endocrine Society clinical practice guideline. *J Clin Endocrinol Metab.* 2018;103(5):1715-1744. PMID: 29562364

Isidori AM, Buvat J, Corona G, et al. A critical analysis of the role of testosterone in erectile function: from pathophysiology to treatment-a systematic review. *Eur Urol.* 2014;65(1):99-112. PMID: 24050791

6 ANSWER: D) Microdissection testicular sperm extraction followed by intracytoplasmic sperm injection

Klinefelter syndrome is the most common chromosomal abnormality in men. While there may be some phenotypic variability, hypergonadotropic hypogonadism characterized by small testes and azoospermia is seen in more than 95% of men with nonmosaic Klinefelter syndrome. While there have been rare case reports of men with Klinefelter syndrome impregnating their partners naturally, this is the exception rather than the rule, and one would not expect the patient to be able to father children without treatment (thus, Answer E is incorrect).

In men with hypogonadotropic hypogonadism, treatment with hCG (Answer B) can increase systemic and intratesticular testosterone levels and, by doing so, stimulate spermatogenesis. However, in the case described, endogenous LH levels are already elevated, so hCG administration would be of no benefit.

With the advent of the technique of microdissection testicular sperm extraction (Answer D) in the late 1990s, fertility options for men with Klinefelter syndrome changed dramatically, and they were no longer limited to use of donor sperm (Answer C) or adoption. Using this technique, normal-sized seminiferous tubules, likely to contain spermatozoa, are selectively removed with microscissors and the removed tissue is immediately examined for the presence of sperm. Sperm are reportedly retrieved in up to 50% of cases. This technique offers affected patients the possibility of biologic paternity when combined with a modification of in vitro fertilization called intracytoplasmic sperm injection, whereby an embryologist directly injects a single sperm into the cytoplasm of an egg.

Because any surviving spermatozoa from men with Klinefelter syndrome originate in euploid germ cells, use of assisted reproduction in these patients is not associated with a higher risk of having a son with Klinefelter syndrome compared with the risk of men with a 46,XY karyotype. There is a case report of a 47,XXY fetus conceived after intracytoplasmic sperm injection of spermatozoa from a patient with Klinefelter syndrome. However, given that Klinefelter syndrome occurs in about 1 in 600 boys in the background population, a few cases of 47,XXY should be expected.

Clomiphene citrate (Answer A) is a selective estrogen receptor modulator that is approved by the US FDA to induce ovulation in women, but it is not approved for use in men. Nonetheless, it is sometimes used off-label to increase testosterone levels in men with hypogonadism, as it is orally active and, unlike testosterone, does not suppress spermatogenesis. Clomiphene can increase testosterone levels in men with hypogonadotropic hypogonadism by reducing estrogen-mediated negative feedback, thus allowing an increase in endogenous LH levels. However, in the patient described who has primary hypogonadism and LH levels that are already elevated, giving clomiphene would be of no benefit.

EDUCATIONAL OBJECTIVE

Counsel patients with Klinefelter syndrome about their fertility potential.

REFERENCE(S)

Gravholt CH, Chang S, Wallentin M, Fedder J, Moore P, Skakkebaek A. Klinefelter syndrome: integrating genetics, neuropsychology, and endocrinology. *Endocr Rev.* 2018;39(4):389-423. PMID: 29438472

Corona G, Pizzocaro A, Lanfranco F, et al; Klinefelter ItaliaN Group (KING). Sperm recovery and ICSI outcomes in Klinefelter syndrome: a systematic review and meta-analysis. *Hum Reprod Update.* 2017;23(3):265-275. PMID: 28379559

7 ANSWER: B) Total testosterone, high or high-normal; free testosterone, low or low-normal; estradiol, high; LH, normal

Gynecomastia is benign enlargement of the male breast due mainly to the proliferation of ductal tissue. Gynecomastia develops when there is an increase in the ratio of estrogen to androgens, with the former having a stimulatory effect on breast tissue, while the latter antagonizes this effect. A small degree of breast enlargement is a relatively common finding, especially in older men, and it generally does not require any workup when asymptomatic. However, breast enlargement that is prominent, painful, progressive, or of recent onset, as in this case, requires thorough evaluation.

The patient described is clinically and biochemically hyperthyroid, a condition known to cause gynecomastia. In men with hyperthyroidism, there is increased hepatic production of SHBG, which results in high levels of total but low or low-normal levels of free testosterone, high estradiol, and normal LH (Answer B). Because of the greater affinity of SHBG for testosterone than for estradiol, there is a relative increase in the amount of free estradiol compared with testosterone. There is also increased aromatization of testosterone to estradiol in extraglandular tissues.

Low serum estradiol with low testosterone and LH levels (Answer A) can be seen with secondary hypogonadism, but this patient's thyroid hormone levels are elevated, indicating his low testosterone is unlikely due to pituitary insufficiency.

High levels of testosterone, estradiol, and LH (Answer D) are typical in patients with partial androgen insensitivity.

A hormone profile characterized by normal testosterone levels, high estradiol, and low LH (Answer C) can be seen in patients with a testicular or extragonadal hCG-secreting tumor. In these patients, hCG stimulates production of both testosterone and estradiol, but because of its stimulatory effect on the aromatase enzyme, there is preferential estradiol production leading to a lower-than-normal testosterone-to-estradiol ratio.

EDUCATIONAL OBJECTIVE

Describe the presentation of gynecomastia due to hyperthyroidism.

REFERENCE(S)

Ali SN, Jayasena CN. Sam AH. Which patients with gynaecomastia require more detailed investigation? *Clin Endocrinol (Oxf).* 2018:88(3):360-363. PMID: 29193251

Narula HS, Carlson HE. Gynaecomastia--pathophysiology, diagnosis and treatment. *Nat Rev Endocrinol.* 2014; 10(11):684-698. PMID: 25112235

Braunstein GD. Clinical practice. Gynecomastia. *N Engl J Med.* 2007;357(12):1229-1237. PMID: 17881754

8 ANSWER: C) Start a GLP-1 receptor agonist, refer to a nutritionist, and encourage lifestyle modifications, including weight-loss goals

This patient is overweight and has low total testosterone levels. Patients who are overweight have low SHBG levels, so in this setting free testosterone concentrations should be used to assess for biochemical hypogonadism. Moreover, he does not have concerns associated with low testosterone (he has normal libido and energy). Thus, neither testosterone therapy (Answer E) nor gonadotropin therapy (Answer D) is appropriate for this patient with obesity and normal free testosterone concentrations.

Weight loss and optimization of glucose management both increase testosterone concentrations, which is important for this patient's long-term fertility. Thus, adding a GLP-1 receptor agonist, referring to a nutritionist, and encouraging lifestyle modifications (Answer C) is the best option. His semen analysis shows sperm production within the reference range even though it is at the lower end of normal; sperm concentrations are highly variable from day to day within an individual.

Administration of clomiphene citrate (Answer B) may mildly increase testosterone concentrations, but it has not been demonstrated to improve semen parameters in men with infertility. Moreover, long-term use of clomiphene citrate, an estrogen antagonist, is likely to have negative effects on bone health and is not recommended.

Cannabis consumption has not been demonstrated to alter fertility or sperm concentrations in men. While this is an area of active investigation, studies to date have not demonstrated that sperm numbers are impacted by occasional cannabis use. Thus, he does not need to be counseled to stop using edibles (Answer A).

EDUCATIONAL OBJECTIVE

Interpret testosterone values in men with obesity and explain how weight loss can raise serum testosterone levels.

REFERENCE(S)

Helo S, Ellen J, Mechlin C, Feustel P, et al. A randomized prospective double-blind comparison trial of clomiphene citrate and anastrozole in raising testosterone in hypogonadal infertile men. *J Sex Med.* 2015;12(8):1761-1769. PMID: 26176805

Anawalt BD. Approach to male infertility and induction of spermatogenesis. *J Clin Endocrinol Metab.* 2013;98(9):3532-3542. PMID: 24014811

Belladelli F, Fallara G, Pozzi E, et al. Effects of recreational cannabis on testicular function in primary infertile men. *Andrology.* 2022 Sep;10(6):1172-1180. PMID: 35868833

9 ANSWER: D) hCG use

This patient has tender gynecomastia. Breast tenderness suggests benign breast growth of recent onset (<6 months). He also has elevated total and free testosterone concentrations, a high estradiol concentration, and low gonadotropin concentrations. This combination can be due to exogenous testosterone, endogenous or exogenous testosterone precursors (eg, dehydroepiandrosterone from an adrenal tumor), and either endogenous hCG (eg, hCG-secreting germ-cell tumor) or exogenous hCG (eg, hCG abuse [Answer D]).

Although chronic hepatitis (Answer B) is commonly associated with elevated SHBG concentrations, the hormone profile in such cases would be a high-normal or elevated total testosterone value but a normal free fraction, so it would not explain this patient's hormone profile.

An estrogen-secreting testicular tumor (Answer C) would cause elevated estradiol concentrations and suppressed gonadotropins, but testosterone levels would not be high.

Finasteride (Answer A) modestly raises serum testosterone concentrations by blocking the conversion of testosterone to dihydrotestosterone, but it would not cause suppressed gonadotropin concentrations.

In men using synthetic anabolic steroids (Answer E), endogenous sex steroid production is suppressed.

EDUCATIONAL OBJECTIVE

Identify the clinical and biochemical features of exogenous testosterone abuse.

REFERENCE(S)

Amory JK, Wang C, Swerdloff RS, et al. The effect of 5alpha-reductase inhibition with dutasteride and finasteride on semen parameters and serum hormones in healthy men [published correction appears in *J Clin Endocrinol Metab.* 2007;92(11):4379]. *J Clin Endocrinol Metab.* 2007;92(5):1659-1665. PMID: 17299062

Braunstein GD. Clinical practice. Gynecomastia. *N Engl J Med.* 2007;357(12):1229-1237. PMID: 17881754

Anawalt BD. Gynecomastia. In: Jameson JL, De Groot LJ, eds. *Endocrinology: Adult and Pediatric.* 7th ed. Philadelphia, PA: Saunders Elsevier; 2015.

10 ANSWER: D) Initiate transdermal testosterone therapy

Twenty to twenty-five percent of men taking highly active antiretroviral therapy for HIV have low total or free testosterone concentrations. Highly active antiretroviral therapy is often associated with increases in SHBG. In men with HIV on highly active antiretroviral therapy, free testosterone should be measured when a borderline total testosterone concentration is noted, and free testosterone should be used as a basis for biochemical hypogonadism. For a trial of testosterone therapy in men with suboptimally controlled hypertension, transdermal testosterone is preferred over oral testosterone undecanoate (Answer C), which has been associated with increases in blood pressure.

Low testosterone in men with HIV is associated with morbidity, and treatment with testosterone is associated with increases in body weight and lean body mass in 3 to 6 months. Dietary counseling alone (Answer E) is insufficient for this patient with hypogonadism.

On the basis of his low free testosterone concentration and persistent weight loss, he meets the threshold for therapy. While 5α-reductase inhibitors (Answer A) may slightly raise testosterone, this would be insufficient to treat his hypogonadism and weight loss.

Megestrol acetate (Answer B) primarily acts as an appetite stimulant and has been trialed in the setting of cancer and HIV cachexia with mixed results. This medication has numerous adverse effects. He is hypogonadal and reports a normal appetite; thus, megestrol should not be first-line therapy.

EDUCATIONAL OBJECTIVE

Recommend a trial of testosterone treatment to improve body composition in hypogonadal men with HIV and unexplained weight loss.

REFERENCE(S)

Pena Dias J, Haberlen SA, Dobs AS, et al. Longitudinal changes in sex hormone–binding globulin in men with HIV. *J Acquir Immune Defic Syndr.* 2021;87(5):1178-1186. PMID: 33990494

Bhasin S, Brito JP, Cunningham GR, et al. Testosterone therapy in men with hypogonadism: an Endocrine Society clinical practice guideline. *J Clin Endocrinol Metab.* 2018;103(5):1715-1744. PMID: 29562364

11 ANSWER: C) Increase the hCG dosage to 1500 international units 3 times weekly

Men with secondary hypogonadism should be treated with exogenous testosterone therapy to achieve physiologic testosterone levels. However, men desiring fertility require gonadotropin therapy to provide stimulus to the testes to support spermatogenesis. In such men, exogenous testosterone therapy should be discontinued and not reintroduced until desired fertility outcomes are achieved.

Gonadotropin therapy is more likely to be successful in men with postpubertal secondary hypogonadism and normal testicular volumes. Gonadotropin therapy is initiated with hCG at dosages of 1000 to 2000 international units 3 times weekly to achieve normal testosterone concentrations, although sometimes lower dosages of hCG are sufficient. In this man, testosterone concentrations are not within the reference range and the hCG dosage should be increased (Answer C) to normalize serum testosterone.

The addition of recombinant FSH (Answer B) should not be considered until after 6 months of hCG therapy.

Clomiphene citrate (Answer A) is an estrogen receptor antagonist that can increase serum testosterone by reducing negative feedback at the pituitary, but this will not be effective in a man without normal gonadotropin production following pituitary adenoma resection.

Initiation of spermatogenesis usually requires approximately 72 days (cycle of sperm maturation); thus, it is too soon for a seminal fluid analysis (Answer D). Furthermore, spermatogenesis requires adequate testosterone for effectiveness. Waiting longer (Answer E) would be inappropriate in this case because the patient is symptomatic and has a low testosterone concentration due to insufficient hCG therapy.

EDUCATIONAL OBJECTIVE

Explain the time course and treatment parameters needed to optimize gonadotropin therapy in patients with secondary hypogonadism.

REFERENCE(S)

Anawalt BD. Approach to male infertility and induction of spermatogenesis. *J Clin Endocrinol Metab.* 2013;98(9):3532-3542. PMID: 24014811

Liu PY, Baker HWG, Jayadev V, Zacharin M, Conway AJ, Handelsman DJ. Induction of spermatogenesis and fertility during gonadotropin treatment of gonadotropin-deficient infertile men: predictors of fertility outcome. *J Clin Endocrinol Metab.* 2009;94(3):801-808. PMID: 19066302

12 **ANSWER: A) Anabolic steroid use**

The fact that this patient is asymptomatic and has elevated hematocrit despite having a hormone profile showing profound hypogonadotropic hypogonadism suggests that he is being exposed to androgens other than testosterone that are not being detected in the testosterone assay. Therefore, use of androgenic anabolic steroids (Answer A) is the most likely cause.

Hereditary hemochromatosis (Answer B), Kallmann syndrome (Answer C), opioid use (Answer D), and prolactinoma (Answer E) would be expected to be associated with symptoms of androgen deficiency given the degree of hypogonadism. In addition, the fact that the patient is normally virilized and has a testicular volume of 10 cc is not consistent with the diagnosis of Kallmann syndrome.

In patients with marked hyperprolactinemia due to a large macroadenoma, serum prolactin levels may be reported as normal unless serial dilution of serum is done to assess for the "hook effect." However, if a prolactinoma (Answer E) were responsible for this patient's hypogonadism, MRI would show a large pituitary adenoma as opposed to the 5-mm lesion seen in this case, which is most likely an incidentaloma.

While opioid use (Answer D) is an increasingly common cause of hypogonadism and could lead to the degree of gonadotropin suppression described in the vignette, it would not explain the patient's lack of symptoms or his elevated hematocrit.

Hereditary hemochromatosis (Answer B) is in the differential diagnosis of acquired hypogonadotropic hypogonadism, but it would not typically cause such profoundly low testosterone and gonadotropin levels. In addition, patients with this disorder are not asymptomatic and usually have other manifestations, including arthralgias, chondrocalcinosis, and hyperpigmentation. Later in the disease course, patients may experience heart failure, cirrhosis, and diabetes. Hemochromatosis is inherited in an autosomal recessive manner and has a prevalence of about 0.4% in populations of northern European descent, but it has much lower clinical penetrance and disease severity is highly variable. Pathogenic variants in the *HFE* gene are responsible, and the most common genotype is homozygosity for the Cys282Tyr (C282Y) variant.

EDUCATIONAL OBJECTIVE

Diagnose anabolic steroid use as a cause of secondary hypogonadism.

REFERENCE(S)

Anawalt BD. Diagnosis and management of anabolic androgenic steroid use. *J Clin Endocrinol Metab.* 2019;104(7):2490-2500. PMID: 30753550

13 ANSWER: C) Sperm cryopreservation before chemotherapy

After 1 year of follow-up, azoospermia is seen in 90% of men with Hodgkin lymphoma who are treated with more than 3 courses of chemotherapy that includes an alkylating agent. The most reliable option for the preservation of male fertility is cryopreservation of sperm before treatment (Answer C). Cryopreservation of human sperm does not decrease its capability for fertilization, and studies have demonstrated successful pregnancies with cryopreserved sperm. Optimal semen collection procedures for cryopreservation include obtaining at least 3 samples after abstinence for a minimum of 48 hours. However, in men with Hodgkin lymphoma, semen analysis is frequently abnormal even before treatment and only 20% to 30% of patients meet traditional criteria for sperm cryopreservation for intrauterine insemination.

Infertility related to chemotherapy is due to loss of spermatogonial stem cells, and the recovery of spermatogenesis occurs via recolonization of the seminiferous tubules by these stem cells. Currently, cryopreservation and subsequent transplant of spermatogonial stem cells (Answer B) is considered experimental.

It has been hypothesized that hormonal suppression and the resulting disruption of gametogenesis (Answer D) renders the gonad less sensitive to damage by the cytotoxic drugs. However, in clinical trials, hormonal suppression with GnRH agonists has not been shown to reliably afford gonadal protection and its use has led to recovery of spermatogenesis in only 20% of patients.

The combination of exogenous testosterone and a progestin (Answer A) has been used in male contraceptive trials but has not been evaluated in the setting of cytotoxic chemotherapy.

Although this patient's testosterone concentration is below normal without a compensatory rise in LH (a pattern often observed during illness), he has plenty of sperm for cryopreservation. Treatment with hCG (Answer E) to increase sperm numbers and increase serum testosterone would delay initiation of cryopreservation and is neither warranted nor beneficial.

EDUCATIONAL OBJECTIVE

Counsel men planning to undergo cytotoxic chemotherapy on the options for fertility preservation.

REFERENCE(S)

Oktay K, Harvey BE, Partridge AH, et al. Fertility preservation in patients with cancer: ASCO clinical practice guideline update. *J Clin Oncol.* 2018;36(19):1994-2001. PMID: 29620997

Ethics Committee of the American Society for Reproductive Medicine. Fertility preservation and reproduction in patients facing gonadotoxic therapies: an Ethics Committee opinion. *Fertil Steril.* 2018;110(3):380-386. PMID: 30098684

Jahnukainen K, Ehmcke J, Hou M, Schlatt S. Testicular function and fertility preservation in male cancer patients. *Best Pract Res Clin Endocrinol Metab.* 2011;25(2):287-302. PMID: 21397199

Levine J, Canada A, Stern CJ. Fertility preservation in adolescents and young adults with cancer. *J Clin Oncol.* 2010;28(32):4831-4841. PMID: 20458029

14 ANSWER: C) *FGFR1*

Once congenital hypogonadotropic hypogonadism has been diagnosed, targeted genetic testing can be considered. In the last decade, considerable advances have been made in unraveling the genetic basis of congenital hypogonadotropic hypogonadism, and to date, pathogenic variants have been identified in approximately 40% of patients. While in familial cases the mode of inheritance can be used to guide genetic testing, most cases of congenital hypogonadotropic hypogonadism are sporadic, as in the patient described in this vignette. However, a careful clinical evaluation can be helpful in prioritizing genetic testing. In an analysis of 219 patients with congenital hypogonadotropic hypogonadism, the following clinical features were highly associated with specific gene defects: synkinesia (*ANOS1* [formerly known as *KAL1*]) (Answer A), dental agenesis (*FGFR1*), digital bony abnormalities including syndactyly (*FGFR1*), and hearing loss (*CHD7*). In the case described where the patient has evidence of syndactyly, genetic testing for an *FGFR1* pathogenic variant (Answer C) would be the appropriate next step.

Pathogenic variants in the *GNRHR* gene (Answer D) cause hypogonadism but not anosmia, syndactyly, or tooth agenesis.

While pathogenic variants in *CHD7* (Answer B) cause Kallmann syndrome, the absence of deafness and the presence of syndactyly and tooth agenesis in this patient make it more likely that the genetic basis for his disease is a pathogenic variant in *FGFR1* rather than in *CHD7*.

Pathogenic variants in *NR0B1* (Answer E) (formerly known as *DAX1*) cause congenital hypogonadotropic hypogonadism and adrenal insufficiency, but do not cause anosmia.

EDUCATIONAL OBJECTIVE

Guide the appropriate workup in a patient with congenital hypogonadotropic hypogonadism.

REFERENCE(S)

Young J. Approach to the male patient with hypogonadotropic hypogonadism. *J Clin Endocrinol Metab.* 2012;97(3):707-718. PMID: 22392951

Costa-Barbosa FA, Balasubramanian R, Keefe KW, et al. Prioritizing genetic testing in patients with Kallmann syndrome using clinical phenotypes. *J Clin Endocrinol Metab.* 2013;98(5):E943-E953. PMID: 23533228

Bailleul-Forestier I, Gros C, Zenaty D, Bennaceur S, Leger J, de Roux N. Dental agenesis in Kallmann syndrome individuals with FGFR1 mutations. *Int J Paediatr Dent.* 2010;20(4):305-312. PMID: 20536592

15 ANSWER: E) Y Chromosome microdeletion

This couple's infertility is due to azoospermia. Absence of sperm in the ejaculate may occur because of an obstruction in the reproductive tract (obstructive azoospermia) or inadequate production of spermatozoa (nonobstructive azoospermia). The volume and pH of the seminal fluid can be used to determine the etiology of a patient's azoospermia.

He has nonobstructive azoospermia based on a normal semen volume and pH. He has normal LH and testosterone levels indicating normal Leydig-cell function, but he has an elevated FSH concentration due to lack of negative feedback from undetectable inhibin B, which suggests a selective defect in the seminiferous tubule compartment of the testis. This presentation is most likely due to a microdeletion in the Y chromosome (Answer E), the second most common genetic cause of male infertility after Klinefelter syndrome. The male-specific region on the long arm of the Y chromosome has a locus known as the azoospermia factor (AZF) that contains genes needed for spermatogenesis. This AZF locus contains 3 regions: AZFa, AZFb, and AZFc. Deletions of the entire AZFa region result in complete atrophy of the tubular compartment, with only Sertoli cells seen on testicular biopsy, making sperm retrieval for intracytoplasmic sperm injection virtually impossible. Large deletions in the AZFb region also result in Sertoli-cell–only syndrome. Pathogenic variants in the AZFc region are the most common and account for 80% of Y chromosome microdeletions. AZFc deletions are compatible with residual spermatogenesis, with oligospermia being a common presentation. These men may be candidates for intracytoplasmic sperm injection. Infertile men who do not have obstructive azoospermia, hypogonadotropic hypogonadism, or a karyotype abnormality should be tested for Y chromosome microdeletions.

Retrograde ejaculation (Answer D) and congenital bilateral absence of the vas deferens (Answer A) are both causes of obstructive azoospermia, so they would not be consistent with this patient's semen analysis. Retrograde ejaculation occurs when semen, which would normally be ejaculated via the urethra, is instead redirected to the bladder. Normally, the sphincter of the bladder contracts before ejaculation, which acts to both inhibit the release of urine and prevent a reflux of seminal fluids into the bladder during ejaculation. Any condition, medication, or surgical procedure that interferes with central control of ejaculation or the autonomic innervation to the seminal tract, can cause ejaculatory dysfunction. Congenital bilateral absence of the vas deferens due to a pathogenic variant in the cystic fibrosis transmembrane conductance regulator gene (*CFTR*) is a relatively frequent cause of infertility in men with obstructive azoospermia. However, given that this patient has a normal semen volume and pH, congenital absence of the vas deferens would not explain his presentation.

Kallmann syndrome (Answer B) is a condition characterized by congenital hypogonadotropic hypogonadism in association with anosmia or hyposmia. This patient's history of normal puberty, normal testicular size, and elevated FSH concentration are not consistent with this condition.

He does not have mosaic Klinefelter syndrome (Answer C) given his normal testicular size and karyotype.

EDUCATIONAL OBJECTIVE

Describe the presentation of Y chromosome microdeletions and outline the differential diagnosis of nonobstructive azoospermia.

REFERENCE(S)

Vogt PH, Edelmann A, Kirsch S, et al. Human Y chromosome azoospermia factors (AZF) mapped to different subregions in Yq11. *Hum Mol Genet.* 1996;5(7):933-943. PMID: 8817327

Pryor JL, Kent-First M, Muallem A, et al. Microdeletions in the Y chromosome of infertile men. *N Engl J Med.* 1997;336(8):534-539. PMID: 9023089

Stahl PJ, Schlegel PN. Genetic evaluation of the azoospermic or severely oligozoospermic male. *Curr Opin Obstet Gynecol.* 2012;24(4):221-228. PMID: 22729088

16 ANSWER: D) Serum prolactin measurement

This patient has secondary hypogonadism (low serum testosterone and inappropriately normal gonadotropin levels). Given that his testes are adult-sized and he is normally virilized, he has acquired secondary hypogonadism after the onset of puberty. The differential diagnosis of postpubertal secondary hypogonadism includes pituitary macroadenoma, Cushing syndrome, hyperprolactinemia, opioid use, and iron-overload syndromes (including hemochromatosis). Given the frequency with which hyperprolactinemia can cause hypogonadotropic hypogonadism, prolactin should be measured (Answer D) in all men with secondary hypogonadism.

In this patient, measurement of late-night salivary cortisol (Answer B) is not indicated because of the absence of any features suggestive of glucocorticoid excess (he has normal weight and blood pressure and no striae or evidence of proximal myopathy).

The major indication for karyotype analysis (Answer A) in men with hypogonadism is to confirm a diagnosis of Klinefelter syndrome, the most common genetic cause of primary hypogonadism. Given that this patient does not have primary hypogonadism, screening for Klinefelter syndrome by karyotyping is not indicated.

Testicular ultrasonography (Answer E) can be helpful in identifying a testicular tumor in a patient with gynecomastia. However, in the case described where there is no gynecomastia and the testes are normal on clinical examination, ultrasonography would not add any useful information.

Pituitary imaging (Answer C) would be premature in the evaluation of hypogonadism without a complete biochemical evaluation. This patient has no evidence of pituitary dysfunction (normal thyroid function) or mass effect and has a low, but not very low, serum testosterone concentration (<150 ng/dL [<5.2 nmol/L]).

EDUCATIONAL OBJECTIVE

Measure prolactin in the evaluation of men with secondary hypogonadism.

REFERENCE(S)

Schlechte JA. Clinical impact of hyperprolactinaemia. *Baillieres Clin Endocrinol Metab.* 1995;9(2):359-366. PMID: 7625989

Bhasin S, Brito JP, Cunningham GR, et al. Testosterone therapy in men with hypogonadism: an Endocrine Society clinical practice guideline. *J Clin Endocrinol Metab.* 2018;103(5):1715-1744. PMID: 29562364

Lipids & Obesity Board Review

Sangeeta Kashyap, MD

1 ANSWER: A) Obtain a coronary artery calcium score

This patient presents to discuss primary prevention. Adults without history of clinical atherosclerotic cardiovascular disease (ASCVD) or diabetes who have an LDL-cholesterol concentration of 70 to 189 mg/dL (1.81-4.90 mmol/L) should be categorized by their 10-year risk of a first hard ASCVD event (ie, fatal and nonfatal myocardial infarction or stroke), as in the 2013 guidelines. However, current guidelines recommend categorizing risk as being low (5%), borderline (5%-7.5%), intermediate (7.5%-20%), or high (>20%). This patient falls into the intermediate-risk category.

One important risk-enhancing factor in this patient is rheumatoid arthritis; the ASCVD 10-year risk may underestimate her overall cardiovascular disease risk.

However, the patient is reluctant to initiate statin therapy and would like to more precisely understand her risk and potential for benefit. This highlights another important aspect of the current guidelines, which is the inclusion of the coronary artery calcium (CAC) score (Answer A) to better refine risk estimation. In adults aged 40 to 75 years without diabetes who have an intermediate 10-year ASCVD risk and for whom the decision about statin therapy is uncertain, determining the CAC score can provide a more precise risk estimate.

If the CAC score is 0, statin treatment may be withheld or delayed, except in patients who smoke cigarettes, have diabetes, and have a family history of premature ASCVD. A CAC score of 1 to 99 favors statin therapy, especially in patients 55 years or older. A CAC score of 100 or greater or at the 75th percentile or greater should lead to statin therapy unless otherwise deferred by the outcome of the clinician-patient risk discussion. Data on the CAC score in patients with rheumatoid arthritis are limited.

This patient desires a more precise risk estimate before making a firm decision on statin therapy, so strongly recommending statin therapy (Answer E) before obtaining a CAC score is incorrect.

Ezetimibe (Answer C) and evolocumab (Answer B) should not be considered first-line treatment for patients at intermediate risk of ASCVD, especially if there is an ongoing discussion about the risk and benefits of statin therapy.

Red yeast rice (Answer D) is available over-the-counter, but it would not be effective.

EDUCATIONAL OBJECTIVE

Explain the role of the coronary calcium score in risk estimation of atherosclerotic cardiovascular disease.

REFERENCE(S)

Nasir K, Bittencourt MS, Blaha MJ, et al. Implications of coronary artery calcium testing among statin candidates according to ACC/AHA cholesterol management guidelines: MESA (Multi-Ethnic Study of Atherosclerosis). *J Am Coll Cardiol.* 2015;66(15):1657-1668. PMID: 26449135

Mahabadi AA, Mohlenkamp S, Lehmann N, et al; Heinz Nixdorf Recall Study Investigators. CAC score improves coronary and CV risk assessment above statin indication by ESC and AHA/ACC primary prevention guidelines. *JACC Cardiovasc Imaging.* 2017;10(2):143-153. PMID: 27665163

2 ANSWER: C) Challenge with another more potent statin such as rosuvastatin

This question highlights the importance of having a clinician-patient risk discussion before starting statin therapy, including the potential for adverse effects. Statin therapy is usually well tolerated and safe, although statin-associated adverse effects are a common challenge. The most frequent adverse effects are statin-associated muscle symptoms (SAMS), with 5% to 20% of patients reporting muscular symptoms in observational studies. Most patients have myalgias with a normal creatine kinase concentration.

Severe SAMS require statin cessation and evaluation. While severe symptoms are rare, clinicians should be aware of such presentations, including statin-associated myositis (elevations of creatine kinase levels with objective muscular weakness), rhabdomyolysis, or statin-associated autoimmune myopathy.

In a patient who developed myalgias without concern for severe SAMS, the initial recommendation is to reassess, discuss, and rechallenge with a statin (preferably rosuvastatin) (Answer C), as most patients are able to tolerate this statin over others. This patient's predisposing factors for SAMS should be assessed, particularly his exercise regimen. A comprehensive assessment and ongoing communication with the patient are essential to prevent ASCVD.

His East Asian ancestry, hypothyroidism, and vigorous exercise regimen are all predisposing factors for SAMS. However, recommending that the patient avoid exercise (Answer A) is not recommended. Other predisposing factors for SAMS are advanced age; female sex; low BMI; excessive alcohol consumption; muscle trauma; comorbidities such as HIV, liver disease, and kidney disease; myopathy; and high-risk medications.

Although statins can cause myositis and rhabdomyolysis, this patient has no clinical evidence suggestive of these conditions. Thus, measuring creatine kinase before restarting a statin (Answer B) is incorrect. However, in patients with severe SAMS and objective muscle weakness, creatine kinase should be measured.

A high-quality randomized controlled trial did not find benefit of coenzyme Q10 (Answer D) for prevention or treatment of SAMS. Therefore, its use for this indication is not currently recommended.

EDUCATIONAL OBJECTIVE

Manage statin-induced myalgias.

REFERENCE(S)

Thompson PD, Panza G, Zleski A, Taylor B. Statin-associated side effects. *J Am Coll Cardiol.* 2016;67(20):2395-2410. PMID: 27199064

Taylor BA, Lorson L, White CM, Thompson PD. A randomized trial of coenzyme Q10 in patients with confirmed stain myopathy. *Atherosclerosis.* 2015:238(2):329-335. PMID: 25545331

3 ANSWER: A) Add inclisiran

An alternative to monoclonal antibodies for PCSK9 lowering are the PCSK9 small interfering RNA molecules (siRNA), which profoundly lower intracellular and extracellular PCSK9 at a lower-dose frequency. Inclisiran (Answer A) can be used as an adjunct to diet and maximally tolerated statin therapy for treatment of heterozygous familial hypercholesterolemia or atherosclerotic cardiovascular disease that requires further LDL-cholesterol lowering in patients with allergic responses to both evolocumab and alirocumab and patients who have difficulty using a pen injector due to arthritis and/or hand weakness. It is a subcutaneous injection administered every 3 months for 2 doses, then every 6 months thereafter. Inclisiran has undergone phase 1, 2, and 3 evaluation, all within the context of the ORION trials. The ORION-9, -10, and -11 phase-3 trials were published in 2020. In all studies, the coprimary end points were the placebo-corrected percentage change in LDL cholesterol from baseline to day 510 and the time-adjusted percentage change in LDL cholesterol from baseline after day 90 and up to day 540. IN ORION-9, 482 adults with heterozygous familial hypercholesterolemia who were treated with maximally tolerated statin dosages were randomly assigned to subcutaneous injections of inclisiran or placebo on days 1, 90, 279, and 450. The mean baseline LDL-cholesterol concentration was 153 mg/dL (3.96 mmol/L). At day 510, inclisiran had reduced LDL cholesterol by 47.9% (95% CI, 42.3%-53.5%) and the corresponding time-adjusted reduction of 44.3% (95% CI, 40.1%-48.5%). Results of the ORION-10 and -11 trials were published together. In these 2 trials, statin-treated patients with cardiovascular disease (CVD) or at high risk were randomly assigned to receive inclisiran or placebo administered by subcutaneous injection on day 1, day 90, and every 6 months over a period of 540 days. In both trials, the mean baseline LDL-cholesterol concentration was approximately 105 mg/dL (2.72 mmol/L). ORION-10 enrolled 1561 patients with CVD. At day 510, inclisiran had reduced LDL cholesterol by 52.3% (95% CI, 48.8%-55.7%) and the corresponding time-adjusted reduction of 53.8% (95% CI, 51.3%-56.2%). ORION-11 enrolled 1617 patients with CVD or who were at high risk. At day 510, inclisiran had reduced LDL cholesterol by 49.9% (95% CI, 46.6%-53.1%) and the corresponding time-adjusted reduction of 49.2% (95% CI, 46.8%-51.6%).

LDL apheresis (Answer D) can be considered in selected patients with severe hypercholesterolemia but only if the LDL-cholesterol concentration remains inadequately controlled with medical therapy. Attempts at better control with other pharmacological agents would be preferred in this situation.

Colesevelam (Answer C) has modest LDL cholesterol–lowering effects and usually requires 6 tablets daily, which is burdensome for patients to consume.

Fenofibrate combined with a statin (Answer E) amplifies risk for statin-induced myalgias, and fenofibrate modestly lowers LDL cholesterol.

Although niacin (Answer B) raises HDL cholesterol, it is not cardioprotective.

EDUCATIONAL OBJECTIVE

Identify indications for use of alternative lipid-lowering agents.

REFERENCE(S)

Ray KK, Landmesser U, Leiter LA, et al. Inclisiran in patients at high cardiovascular risk with elevated LDL cholesterol. *N Engl J Med.* 2017;376(15):1430-1440. PMID: 28306389

Raal FJ, Kallend D, Ray KK, et al; ORION-9 Investigators. Inclisiran for the treatment of heterozygous familial hypercholesterolemia. *N Engl J Med.* 2020;382(16):1520-1530. PMID: 32197277

Ray KK, Wright RS, Kallend D, et al; ORION-10 and ORION-11 Investigators. Two phase 3 trials of inclisiran in patients with elevated LDL cholesterol. *N Engl J Med.* 2020;382(16):1507-1519. PMID: 32187462

Wright RS, Ray KK, Raal FJ, et al; ORION Phase III Investigators. Pooled patient-level analysis of inclisiran trials in patients with familial hypercholesterolemia or atherosclerosis. *J Am Coll Cardiol.* 2021;77(9):1182-1193. PMID: 33663735

4 ANSWER: E) Semaglutide

Semaglutide 1.0 mg, once-weekly subcutaneous injection, was first approved as a treatment for type 2 diabetes in 2017. Semaglutide 2.4 mg administered as a once-weekly, subcutaneous injection (Answer E), was approved for long-term weight management by the FDA in 2021, by the UK Medicine and Health Products Regulations Agency in 2021, and by the European Medicines Agency's Committee for Medicinal Products for Human Use in 2022. The average placebo-subtracted weight loss for semaglutide is 28.0 lb (12.7 kg). Semaglutide has generated much scientific, clinical, and public excitement and interest. Orlistat, semaglutide, and liraglutide can be used in selected patients who have chronic kidney disease. In exploratory analyses, semaglutide has demonstrated kidney-protective effects. These effects are most evident in patients with preexisting chronic kidney disease. Semaglutide is not excreted by the kidneys, so dosage reduction with impaired kidney function is not necessary. Rare cases of acute kidney injury have been reported in patients with chronic kidney disease stage 3b-4, and caution should be used in patients with later-stage chronic kidney disease. The FLOW study (https://clinicaltrials.gov/study/NCT03819153) is currently ongoing and will prospectively assess the effects of semaglutide 1.0 mg on kidney outcomes in patients with type 2 diabetes and chronic kidney disease. Kidney function should be monitored in treated patients, especially those with severe gastrointestinal adverse effects, as these may result in dehydration. Dehydration should be prevented and treated to reduce risk of acute kidney injury.

Cellulose and citric acid hydrogel (Answer A) is not systemically absorbed and is thus approved for individuals with any glomerular filtration rate. However, it is less effective for weight loss than semaglutide.

Orlistat (Answer C) results in some weight loss because it is a lipase inhibitor and has no systemic absorption, but it is less effective than semaglutide.

Both naltrexone/bupropion (Answer B) and phentermine/topiramate (Answer D) are excreted through the kidneys and would be contraindicated in this patient.

EDUCATIONAL OBJECTIVE

Prescribe antiobesity medications in the setting of chronic kidney disease.

REFERENCE(S)

Garvey WT, Mechanick JI, Brett EM, et al; Reviewers of AACE/ACE Obesity Clinical Practice Guidelines. American Association of Clinical Endocrinologists and American College of Endocrinology comprehensive clinical practice guidelines for medical care of patients with obesity. *Endocr Pract.* 2016;22(Suppl 3):1-203. PMID: 27219496

Shaman AM, Bain SC, Bakris GL, et al. Effect of the glucagon-like peptide-1 receptor agonists semaglutide and liraglutide on kidney outcomes in patients with type 2 diabetes: pooled analysis of SUSTAIN 6 and LEADER. *Circulation.* 2022;145(8):575-585. PMID: 34903039

Leehey DJ, Rahman MA, Borys E, Picken MM, Clise CE. Acute kidney injury associated with semaglutide. *Kidney Med.* 2021;3(2):282-285. PMID: 33851124

US Government Accountability Office. Obesity Drugs: Few Adults Used Prescription Drugs for Weight Loss and Insurance Coverage Varied. 2019. https://www.gao.gov/products/gao-19-577. Accessed April 2024.

American Diabetes Association Professional Practice Committee. 8. Obesity and weight management for the prevention and treatment of type 2 diabetes: standards of care in diabetes-2024. *Diabetes Care.* 2024;47(Suppl 1):S145-S157. PMID: 38078578

5 ANSWER: C) Increased dietary carbohydrate-to-protein ratio

Night eating syndrome is classically characterized by the triad of morning anorexia, evening hyperphagia, and insomnia. It is associated with nocturnal food consumption, increased carbohydrate-to-protein ratio (7:1) (Answer C), and consumption of 25% to 50% of daily calories after the evening meal. Night eating syndrome is a form of disordered eating associated with overweight and obesity. While this disorder also occurs in persons without obesity, it is associated with weight gain over time and higher risk of diabetes and other metabolic dysfunction. Night eating syndrome is also associated with higher risk of psychopathology, including mood, anxiety, and sleep problems, than the risk in individuals with similar weight status who do not have disordered eating. Treatment for night eating syndrome includes cognitive behavior therapy, selective serotonin reuptake inhibitors, progressive muscle relaxation, and bright light therapy.

Night eating syndrome is characterized by insomnia, not excessive sleep (Answer A).

Purging behavior (Answer D) is associated with binge eating disorder and not night eating syndrome.

Increased caffeine intake (Answer B) is not characteristic of night eating syndrome.

Sense of lack of control with overeating throughout the day (Answer E) is not characteristic of night eating syndrome.

EDUCATIONAL OBJECTIVE

Describe weight gain and other characteristics associated with night eating syndrome.

REFERENCE(S)

Allison KC, Tarves EP. Treatment of night eating syndrome. *Psychiatr Clin North Am.* 2011:34(4):785-796. PMID: 22098804

6 ANSWER: C) Orlistat

Orlistat (Answer C) is an inhibitor of pancreatic lipase. The result of this inhibition is that about 30% of the daily ingested fat intake is not absorbed. This leads to a 200-calorie deficit per day in an individual who consumes a diet of 2000 calories per day with 30% of calories as fat. The most common adverse effects of orlistat are gastrointestinal, such as fatty or oily stools, more frequent defecation, and fecal incontinence. Another adverse effect is a slight reduction in absorption of fat-soluble vitamins, although not generally outside the reference range. Orlistat can impair levothyroxine absorption. Administration of these medications should be spaced apart by 4 or more hours.

Bupropion (Answer A), naltrexone (Answer B), and phentermine (Answer D) do not interfere with levothyroxine absorption.

EDUCATIONAL OBJECTIVE

Identify weight-loss drug interactions with other medications.

REFERENCE(S)

Manu P, Lăcătușu C-M, Rogozea LM, Cernea S. Pharmacological management of obesity: a century of expert opinions in Cecil Textbook of Medicine. *Am J Ther.* 2022;29(4):e410-e424. PMID: 35687055

7 ANSWER: E) Type 2 diabetes

Most patients with metabolic dysfunction-associated steatotic liver disease (MASLD) are diagnosed in their 40s or 50s. Thus, this patient's age (Answer A) is not her strongest risk factor.

Study findings vary regarding the sex distribution of MASLD, with some suggesting it is more common in women, especially after menopause due to weight gain, and others suggesting it is more common in men. However, menopause status (Answer C) is a weaker recognized risk factor than type 2 diabetes (Answer E).

Metabolic syndrome related to obesity (Answer B) is a risk factor for liver steatosis, and patients with type 2 diabetes are particularly at increased risk of metabolic dysfunction-associated steatohepatitis (MASH). Obesity is not always linked to insulin resistance and MASLD. A recent study found 1 of 6 people with type 2 diabetes had liver fibrosis. Liver fibrosis increases the risk of cardiometabolic complications and worsens type 2 diabetes. All patients with type 2 diabetes should be screened for MASLD with FIB-4.

Obstructive sleep apnea (Answer D) is associated with obesity and insulin resistance but is not necessarily linked with increased risk of MASLD.

EDUCATIONAL OBJECTIVE

Identify risk factors for metabolic dysfunction-associated steatohepatitis.

REFERENCE(S)

Vernon G, Baranova A, Younossi ZM. Systematic review: the epidemiology and natural history of non-alcoholic fatty liver disease and non-alcoholic steatohepatitis in adults. *Aliment Pharmacol Ther.* 2011;34(3):274-285. PMID: 21623852

Lazo M, Hernaez R, Eberhardt MS, et al. Prevalence of nonalcoholic fatty liver disease in the United States: the Third National Health and Nutrition Examination Survey, 1988-1994. *Am J Epidemiol.* 2013;178(1):38-45. PMID: 23703888

Browning JD, Szczepaniak LS, Dobbins R, et al. Prevalence of hepatic steatosis in an urban population in the United States: impact of ethnicity. *Hepatology.* 2004;40(6):1387-1395. PMID: 1556557

8 ANSWER: B) Enhancement of GABA activity and sodium channels

Topiramate alters the taste of carbonated beverages due to carbonic anhydrase inhibition and may be used for soda aversion. The exact mechanism of topiramate-induced weight loss is still unclear, although an anorectic action has been postulated following carbonic-anhydrase inhibition on taste and the activation of γ-aminobutyric acid (GABA)-A receptor in the lateral hypothalamus known to interact with leptin pathway (thus, Answer B is correct and Answers A, C, and D are incorrect). The incorrect options do not accurately describe mechanisms of appetite suppression related to topiramate but are associated with other therapeutic agents.

EDUCATIONAL OBJECTIVE

Explain topiramate's mechanism of action.

REFERENCE(S)

Wajid I, Vega A, Thornhill K, et al. Topiramate (Topamax): evolving role in weight reduction management: a narrative review. *Life (Basel).* 2023;13(9):1845. PMID: 37763249

9 ANSWER: D) Start naltrexone, bupropion, or a GLP-1 receptor agonist

Data from the SOS and LABS-2 cohorts demonstrate that weight regain following metabolic and bariatric surgery (MBS) is not uncommon, and it affects patients to varying degrees depending on the type of surgery performed. Although alcohol use disorder is most commonly associated with Roux-en-Y gastric bypass, this disorder can occur in patients who have undergone other bariatric procedures, including sleeve gastrectomy and lap-banding. Weight regain after MBS is multifactorial and attributable to surgical, physiological, and patient factors and is often exacerbated with alcohol use due to increased caloric intake.

Multiple studies have shown that patients who undergo MBS are at increased risk of developing alcohol use disorder. The American Society for Metabolic and Bariatric Surgery position statement on alcohol use before and after bariatric surgery recommends screening for alcohol intake both before and after MBS. Patients with marked weight regain of unclear etiology after MBS should be asked about alcohol intake. Underreporting of alcohol consumption is not uncommon. An elevated γ-glutamyltransferase level or abnormal liver enzymes can be indicators of alcohol use. The presence of depression and anxiety exacerbated by life stressors often accompanies excessive alcohol intake.

Some antiobesity medications that affect appetite regulation also have favorable effects to limit excessive alcohol intake. These agents include naltrexone, bupropion, and some GLP-1 receptor agonists, including exenatide and liraglutide (Answer D).

There are no standard addiction scores (Answer A). However, patients with alcohol use disorder may have other addictive behaviors.

Referring the patient to a social worker (Answer B) would not directly address the alcohol addiction.

Supplementation with calcium, magnesium, and vitamin D (Answer C) would not specifically correct the alcohol addiction issues.

EDUCATIONAL OBJECTIVE

Address alcohol use disorder in patients who have undergone bariatric surgery.

REFERENCE(S)

King WC, Chen J, Mitchell JE, et al. Prevalence of alcohol use disorders before and after bariatric surgery. *JAMA.* 2012;307(23):2516-2525. PMID: 22710289

White GE, Boles RE, Courcoulas AP, et al. A prospective cohort of alcohol use and alcohol-related problems before and after metabolic and bariatric surgery in adolescents. *Ann Surg.* 2023;278(3):e519-e525. PMID: 36538630

10 ANSWER: D) Red yeast rice

Many supplements have been used to lower cholesterol. Red yeast rice (Answer D) and red yeast rice extract have been used historically in China to lower cholesterol. Red yeast rice is produced by fermentation of a fungus (*Monascus purpureus*) grown on rice, which makes a substance called monacolin K (similar to lovastatin) that lowers total and LDL cholesterol by competitively binding HMG-CoA reductase with very high affinity (as statins do). A byproduct is a red pigment that gives the rice its red color. Several small studies of short duration (1-12 months) have demonstrated its lipid-lowering effects, and a meta-analysis of 13 trials showed a significant reduction in both total and LDL cholesterol. In a placebo-controlled trial for secondary prevention in 5000 patients in China, red yeast rice taken for 4.5 years showed a 45% relative risk reduction in nonfatal myocardial infarction and cardiovascular death compared with placebo (5.7% vs 10.4%) and a 35% reduction in cardiovascular death, which suggests some efficacy. In general, data have not reached sufficient quality such that red yeast rice can be recommended from an evidence-based perspective compared with the amount of data on FDA-approved statin medications. Since this patient is statin intolerant, the use of a supplement that has a similar mechanism of action as statin medications (ie, HMG-CoA reductase inhibition) would likely convey similar adverse effects.

The supplement berberine (Answer A), an alkaloid derived from the bark of a shrub found in the Himalayas called *Berberis aristata,* is thought to lower cholesterol by inhibiting PSCK9 production (thus functioning like a PCSK9 inhibitor antibody) and by stimulating AMPK.

Folate (Answer C) functions to lower methylate homocysteine, but treatment with folate has failed to show beneficial effects on cardiovascular disease.

Coenzyme Q10 (Answer B) is an antioxidant supplement that is believed to be beneficial due to its ability to prevent LDL oxidation, but which is depleted by HMG-CoA reductase inhibitor therapy (ie, by statin use). Many people anecdotally feel that taking coenzyme Q10 helps to avoid myalgias and fatigue while taking statin medications, although high-quality evidence from randomized placebo-controlled trials does not support this belief. The above supplements do not have the same mechanism of action as statins (inhibition of HMG-CoA reductase) and therefore would not be expected to cause similar adverse effects.

Vitamin D (Answer E) has no effect on cardiovascular risk factors.

EDUCATIONAL OBJECTIVE

List commonly used supplements to lower cholesterol and describe their mechanisms of action.

REFERENCE(S)

Gerards MC, Terlou RJ, Yu H, Koks CH, Gerdes VE. Traditional Chinese lipid-lowering agent red yeast rice results in significant LDL reduction but safety is uncertain - systematic review and meta-analysis. *Atherosclerosis.* 2015;240(2):415-423. PMID: 25897793

Fogacci F, Banach M, Mikhailidis DP, et al; Lipid and Blood Pressure Meta-Analysis Collaboration (LBPMC) Group; International Lipid Expert Panel (ILEP). Safety of red yeast rice supplementation: a systematic review and meta-analysis of randomized controlled trials. *Pharmacologic Res.* 2019;143:1-16. PMID: 30844537

Li Y, Jiang L, Jia Z, Xin W, Yang S, Yang Q, Wang L. A meta-analysis of red yeast rice: an effective and relatively safe alternative approach for dyslipidemia. *PLoS One.* 2014;9(6):e98611. PMID: 24897342

Lu Z, Kou W, Du B, et al. Effect of Xuezhikang, an extract from red yeast Chinese rice, on coronary events in a Chinese population with previous myocardial infarction. *Am J Cardiol.* 2008;101(12):1689-1693. PMID: 18549841

Barrios V, Escobar C, Cicero AF, et al. A nutraceutical approach (Armolipid Plus) to reduce total and LDL cholesterol in individuals with mild to moderate dyslipidemia: review of the clinical evidence. *Atheroscler Suppl.* 2017;24:1-15. PMID: 27998714

11 ANSWER: C) Lipoprotein (a) measurement

This patient has a first-degree relative with premature heart disease who sustained a myocardial infarction at age 45 years before being treated with lipid-lowering therapy. This history puts the patient at risk of early cardiovascular disease, possibly due to familial hyperlipidemia. Familial hyperlipidemia is a relatively common genetic disorder affecting 1 in 250 to 500 persons depending on the population. The American Heart Association recommends high-intensity statin treatment for individuals with an LDL-cholesterol concentration greater than 190 mg/dL (>4.92 mmol/L) due to the very high likelihood that they have familial hyperlipidemia and are at very high cardiovascular risk. However, some patients with familial hyperlipidemia may have LDL-cholesterol concentrations less than 190 mg/dL (<4.92 mmol/L) as well, depending on their lifestyle habits (diet and exercise). Even patients with familial hyperlipidemia can lower their LDL cholesterol through lifestyle changes, as this patient did by adopting a vegan diet. Although she lowered her LDL cholesterol by approximately 27%, her LDL-cholesterol concentration remains above 100 mg/dL (>2.59 mmol/L), and her triglycerides are also above target according to the 2018 American Heart Association/American College of Cardiology cholesterol management guidelines.

Other conditions can place patients at high risk of premature cardiovascular disease. Elevated lipoprotein (a) (Answer C), a highly atherogenic lipoprotein, is also associated with very high cardiovascular disease risk, as well as aortic stenosis. Lipoprotein (a) is produced by the liver, and levels are predominantly genetically inherited. Lipoprotein (a) is a large lipoprotein in which apolipoprotein (a) is attached covalently to apolipoprotein B. Lipoprotein (a) may be modestly elevated in familial hyperlipidemia, but it is an independent risk factor for atherosclerotic disease. Persons with a lipoprotein (a) level in the upper tertile have increased risk of cardiovascular disease (odds ratio, 1.7; 95% CI, 1.4-1.9) compared with persons whose concentration is in the lower tertile. Elevated lipoprotein (a) is a strong indication for aggressive lipid lowering through available pharmacologic options in addition to lifestyle modification and a low-cholesterol diet to target a non–HDL-cholesterol concentration less than 100 mg/dL (<2.59 mmol/L) (LDL cholesterol <70 mg/dL [<1.81 mmol/L]). New therapeutic agents are in development that target lipoprotein (a) and effectively lower it in a dose-dependent manner. However, longer trials are needed to demonstrate a reduction in cardiovascular events with these compounds.

Current guidelines recommend screening for lipoprotein (a) in individuals at very high cardiovascular risk and those with a history of premature cardiovascular disease, a first-degree relative with premature cardiovascular disease or known lipoprotein (a) elevation, progressive cardiovascular disease despite maximal LDL-cholesterol lowering, or borderline 10-year cardiovascular risk with need for additional information to inform treatment decisions.

The 2018 American Heart Association guidelines recommend intensified lifestyle modification if triglycerides are greater than 150 mg/dL (>1.70 mmol/L) and consideration of additional lipid-lowering therapy if triglycerides are persistently greater than 175 mg/dL (>1.98 mmol/L) in patients at high cardiovascular risk, particularly in the setting of diabetes, which this patient does not have. For triglycerides in this range, therapy should start with a statin.

Non–HDL cholesterol is considered a marker of cardiovascular risk that includes all atherogenic particles, including triglyceride-rich particles, but it would not add any additional information. Thus, measuring non-HDL cholesterol (Answer D) is incorrect. Similarly, measurement of apolipoprotein B (Answer A) would also provide a measure of additional atherogenic triglyceride-rich lipoproteins, as apolipoprotein B is a structural component of all of them. Its measurement would not add additional information to what is already available in her lipid profile since her LDL-cholesterol and triglyceride concentrations are listed. Her triglycerides could be a secondary target clinically as they are above target for optimal cholesterol profiles.

Circulating chylomicrons (Answer B) relate to dietary fat ingestion, and severe elevations increase risk for pancreatitis. This patient's triglyceride concentration is less than 400 mg/dL (<4.52 mmol/L), which makes chylomicronemia syndrome unlikely.

Nuclear magnetic resonance spectroscopy (Answer E) gives information about particle size and concentration. Nuclear magnetic resonance spectroscopy typically provides information on lipoprotein profiles notable for high concentrations of small, dense LDL particles that are typical of an insulin-resistant phenotype associated with type 2 diabetes. This patient does not have diabetes. Nuclear magnetic resonance spectroscopy is not likely to provide additional insight into her risk of cardiovascular disease beyond her cholesterol profile with elevated LDL cholesterol.

EDUCATIONAL OBJECTIVE

Determine when measurement of lipoprotein (a) is indicated in the assessment of cardiovascular risk.

REFERENCE(S)

Danesh J, Collins R, Peto R. Lipoprotein(a) and coronary heart disease. Meta-analysis of prospective studies. *Circulation.* 2000;102(10):1082-1085. PMID: 10973834

Ma L, Chan DC, Ooi EMM, Marcovina SM, Barrett PHR, Watts GF. Apolipoprotein(a) kinetics in statin-treated patients with elevated plasma lipoprotein(a) concentration. *J Clin Endocrinol Metab.* 2019;104(12):6247-6255. PMID: 31393573

Tsimikas S, Karwatowska-Prokopczuk E, Gouni-Berthold I, et al; AKCEA-APO(a)-LRx Study Investigators. Lipoprotein(a) reduction in persons with cardiovascular disease. *N Engl J Metab.* 2020;382(3):244-255. PMID: 31893580

Grundy SM, Stone NJ, Bailey AL, et al. 2018 AHA/ACC/AACVPR/AAPA/ABC/ACPM/ADA/AGS/APhA/ASPC/NLA/PCNA guideline on the management of blood cholesterol. *Circulation.* 2019;139(25):e1082-e1143. PMID: 30586774

12 ANSWER: E) Microsomal triglyceride transfer protein (*MTTP*)

Hypolipidemia can be genetic or acquired. Acquired disorders include malignancy (colorectal and prostate cancer, leukemias, myeloma), malabsorption (pancreatic exocrine insufficiency, celiac disease, post bowel surgery), infection (giardiasis, tuberculosis, schistosomiasis), and severe or critical illness. This patient was diagnosed as an infant, which is most consistent with an inherited disorder. Her very low total cholesterol concentration (<50 mg/dL [<1.30 mmol/L]) with undetectable LDL cholesterol and apolipoprotein B suggests severe hypolipidemia from alterations in genes regulating lipid metabolism. This patient has abetalipoproteinemia, a rare autosomal recessive disorder (1 in 1 million persons) caused by microsomal triglyceride transfer protein (MTTP) deficiency. Multiple variants in the *MTTP* gene (Answer E) cause MTTP deficiency. MTTP is produced in the liver and intestines where it is crucial for the formation of apolipoprotein B–containing lipoproteins in the endoplasmic reticulum through transfer of triglyceride or phospholipids. The absence of MTTP results in no synthesis or secretion of apolipoprotein B into the circulation where it is undetectable. Lack of MTTP in intestinal cells impairs chylomicron formation and severe malabsorption of fat and fat-soluble vitamins (A, D, E, and K). If not diagnosed early and treated aggressively, the severe vitamin deficiencies can lead to a range of complications, including retinal degeneration and blindness, degenerative neurologic disorders, anemias, and osteoporosis. Affected patients are treated with high-dosage oral supplements, as well as intravenous infusion of lipids and vitamins.

Two other rare genetic disorders in the differential diagnosis of severe hypolipidemias are the homozygous form familial hypobetalipoproteinemia and chylomicron retention syndrome (Anderson disease). Familial hypobetalipoproteinemia is a disorder of low cholesterol due to defective apolipoprotein B. The heterozygous form of familial hypobetalipoproteinemia occurs in 1 in 500 persons and is characterized by a cholesterol concentration less than 100 mg/dL (<2.59 mmol/L), or half of typical values but not severely low levels less than 50 mg/dL (<1.30 mmol/L). Affected patients are generally asymptomatic and identified with screening lipid profiles. The homozygous form is rare and presents with very low cholesterol levels and a clinical presentation similar to that of abetalipoproteinemia, although the defect is in the *APOB* gene and not in the *MTTP* gene. Chylomicron retention syndrome (Anderson disease) is a rare autosomal recessive disorder due to pathogenic variants in the *SAR1B* gene. In this disorder, chylomicrons cannot be secreted from the intestines, which results in very low circulating cholesterol and triglycerides with a clinical presentation similar to that of abetalipoproteinemia. Neither of these severe forms of hypolipidemias were presented as an option in this vignette.

Lipoprotein lipase deficiency (Answer D) is a primary hypertriglyceridemia disorder with severely elevated triglycerides (>1000 mg/dL [>11.30 mmol/L]), not low cholesterol. Lipoprotein lipase is located on endothelial cells where it hydrolyzes triglycerides from chylomicrons and VLDL particles, effectively clearing triglyceride. The absence of lipoprotein lipase activity results in very high triglycerides.

Apolipoprotein CII (Answer B) is a cofactor of lipoprotein lipase, and its deficiency leads to very high triglycerides (>1000 mg/dL [>11.30 mmol/L]).

Apolipoprotein A1 (Answer A) is an important protein for HDL cholesterol, and its absence leads to very low HDL cholesterol but not low LDL cholesterol or low triglycerides.

Cholesterol ester transfer protein (Answer C) transfers cholesterol esters from HDL to VLDL, IDL, and remnant particles in exchange for triglyceride, essentially clearing HDL cholesterol. The absence of cholesterol ester transfer protein results in high circulating levels of HDL cholesterol with concentrations usually greater than 100 mg/dL (>2.59 mmol/L).

EDUCATIONAL OBJECTIVE

Describe the causes of hypolipidemias and key management considerations.

REFERENCE(S)

Welty FK. Hypobetalipoproteinemia and abetalipoproteinemia: liver disease and cardiovascular disease. *Curr Opin Lipidol.* 2014;31(2):49-55. PMID: 32039990

Olsson AG, Angelin B, Assmann G, et al. Can LDL cholesterol be too low? Possible risks of extremely low levels. *J Intern Med.* 2017;281(6):281-534. PMID: 28295777

Sharp D, Blinderman L, Combs KA, et al. Cloning and gene defects in microsomal triglyceride transfer protein associated with abetalipoproteinaemia. *Nature.* 1993;365(6441):65-69. PMID: 8361539

Wetterau JR, Aggerbeck LP, Bouma ME, et al. Absence of microsomal triglyceride transfer protein in individuals with abetalipoproteinemia. *Science.* 1992;258(5084):999-1001. PMID: 1439810

Peretti N, Sassolas A, Roy CC, et al. Guidelines for the diagnosis and management of chylomicron retention disease based on a review of the literature and experience of the two centers. *Orphanet J Rare Dis.* 2010;5:24. PMID: 20920215

13 ANSWER: B) Colesevelam

This patient most likely has heterozygous familial hyperlipidemia (FH) with an LDL-cholesterol concentration of 300 mg/dL (7.77 mmol/L) before pregnancy. This diagnosis puts her at very high risk for cardiovascular disease. All adults with familial hyperlipidemia and LDL-cholesterol concentrations greater than 190 mg/dL (>4.92 mmol/L) should be started on lipid-lowering therapy with a high-intensity statin followed by additional medications as needed to target at least a 50% reduction in LDL cholesterol and ideally an LDL-cholesterol concentration less than 100 mg/dL (<2.59 mmol/L). A long-term study of children with genetically confirmed FH treated with statins for an average of 20 years showed less subclinical atherosclerosis as indicated by carotid intima-media thickness measurement and reduced cardiovascular disease compared with their affected parents and unaffected siblings. Women of reproductive age who have FH should be counseled regarding treatment during pregnancy and lactation. In a 40-year observational cohort study of the Medical Birth Registry of Norway (1967-2006), there was no increased risk of preterm delivery (<37 weeks), low birth weight (<2500 g), or congenital malformations in 1869 women with FH compared with outcomes of other women. Women of reproductive age who have FH should be treated with lipid-lowering treatment with cessation of statins and/or other lipid-lowering medications 3 months before planned conception. All lipid-lowering therapy is recommended to be stopped during pregnancy due to risk to the fetus. Cholesterol levels increase by approximately one-third during pregnancy, including LDL cholesterol.

Breastfeeding presents another challenge, although cholesterol levels generally return to prepregnancy levels over time while lactating. Lipid-lowering medication is generally not recommended while breastfeeding, including any intensity statin and PCSK9 inhibitors (Answers A, C, D, and E). However, the time without lipid-lowering therapy in the context of term pregnancy and lactation can extend to 2 years with high circulating LDL-cholesterol levels in patients with FH. If lipid-lowering therapy is going to be started, bile-acid resins such as colesevelam (Answer B) can be initiated while breastfeeding. For patients with severely elevated levels or homozygous FH, apheresis has been used in some patients to remove LDL cholesterol during pregnancy and lactation, but this was not a choice presented in this vignette.

EDUCATIONAL OBJECTIVE

Manage heterozygous familial hyperlipidemia in women of reproductive age.

REFERENCE(S)

Arnett DK, Blumenthal RS, Albert MA, et al. 2019 ACC/AHA guideline on the primary prevention of cardiovascular disease: a report of the American College of Cardiology/American Heart Association Task Force on Clinical Practice Guidelines. *J Am Coll Cardiol.* 2019;74(10):1376-1414. PMID: 30894319

Luirink IK, Wiegman A, Kusters DM, et al. 20-year follow-up of statins in children with familial hyperlipidemia. *N Engl J Metab.* 2019;381(16):1547-1556. PMID: 31618540

Toleikyte I, Retterstol K, Leren TP, Iversen PO. Pregnancy outcomes in familial hypercholesterolemia: a registry-based study. *Circulation.* 2011;124(15):1606-1614. PMID: 21911783

deGoma EM, Ahmad ZS, O'Brien EC, et al. Treatment gaps in adults with heterozygous familial hypercholesterolemia in the United States: data from the CASCADE-FH Registry. *Circ Cardiovasc Genet.* 2016;9(3):240-249. PMID: 27013694

14 ANSWER: B) 48-year-old patient; hemoglobin A_{1c} of 7.0% (53 mmol/mol); 4-year duration of diabetes; metformin; Roux-en-Y gastric bypass

Gastric bypass and sleeve gastrectomy result in remission of type 2 diabetes for up to 5 years in randomized controlled trials of metabolic surgery vs medical treatment. The preoperative predictors of diabetes remission include shorter duration of diabetes, younger age, lower hemoglobin A_{1c} level, oral agent vs insulin use, and type of surgery (Roux-en-Y gastric bypass is the most effective). Compared with sleeve gastrectomy, Roux-en-Y gastric bypass results in higher rates of biochemical remission. Laparoscopic gastric banding results in a similar rate of remission to that of metformin when used in patients with new-onset type 2 diabetes. The patient described in Answer B depicts the optimal clinical characteristics: younger age, shorter duration of diabetes, well-controlled diabetes on an oral agent, and Roux-en-Y gastric bypass.

EDUCATIONAL OBJECTIVE

Identify predictors of diabetes remission following bariatric surgery.

REFERENCE(S)

Still CD, Wood GC, Benotti P, et al. Preoperative prediction of type 2 diabetes remission after Roux-en-Y gastric bypass surgery: a retrospective cohort study. *Lancet Diabetes Endocrinol.* 2013;2(1):38-45. PMID: 24579062

Schauer PR, Burguera B, Ikramuddin S, et al. Effect of laparoscopic Roux-en Y gastric bypass on type 2 diabetes mellitus. *Ann Surg.* 2003;238(4):467-484. PMID: 14530719

Brethauer SA, Aminian A, Romero-Talamás H, et al. Can diabetes be surgically cured? Long-term metabolic effects of bariatric surgery in obese patients with type 2 diabetes mellitus. *Ann Surg.* 2013;258(4):628-637. PMID: 24018646

Xiang AH, Trigo E, Martinez M, et al; RISE Consortium; RISE Collaborators. Impact of gastric banding versus metformin on beta-cell function in adults with impaired glucose tolerance or mild type 2 diabetes. *Diabetes Care.* PMID: 30282699

15 ANSWER: A) Reduced total daily energy expenditure; reduced resting metabolic rate; reduced exercise energy expenditure

Weight loss from diet and exercise is often followed by weight regain. In response to a hypocaloric diet, an energy deficit occurs, which causes increased hunger and reduced energy expenditure. The difference between energy desired and energy required is termed the energy gap. With weight loss that results in lower BMI and body surface area, there is a reduction in energy expenditure, resting metabolic rate, and total daily expenditure. On the expenditure side, diet-induced weight loss reduces total daily energy expenditure because of a lower resting metabolic rate and the thermic effect of food, and it often decreases exercise energy expenditure and nonexercise activity thermogenesis. Increased hunger and decreased energy expenditure can readily promote weight regain.

Thus, Answer A correctly identifies the features of metabolic adaptation following weight loss.

EDUCATIONAL OBJECTIVE

Identify metabolic adaptation to weight loss and factors that promote weight gain following caloric restriction.

REFERENCE(S)

Melby CL, Paris HL, Foright RM, Peth J. Attenuating the biologic drive for weight regain following weight loss: must what goes down always go back up? *Nutrients.* 2017;9(5):468. PMID: 28481261

16 ANSWER: B) Worsened dietary adherence; no difference in weight loss; no difference in triglycerides; no difference in blood pressure

Short-term, uncontrolled studies have shown that alternate-day fasting results in improved weight loss, increased insulin sensitivity, and improved lipid profiles. However, a recent randomized controlled trial that compared alternate-day fasting with restricted daily caloric intake in adults with obesity (average BMI = 34 kg/m^2) did not show any difference in weight loss or lipid profiles. Dietary adherence was, in fact, worse in the alternate-day fasting group vs the restricted daily caloric intake group. Thus, the expected pattern of alternate-day fasting is best depicted in Answer B.

EDUCATIONAL OBJECTIVE

List the clinical outcomes of intermittent fasting for weight loss.

REFERENCE(S)

Trepanowski JF, Kroeger CM, Barnosky A, et al. Effect of alternate-day fasting on weight loss, weight maintenance, and cardioprotection among metabolically healthy obese adults: a randomized clinical trial. *JAMA Intern Med.* 2017;177(7):930-938. PMID: 28459931

Sutton EF, Beyl R, Early KS, Cefalu WT, Ravussin E, Peterson CM. Early time-restricted feeding improves insulin sensitivity, blood pressure, and oxidative stress even without weight loss in men with prediabetes. *Cell Metab.* 2018;27(6):1212-1221. PMID: 29754952

17 ANSWER: C) Pravastatin, 10 mg daily, and reevaluate in 3 months

The incidence of statin-induced new-onset diabetes is higher in patients with impaired fasting glucose and elevated BMI and usually occurs with more potent statins (eg, rosuvastatin vs pravastatin). Thus, the best course of action is to start with pravastatin and reevaluate this patient for hyperglycemia in 3 months (Answer C). There is no evidence to suggest that metformin treatment before initiation of a statin (Answer B) or concomitant use of metformin and pravastatin (Answer A) lowers the risk of statin-induced new-onset diabetes. Post hoc evaluation of previously reported statin trials shows a small increase in the risk of developing new-onset diabetes, which is associated with all statins. Potential mechanisms include reduced insulin secretion and reduced insulin sensitivity.

The JUPITER trial (Justification for Use of Statins in Prevention: An Intervention Trial Evaluating Rosuvastatin), a primary prevention trial in which 17,802 patients were randomly assigned to receive rosuvastatin, 20 mg daily, or placebo over a 1.9-year period, showed an overall 27% increase in investigator-reported diabetes in patients treated with rosuvastatin compared with placebo and a moderate but significant increase in median hemoglobin A_{1c} levels in the rosuvastatin arm. Almost all of the excess risk occurred in participants with baseline evidence of impaired fasting glucose. There were 134 vascular events or deaths avoided for every 54 new cases of diabetes. The statin benefit was as good in those who developed diabetes as in the trial as a whole. Given that rosuvastatin (Answer D) was initially implicated in causing an increased risk of diabetes, it should not be prescribed for this patient.

Further studies have identified additional risk factors in statin-treated patients at risk for developing diabetes, including elevated plasma glucose, triglycerides, BMI higher than 30 kg/m^2, and presence of hypertension.

EDUCATIONAL OBJECTIVE

Identify the adverse effect of new-onset diabetes in patients treated with statins.

REFERENCE(S)

Ruscica M, Macchi C, Morlotti B, Sirtori CR, Magni P. Statin therapy and related risk of new-onset type 2 diabetes mellitus. *Eur J Intern Med.* 2014;25(5):401-406. PMID: 24685426

Ridker PM, Pradhan A, MacFadyen JG, Libby P, Glynn RJ. Cardiovascular benefits and diabetes risks of statin therapy in primary prevention: an analysis from the JUPITER trial. *Lancet.* 2012;380(9841):565-571. PMID: 22883507

18 ANSWER: D) Significant improvement in quality of life, depression, and sleep apnea

The Look AHEAD trial compared the effect of intensive lifestyle intervention with a control standard regimen of diabetes support and education among patients with type 2 diabetes and a BMI greater than 25 kg/m^2. At a median follow-up of almost 10 years, there was no significant difference between the 2 groups in cardiovascular morbidity and mortality (thus, Answer B is incorrect). Initial mean weight loss in the intervention group was 8.6% at 12 months. This was followed by weight regain through year 5 and then a subsequent gradual decrease in weight, resulting in an average weight loss of 6.0% at the end of the trial. The weight loss is not expected to be durable (thus, Answer E is incorrect). The control group had gradual but consistent weight loss throughout the study, resulting in an average weight loss of 3.5% at the end of the trial. The intervention group also had greater improvements in fitness, particularly at 1 year, along with improved obesity-related comorbidities such as reduced depression, decreased medication use, and improved quality of life (thus, Answer D is correct). Even minor weight loss is associated with improved hemoglobin A_{1c} levels, but few study participants experienced complete remission of diabetes and withdrawal of antidiabetes medications (thus, Answer A is incorrect). No reduction in visceral fat was noted (thus, Answer C is incorrect).

EDUCATIONAL OBJECTIVE

Describe the clinical effect of weight loss induced by intensive diet and exercise on mortality from cardiovascular disease and cardiovascular risk factors in patients with type 2 diabetes and overweight or obesity.

REFERENCE(S)

Look AHEAD Research Group, Wing RR, Bolin P, et al. Cardiovascular effects of intensive lifestyle intervention in type 2 diabetes [published correction appears in *N Engl J Med.* 2014;370(19):1866]. *N Engl J Med.* 2013;369(2):145-154. PMID: 23796131

19 ANSWER: E) Vitamin E, 800 international units daily

Metabolic dysfunction-associated steatotic liver disease (MASLD), the most common cause of chronic liver disease in the western world, encompasses a histologic spectrum of liver disease ranging from simple steatosis to metabolic dysfunction-associated steatohepatitis (MASH), which can progress to cirrhosis and liver cancer. In the United States, the prevalence of MASLD and MASH is estimated to be 17% to 33% and 5.7% to 17%, respectively. The disease is closely associated with obesity and diabetes and, due to their ongoing epidemics, the prevalence of MASLD both in adults and children is likely to increase over time and continues to be a serious public health burden. Currently, there is no definitive treatment. MASH is characterized histologically by the presence of hepatic steatosis, lobular inflammation, and hepatocyte ballooning. Although the precise mechanism underlying disease progression from steatosis alone to MASH remains poorly understood, it is believed that oxidative stress has a central role contributing to hepatocellular injury. Thus, an effective therapeutic strategy is to target reduction in oxidative stress in patients with this disease.

In the PIVENS trial (Pioglitazone versus Vitamin E versus Placebo for the Treatment of Nondiabetic Patients with Nonalcoholic Steatohepatitis), vitamin E therapy (Answer E) demonstrated significant improvement in steatosis, inflammation, ballooning, and resolution of steatohepatitis in adult patients with aggressive MASH who did not have diabetes or cirrhosis.

Pioglitazone (Answer C) has some benefits for MASLD and MASH in patients with type 2 diabetes, but the patient in this vignette does not have diabetes.

Vitamin D (Answer D) has no established role in the treatment of MASH.

Metformin use (Answer B) is not associated with improvement in nonalcoholic steatohepatitis.

Although atorvastatin (Answer A) is indicated for lowering cardiovascular disease risk, it does not improve nonalcoholic steatohepatitis.

EDUCATIONAL OBJECTIVE

Recommend vitamin E in the management of metabolic dysfunction-associated steatotic liver disease in patients with obesity who do not have diabetes.

REFERENCE(S)

Sanyal AJ, Chalasani N, Kowdley KV, et al; NASH CRN. Pioglitazone, vitamin E, or placebo for nonalcoholic steatohepatitis. *N Engl J Med.* 2010;362(18):1675-1685. PMID: 20427778

McCullough AJ. Pathophysiology of nonalcoholic steatohepatitis. *J Clin Gastroenterol.* 2006;40(Suppl 1):S17-S29. PMID: 16540762

20 ANSWER: A) Dietary modification and acarbose

Postbariatric hypoglycemia is a rare complication of bariatric surgery that is occurring more frequently. Affected individuals present at least 6 months postoperatively with frequent postprandial episodes of hypoglycemia accompanied by adrenergic and/or neuroglycopenic signs and symptoms, including altered mental status, vision changes, motor incoordination, loss of consciousness, and seizures. While the underlying physiology is incompletely understood, the presence of inappropriately high insulin secretion after oral ingestion of nutrients is well established. Hyperinsulinemia occurs in response to oral, but not intravenous, glucose, which points to enteroinsular-axis overstimulation and an exaggerated incretin effect. Plasma concentrations of GLP-1 secreted by L cells in response to luminal nutrient stimulation are markedly elevated after meal intake. GLP-1 hypersecretion and hyperinsulinemic hypoglycemia are fully reversible by restoring the original route of nutrient transit via gastrostomy tube feeding into the remnant stomach. This suggests that altered nutrient transit with foregut bypass and hindgut stimulation potentiates hypoglycemia via GLP-1 secretion.

In this vignette, the Whipple triad has been fulfilled and there is symptomatic hypoglycemia in response to a mixed-meal challenge. The initial treatment of hypoglycemia is dietary counseling to assist the patient eliminate refined starches and replace them with high-fiber, low–glycemic index foods. However, dietary modification alone is not sufficient for this patient with frequent hypoglycemia, and the use of a glucosidase inhibitor such as acarbose would reduce glucose absorption and decrease the postprandial insulin response. Thus, recommending both dietary modification and acarbose (Answer A) would be the best initial treatment. Other agents such as diazoxide and octreotide have been used if initial treatment with acarbose is suboptimal.

There is no role for reversal of gastric bypass (Answer E) in treating this condition. Placement of a gastrostomy tube to reverse nutrient ingestion through the intact alimentary tract has been shown to reverse post–gastric bypass hypoglycemia.

A ketogenic diet (Answer B) has no role in the treatment of post–gastric bypass hypoglycemia.

Although liraglutide (Answer C) is a GLP-1 receptor agonist that slows the motility of the gastrointestinal tract and nutrient absorption and has been shown in case reports to be beneficial in treating hypoglycemia in patients who have undergone bariatric surgery, there are no trials documenting its efficacy in patients with post–gastric bypass hypoglycemia.

Use of a β-adrenergic blocker such as propranolol (Answer D) may mask the adrenergic response to hypoglycemia and has no role in this case.

A multicenter trial of exendin 9-36 (GLP-1 antagonist) has shown that it reduces hypoglycemia, but it is not available for commercial use.

EDUCATIONAL OBJECTIVE

Treat post–gastric bypass hypoglycemia.

REFERENCE(S)

Kellogg TA, Bantle JP, Leslie DB, et al. Postgastric bypass hyperinsulinemic hypoglycemia syndrome: characterization and response to a modified diet. *Surg Obes Relat Dis.* 2008;4(4):492-499. PMID: 18656831

Suhl E, Anderson-Haynes S-E, Mulla C, Patti M-E. Medical nutrition therapy for post-bariatric hypoglycemia: practical insights. *Surg Obes Relat Dis.* 2017;13(5):888-896. PMID: 28392017

Craig CM, Lawler HM, Lee CJE, et al. PREVENT: a randomized, placebo-controlled crossover trial of avexitide for treatment of postbariatric hypoglycemia. *J Clin Endocrinol Metab.* 2021;106(8):e3235-e3248. PMID: 33616643

21 ANSWER: D) Paroxetine

The effect of antidepressants on weight depends on the specific medication prescribed and the length of treatment. Short-term treatment for 2 to 3 months with selective serotonin reuptake inhibitors (SSRIs) usually causes little or no weight change. However, treatment with SSRIs for longer periods may result in significant weight gain. In some cases, it is not clear whether this is a true medication adverse effect or the result of recovery from depression and reversal of undesired weight loss. Evidence suggests that both bupropion (Answer B) and fluoxetine (Answer C) may be the least problematic SSRIs regarding undesired weight gain. Bupropion leads to weight loss and is used in combination with naltrexone for weight loss. Paroxetine (Answer D) may be the most problematic. In 6% of patients, paroxetine leads to weight gain ranging from 1.6% to 3.6% of baseline body weight. Venlafaxine (Answer E) and amitriptyline (Answer A) are considered to be weight neutral or to promote weight loss.

Most studies on this topic have evaluated patients who have major depressive disorder. It is not clear whether weight change caused by SSRIs differs according to demographic profiles such as age or sex. A review found that weight gain during treatment with SSRIs may be due to remission of major depression, improved appetite, increased carbohydrate craving, and changes in serotonin 2C receptor activity. Conversely, weight loss during acute SSRI treatment may be related to poor appetite at the beginning of treatment.

Weight gain due to long-term treatment with SSRIs may lead to diabetes. A nested case-control study of patients with depression found that use of moderate to high daily dosages of SSRIs for periods longer than 24 months is associated with a significant 2-fold increased risk of developing diabetes compared with not using antidepressants (incidence rate ratio: 2.06; 95% CI, 1.20-3.52). Analysis of individual antidepressants found an increased risk estimate for paroxetine (incidence rate ratio: 1.33; 95% CI, 1.02-1.73), suggesting the possibility that the increased risk associated with SSRIs might have primarily been due to this specific agent.

EDUCATIONAL OBJECTIVE

Identify antidepressant medications associated with weight gain.

REFERENCE(S)

Uher R, Farmer A, Henigsberg N, et al. Adverse reactions to antidepressants. *Br J Psychiatry.* 2009;195(3):202-210. PMID: 19721108

de Jonghe F, Ravelli DP, Tuynman-Qua H. A randomized, double-blind study of fluoxetine and maprotiline in the treatment of major depression. *Pharmacopsychiatry.* 1991;24(2):62-67. PMID: 1852793

Wade A, Michael Lemming O, Bang Hedegaard K. Escitalopram 10 mg/day is effective and well tolerated in a placebo-controlled study in depression in primary care. *Int Clin Psychopharmacol.* 2002;17(3):95-102. PMID: 11981349

22 ANSWER: A) Avoid pregnancy (with use of an intrauterine device) until she is weight stable

More than 80% of bariatric procedures are performed in women, and approximately half of these procedures are performed in reproductive-aged women. Thus, it has become increasingly common for women who have undergone bariatric surgery to present for preconception counseling or prenatal care. A joint 2013 clinical practice guideline by the American Association of Clinical Endocrinologists, the Obesity Society, and the American Society for Metabolic and Bariatric Surgery recommends that women avoid conception for 12 to 18 months after bariatric surgery because this time frame is when women are actively losing the most weight. This delay is done in an effort to optimize weight loss and reduce the potentially adverse effect of postbariatric surgical nutritional deficiencies. Procedures that create malabsorption, such as biliopancreatic diversion, jejunoileal bypass, or Roux-en-Y bypass, may interfere with the absorption of oral contraceptives (Answer B), thereby reducing their effectiveness. Thus, an intrauterine device (Answer A) is a preferable method of contraception.

As discussed, pregnancy during the time of active weight loss after bariatric surgery is not recommended (thus, Answers C, D, and E are incorrect). Breastfeeding is not contraindicated following bariatric surgery. Monitoring nutritional status (ie, prealbumin levels) and micronutrient levels (especially iron, ferritin, vitamin B_{12}, calcium, PTH, 25-hydroxyvitamin D) is essential after gastric bypass, as well as before, during, and after pregnancy.

EDUCATIONAL OBJECTIVE

Provide pregnancy counseling to women who have undergone bariatric surgery.

REFERENCE(S)

Mechanick JI, Youdim A, Jones DB, et al, American Association of Clinical Endocrinologists, Obesity Society, American Society for Metabolic & Bariatric Surgery. Clinical practice guidelines for the peroperative nutritional, metabolic, and nonsurgical support of the bariatric surgery patient—2013 update: cosponsored by American Association of Clinical Endocrinologists, the Obesity Society, and American Society for Metabolic & Bariatric Surgery. *Endocr Pract.* 2013;19(2):337-372. PMID: 23529351

American College of Obstetricians and Gynecologists. ACOG practice bulletin No. 105: bariatric surgery and pregnancy. *Obstet Gynecol.* 2009;113(6):1405-1413. PMID: 19461456

23 ANSWER: B) Refer him for nutritional counseling to reduce his intake of saturated fat and alcohol

This patient has metabolic syndrome without diabetes. He is at intermediate risk for atherosclerotic cardiovascular disease with moderate hypertriglyceridemia in the range of 300 to 500 mg/dL (3.39-5.65 mmol/L) and an LDL-cholesterol level at target. Hypertriglyceridemia in this range is considered atherogenic and warrants attention. The initial approach should consist of general measures, which include diet, exercise, weight loss, and assessment of secondary causes of hypertriglyceridemia (ie, hypothyroidism, medications) (Answer B).

For moderate hypertriglyceridemia, targets include less than 6% of calories from added sugar, less than 30% to 35% of calories from total dietary fat, and 2 or fewer alcoholic drinks per day for men and 1 or fewer per day for women. For moderate to severe hypertriglyceridemia, targets include less than 5% of calories from added sugar, less than 20% to 25% of calories from total dietary fat, and alcohol abstinence. For patients with glucose intolerance or diabetes and high risk of atherosclerotic cardiovascular disease, moderate hypertriglyceridemia should not be treated with niacin (Answer E), as it can worsen glucose tolerance.

Fenofibrate (Answer D) is recommended for patients with severe hypertriglyceridemia (>1000 mg/dL [>11.30 mmol/L]) to avoid pancreatitis.

Changing atorvastatin to rosuvastatin (Answer A) would not significantly lower this patient's triglyceride levels.

The efficacy of triglyceride lowering in decreasing risk of atherosclerotic cardiovascular disease has not been established, in contrast to the established risk reduction with lowering LDL cholesterol.

Also, LDL-cholesterol levels may underrepresent cardiovascular risk in patients with hypertriglyceridemia. High triglyceride levels are associated with small, dense cholesterol-depleted LDL particles that may not be captured by LDL-cholesterol measurement. Non-HDL cholesterol and apolipoprotein B concentrations are better measures of excess concentrations of atherogenic lipoproteins in patients with moderate and severe hypertriglyceridemia.

EDUCATIONAL OBJECTIVE

Manage hypertriglyceridemia in patients with moderate risk of atherosclerotic cardiovascular disease.

REFERENCE(S)

Virani SS, Morris PB, Agarwala A, et al. 2021 ACC expert consensus decision pathway on the management of ASCVD risk reduction in patients with persistent hypertriglyceridemia: a report of the American College of Cardiology Solution Set Oversight Committee. *J Am Coll Cardiol.* 2021;78(9):960-993. PMID: 34332805

Ballantyne CM, Grundy SM, Oberman A, et al. Hyperlipidemia: diagnostic and therapeutic perspectives. *J Clin Endocrinol Metab.* 2000;85(6):2089-2112. PMID: 10852435

Gotto AM Jr. Hypertriglyceridemia: risks and perspectives. *Am J Cardiol.* 1992;70(19):19H-25H. PMID: 1466313

24 ANSWER: B) Start bempedoic acid

This patient presents for treatment of secondary cardiovascular disease risk and has an elevated LDL-cholesterol level that does not meet target (<55 mg/dL [<1.42 mmol/L]). He is not tolerant of PCSK9 inhibitors. Bempedoic acid (Answer B) is an inhibitor of adenosine triphosphate citrate lyase, an enzyme upstream of 3-hydroxy-3-methylglutaryl-CoA reductase (the target of statins) in the cholesterol biosynthesis pathway.

Two randomized controlled trials that evaluated the safety and LDL-cholesterol–lowering efficacy of this drug have been published. In both trials, patients with either established cardiovascular disease or heterozygous familial hypercholesterolemia were randomly assigned to bempedoic acid (180 mg once daily) or placebo in a 2:1 ratio and followed up for 52 weeks. The CLEAR Harmony trial enrolled 2230 patients taking maximally tolerated dosages of a statin (6.6% taking low-intensity statin therapy, 43.5% taking moderate-intensity statin therapy, and 49.9% taking high-intensity statin therapy). The baseline LDL-cholesterol concentration had to be above 70 mg/dL (>1.81 mmol/L). The primary end point of safety (any adverse event) was similar in the 2 groups who were randomly assigned to placebo vs bemepdoic acid (78.5% vs 78.7%, respectively), as was the end point of serious adverse events. At week 12, bempedoic acid reduced the mean LDL-cholesterol concentration by 19.2 mg/dL (0.50 mmol/L), representing a change of −16.5% from baseline (difference vs placebo in change from baseline, −18.1%; $P < .001$). There was a trend toward a greater LDL-cholesterol–lowering response of bempedoic acid in patients receiving a low- to moderate-intensity statin (−20.0%) compared with those receiving a high-intensity statin (−17.5%). The CLEAR Wisdom trial enrolled 779 patients receiving maximally tolerated lipid-lowering therapies and whose baseline LDL-cholesterol concentration was at least 100 mg/dL (≥2.59 mmol/L). The primary efficacy end point of the percentage change in LDL cholesterol from baseline to week 12 was significantly lower with bempedoic acid than with placebo (−15.1% vs −2.4%; 97.6 mg/dL vs 122.8 mg/dL, respectively). Adverse events included elevated uric acid in a higher percentage of patients receiving active treatment. Measuring serum uric acid and stabilizing patients with active gout before starting bempedoic acid is advised.

The other lipid-lowering agents listed—fenofibrate (Answer C), niacin (Answer D), and omega-3 fatty acids (Answer E)—have not been shown to reduce MACE outcomes (major adverse cardiovascular event outcomes) in patients in secondary prevention.

Changing atorvastatin to rosuvastatin (Answer A) would not result in more incremental LDL-cholesterol lowering that is needed to achieve this patient's target concentration.

EDUCATIONAL OBJECTIVE

Explain the benefits of bempedoic acid in patients with familial hypercholesterolemia.

REFERENCE(S)

Ray KK, Bays HE, Catapano AL, et al; CLEAR Harmony Trial. Safety and efficacy of bempedoic acid to reduce LDL cholesterol. *N Engl J Med.* 2019;380(11):1022-1032. PMID: 30865796

Goldberg AC, Leiter LA, Stroes ESG, et al. Effect of bempedoic acid vs placebo added to maximally tolerated statins on low-density lipoprotein cholesterol in patients at high risk for cardiovascular disease: the CLEAR Wisdom Randomized Clinical Trial. *JAMA.* 2019;322(18):1780-1788. PMID: 31714986

25 ANSWER: E) Tirzepatide

Tirzepatide (Answer E) is a long-acting dual GLP-1 receptor agonist with structural modifications to reduce renal clearance and decrease degradation by DPP-4, resulting in slower degradation and allowing for once-weekly subcutaneous or once-daily oral dosing. Tirzepatide is approved for patients with overweight who do not have type 2 diabetes, and it results in significant weight loss compared with that observed with placebo. It also confers benefits in terms of risk of diabetes, liver steatosis, and cardiovascular disease.

Semaglutide (Answer D) also reduces liver injury from metabolic dysfunction-associated steatohepatitis in overweight patients. All GLP-1 receptor agonists slow gastric emptying and can cause nausea. They are contraindicated in pregnancy, in patients with a personal or family history of medullary thyroid cancer, and in patients with a history of pancreatitis. Greater weight loss is noted with tirzepatide vs semaglutide in head-to-head trials.

Orlistat (Answer B) induces some weight loss but has not been shown to alter cardiovascular disease risk or liver fat levels.

Phentermine (Answer C) is a stimulant and appetite suppressant that leads to weight loss without other benefits.

Bupropion (Answer A) reduces appetite and induces weight loss, but it does not have benefits with respect to cardiovascular disease or liver fat levels.

EDUCATIONAL OBJECTIVE

Explain the benefits of GLP-1 receptor agonists for weight loss.

REFERENCE(S)

Aronne LJ, Sattar N, Horn DB, et al; SURMOUNT-4 Investigators. Continued treatment with tirzepatide for maintenance of weight reduction in adults with obesity: the SURMOUNT-4 Randomized Clinical Trial. *JAMA.* 2024;331(1):38-48. PMID: 38078870

le Roux CW, Hankosky ER, Wang D, et al. Tirzepatide 10 and 15 mg compared with semaglutide 2.4 mg for the treatment of obesity: an indirect treatment comparison. *Diabetes Obes Metab.* 2023;25(9):2626-2633. PMID: 37344384

26 ANSWER: B) Calculate FIB-4 score and consider liver elastography

Metabolic dysfunction-associated steatotic liver disease commonly occurs in patients with type 2 diabetes, and approximately 15% of patients with type 2 diabetes in general endocrinology clinics have evidence of inflammation and fibrosis as determined by liver biopsy. Screening for metabolic dysfunction-associated steatohepatitis (Answer B) is critical in overweight patients with type 2 diabetes because liver steatosis can progress to liver cirrhosis and hepatocellular carcinoma. Liver scores to assess liver injury are validated, noninvasive screening measures. Several liver scores are used clinically; if the FIB-4 score is abnormal, then assessment with vibration-controlled transient elastography or other imaging can be recommended. FIB-4 uses the clinical parameters of age, AST, ALT, and platelets. A FIB-4 index greater than 3.25 indicates suspicion for liver scarring and warrants additional testing. A FIB-4 index less than 1.45 has a negative predictive value of 94.7% to exclude severe fibrosis with a sensitivity of 74.3%. A FIB-4 index higher than 3.25 has a positive predictive value of 82.1% for confirming the existence of significant fibrosis (F3-F4) with a specificity of 98.2%.

Metabolic dysfunction-associated steatotic liver disease/metabolic dysfunction-associated steatohepatitis can be present even when liver transaminase levels are normal (thus, Answer D is incorrect).

Although it is important to check for secondary causes of liver fibrosis (Answer A), this choice does not best address direct assessment for nonalcoholic steatohepatitis. In patients with an abnormal liver score and/or imaging, secondary causes of liver disease should be evaluated.

Liver ultrasonography (Answer C) can detect steatosis but does not assess for fibrosis. Liver biopsy is the gold standard for diagnosing metabolic dysfunction-associated steatohepatitis. There is insufficient evidence to recommend use of vitamin E in patients with diabetes. However, some antidiabetes agents (pioglitazone, liraglutide, and semaglutide) have been shown to reduce features of metabolic dysfunction-associated steatohepatitis in patients with diabetes.

EDUCATIONAL OBJECTIVE

Assess for metabolic dysfunction-associated steatohepatitis in patients with type 2 diabetes.

REFERENCE(S)

Angulo P, Keach JC, Batts KP, Lindor KD. Independent predictors of liver fibrosis in patients with nonalcoholic steatohepatitis. *Hepatology.* 1999;30(6):1356-1362. PMID: 10573511

Dixon JB, Bhathal PS, O'Brien PE. Nonalcoholic fatty liver disease: predictors of nonalcoholic steatohepatitis and liver fibrosis in the severely obese. *Gastroenterology.* 2001;121(1):91-100. PMID: 11438497

Angulo P, Hui JM, Marchesini G, et al. The NAFLD fibrosis score: a noninvasive system that identifies liver fibrosis in patients with NAFLD. *Hepatology.* 2007;45(4):846-854. PMID: 1739350

Pituitary Board Review

John David Carmichael, MD

1 ANSWER: D) Increase levothyroxine to 125 mcg daily because the free T_4 concentration is in the lower half of the reference range

This patient's case demonstrates progressive loss of pituitary function after radiation for residual pituitary adenoma. A year following radiation, she was diagnosed with GH deficiency, which was treated. Subsequently, she had progressive loss of gonadotropin function and then thyroid function. It is clear from the description that her adrenal axis remains intact. Her levothyroxine dosage should be increased to 125 mcg daily because the free T_4 concentration is in the lower half of the reference range (Answer D). In the setting of a pituitary tumor, the TSH concentration is not helpful in the titration of thyroid hormone (thus, Answers B and E are incorrect). Monitoring relies on T_4 values, and the free T_4 concentration is the most accurate. Patients with central hypothyroidism are frequently underdosed, and free T_4 levels are in the lower half or below the reference range. It is best to target free T_4 in the upper half of the reference range (thus, Answer A is incorrect).

While suppression of TSH is very common in treated central hypothyroidism, suppression is not the goal for thyroid replacement dosing, and the levothyroxine dosage should not be decreased in the face of a low TSH value (Answer B).

Targeting the upper half of the free T_4 reference range is optimal, and while oral estrogen may increase the total T_4 value, it would not artifactually lower the free T_4 laboratory result (Answer C).

EDUCATIONAL OBJECTIVE

Guide optimal replacement of thyroid hormone in central hypothyroidism in a patient with hypopituitarism.

REFERENCE(S)

Persani L. Clinical review: Central hypothyroidism: pathogenic, diagnostic, and therapeutic challenges. *J Clin Endocrinol Metab.* 2012;97(9):3068-3078. PMID: 22851492

Kaminski J, Junior CM, Pavesi H, Drobrzenski B, Amaral GMD. Effects of oral versus transdermal estradiol plus micronized progesterone on thyroid hormones, hepatic proteins, lipids, and quality of life in menopausal women with hypothyroidism: a clinical trial. *Menopause.* 2021;28(9):1044-1052. PMID: 34183565

2 ANSWER: B) Formal testing of visual fields by an ophthalmologist

This patient has an incidentally discovered pituitary adenoma. Although he is asymptomatic, the tumor size and the degree of extension warrant further workup. The best next step is to fully assess this tumor's impact via formal visual field testing by an ophthalmologist (Answer B).

For individuals with incidental pituitary adenomas, guidance from published clinical guidelines is to screen for hypercortisolemia (Answer A) only in the setting of clinical symptoms.

This patient may require surgery (Answer C), but the first priority is to determine whether he has a visual field defect.

If the tumor were larger and the symptoms suggested that hyperprolactinemia were causing interference with gonadal function, then repeating the prolactin measurement with serial dilutions (Answer E) could be considered. Serial dilutions can help to eliminate the hook effect, a laboratory error induced by oversaturation of the antibodies used for assessment of the serum prolactin concentration.

Given the current finding of optic chiasm compression, recommending observation with follow-up MRI in 6 months (Answer D) is inadequate and could jeopardize vision recovery.

EDUCATIONAL OBJECTIVE

Guide the evaluation of incidental pituitary adenomas.

REFERENCE(S)

Freda PU, Beckers AM, Katznelson L, Molitch ME, Montori VM, Post KD, Vance ML; Endocrine Society. Pituitary incidentaloma: an Endocrine Society clinical practice guideline. *J Clin Endocrinol Metab.* 2011;96(4):894-904. PMID: 21474686

Raverot V, Perrin P, Chanson P, Jouanneau E, Brue T, Raverot G. Prolactin immunoassay: does the high-dose hook effect still exist? *Pituitary.* 2022;25(4):653-657. PMID: 35793045

Chanson P, Raverot G, Castinetti F, Cortet-Rudelli C, Galland F, Salenave S; French Endocrinology Society non-functioning pituitary adenoma work-group. Management of clinically non-functioning pituitary adenoma. *Ann Endocrinol (Paris).* 2015;76(3):239-247. PMID: 26072284

Giraldi E, Allen JW, Ioachimescu AG. Pituitary incidentalomas: best practices and looking ahead. *Endocr Pract.* 2023;29(1):60-68. PMID: 36270609

3 ANSWER: C) Pituitary hyperplasia

This case demonstrates pituitary hyperplasia (Answer C), a commonly noted incidental finding on pituitary imaging in young women of reproductive age. The hallmark of pituitary hyperplasia is an increase in pituitary size with homogeneous tissue enhancement. Individuals with pituitary hyperplasia have no findings of pituitary dysfunction.

Rathke cleft cyst (Answer E) is characteristically a cystic lesion located between the anterior and posterior lobes of the pituitary. It is also a common incidental finding, usually without associated pituitary dysfunction. Rathke cleft cysts can grow to a large size and cause pituitary dysfunction that may require surgical intervention.

Pituitary macroadenomas (Answer D) typically demonstrate nonenhancement compared with a normal pituitary gland. Macroadenomas are usually identifiable as discrete masses that are distinct from the normal gland, and they are typically accompanied by pituitary dysfunction.

Lymphocytic hypophysitis (Answer A) is often associated with pregnancy or the postpartum stage, but it is more frequently noted to be an adverse effect of checkpoint inhibitor chemotherapy. The hallmark of lymphocytic hypophysitis is homogeneous bright enhancement with characteristic clinical findings of central adrenal insufficiency followed by central hypothyroidism and other pituitary deficiencies.

Parasellar meningioma (Answer B) usually appears as a mass in the margins of the sella, and it can be identified by the sign of a dural tail.

EDUCATIONAL OBJECTIVE

Identify the etiology of a pituitary incidentaloma based on history and MRI findings.

REFERENCE(S)

Jipa A, Jain V. Imaging of the sellar and parasellar regions. *Clin Imaging.* 2021;77:254-275. PMID: 34153590

Chanson P, Daujat F, Young J, Bellucci A, Kujas M, Doyon D, Schaison G. Normal pituitary hypertrophy as a frequent cause of pituitary incidentaloma: a follow-up study. *J Clin Endocrinol Metab.* 2001;86(7):3009-3015. PMID: 11443160

Freda PU, Beckers AM, Katznelson L, Molitch ME, Montori VM, Post KD, Vance ML; Endocrine Society. Pituitary incidentaloma: an Endocrine Society clinical practice guideline. *J Clin Endocrinol Metab.* 2011;96(4):894-904. PMID: 21474686

Giraldi E, Allen JW, Ioachimescu AG. Pituitary Incidentalomas: best practices and looking ahead. *Endocr Pract.* 2023;29(1):60-68. PMID: 36270609

4 ANSWER: A) Assessment for adrenal insufficiency now and then annually with stimulation testing (likely *PROP1* pathogenic variant)

This patient presents with a progressive pattern of pituitary hormone deficiencies caused by *PROP1*-related combined pituitary hormone deficiencies, which is characterized by deficiencies of GH, TSH, gonadotropins, prolactin, and sometimes ACTH. *PROP1* pathogenic variants are the most common cause of genetic combined pituitary hormone deficiencies, and they result in the most variable presentation. Deficiencies caused by *PROP1* pathogenic variants are not apparent at birth, but are discovered due to short stature, with TSH deficiency coming to light after GH replacement in many cases. LH and FSH deficiencies are typically identified at puberty. ACTH deficiency, if it develops, is typically identified in late adolescence or adulthood. Therefore, this patient requires screening to assess for the possible development of adrenal insufficiency now and then annually thereafter (Answer A).

TPIT pathogenic variants (Answer B) present with isolated adrenal insufficiency at birth, which does not fit the clinical presentation here.

Combined deficiencies from *POU1F1* pathogenic variants (Answer E) (formerly known as *PIT1)* present similarly, but with adrenal and gonadal function preserved.

Patients with genetic causes of their combined pituitary hormone deficiencies do not require retesting as adults. Patient education is the key to identifying adrenal insufficiency, as testing periodically can lead to a delay in diagnosis. However, empiric treatment (Answer D) to prevent possible untoward events of incipient adrenal insufficiency, especially when its development is not a certainty, is not warranted.

EDUCATIONAL OBJECTIVE

Guide management of combined pituitary hormone deficiencies based on genetic etiology.

REFERENCE(S)

Yuen KCJ, Biller BMK, Radovick S, Carmichael JD, Jasim S, Pantalone KM, Hoffman AR. American Association of Clinical Endocrinologists and American College of Endocrinology guidelines for management of growth hormone deficiency in adults and patients transitioning from pediatric to adult care. *Endocr Pract.* 2019;25(11):1191-1232. PMID: 31760824

Cerbone M, Dattani MT. Progression from isolated growth hormone deficiency to combined pituitary hormone deficiency. *Growth Horm IGF Res.* 2017;37:19-25. PMID: 29107171

Prince KL, Walvoord EC, Rhodes SJ. The role of homeodomain transcription factors in heritable pituitary disease. *Nat Rev Endocrinol.* 2011;7(12):727-737. PMID: 21788968

Bertko E, Klammt J, Dusatkova P, et al. Combined pituitary hormone deficiency due to gross deletions in the POU1F1 (PIT-1) and PROP1 genes. *J Hum Genet.* 2017;62(8):755-762. PMID: 28356564

5 ANSWER: E) Sheehan syndrome with infarction of normal pituitary during childbirth

Empty sella, which is a radiological finding and not a syndrome, can be broken down into 2 major categories: primary empty sella and secondary empty sella. In most cases, empty sella is not associated with pituitary dysfunction. There are exceptions to this, including empty sella arising from infarction of pituitary tissue (apoplexy), genetic defects causing hypoplasia or aplasia of the pituitary, and late stages of hypophysitis. The cause of this patient's empty sella is Sheehan syndrome with infarction of the normal pituitary gland during childbirth (Answer E). During pregnancy, the pituitary doubles in size. At the time of delivery, if there is extensive blood loss, infarction of the enlarged gland can result in infarction of the hyperplastic tissue. This can cause empty sella after the acute event has subsided. Pituitary hormone recovery is highly variable. Typically, patients come to medical attention earlier; however, this patient was not diagnosed for several years after the event. Primary empty sella typically results from laxity of the diaphragma sella with cerebrospinal fluid filling the sella and compressing the normal gland. Empty sella is commonly associated with increased intracranial pressure from pseudotumor cerebri (Answer C). Individuals with pseudotumor cerebri typically have obesity, and their presentation is accompanied by other findings, including papilledema and other neurologic or radiologic findings associated with increased intracranial pressure. This patient has none of these findings.

It would be unusual for apoplexy (Answer A) to completely resolve a pituitary macroadenoma or not leave a remnant. Typically, a pituitary macroadenoma would have caused sellar enlargement, a finding not observed in this case.

Ruptured Rathke cleft cyst (Answer D) is an unusual finding that may have similar characteristics as those of pituitary tumor apoplexy or Sheehan syndrome. When found, it is often accompanied by xanthogranulomatous tissue, for which there is no evidence on this patient's MRI.

PROP1 pathogenic variants (Answer B) may result in a hypoplastic gland and empty sella, but they are usually associated with pituitary dysfunction before puberty, and they typically result in infertility.

EDUCATIONAL OBJECTIVE

Determine the etiology of empty sella.

REFERENCE(S)

Giustina A, Aimaretti G, Bondanelli M, et al. Primary empty sella: why and when to investigate hypothalamic-pituitary function. *J Endocrinol Invest.* 2010;33(5):343-346. PMID: 20208457

Carosi G, Brunetti A, Mangone A, et al. A multicenter cohort study in patients with primary empty sella: hormonal and neuroradiological features over a long follow-up. *Front Endocrinol (Lausanne).* 2022;13:925378. PMID: 35813618

Auer MK, Stieg MR, Crispin A, Sievers C, Stalla GK, Kopczak A. Primary empty sella syndrome and the prevalence of hormonal dysregulation. *Dtsch Arztebl Int.* 2018;115(7):99-105. PMID: 29510819

6 ANSWER: C) Macroprolactin

The differential diagnosis for oligomenorrhea includes hyperprolactinemia, polycystic ovary syndrome, and hypothyroidism. This patient has some features of mild polycystic ovary syndrome. The important aspects of her evaluation are the negative MRI and the absence of galactorrhea. Assessment of macroprolactin (Answer C) would be helpful in this case because it would distinguish between oligomenorrhea due to polycystic ovary syndrome and oligomenorrhea associated with hyperprolactinemia. Macroprolactin is a complex of immunoglobulin-bound prolactin, which is biologically inert, and it is typically found in asymptomatic patients with elevated serum prolactin. Distinguishing polycystic ovary syndrome from hyperprolactinemia is important.

Prolactin measurement with serial dilutions (Answer D) is helpful to identify the hook effect, but this is reserved for the evaluation of large pituitary masses in patients with a normal prolactin concentration.

Her thyroid function test results are consistent with subclinical hypothyroidism, and measurement of TPO antibodies (Answer E) may be helpful for decision-making regarding treatment plans, but this is not the first priority in her diagnostic workup.

DHEA-S measurement (Answer A) may help to fully evaluate her androgen-related symptoms, but since her total testosterone is already mildly elevated, there is enough androgen-related information and a DHEA-S value would not be helpful.

While measurement of IGF-1 (Answer B) may be helpful if a co-secreting adenoma (secreting both prolactin and GH) were suspected, the negative MRI makes this possibility very unlikely.

EDUCATIONAL OBJECTIVE

Distinguish polycystic ovary syndrome from hyperprolactinemia in a patient with oligomenorrhea.

REFERENCE(S)

Melmed S, Casanueva FF, Hoffman AR, et al; Endocrine Society. Diagnosis and treatment of hyperprolactinemia: an Endocrine Society clinical practice guideline. *J Clin Endocrinol Metab.* 2011;96(2):273-288. PMID: 21296991

Petersenn S, Fleseriu M, Casanueva FF, et al. Diagnosis and management of prolactin-secreting pituitary adenomas: a Pituitary Society international Consensus Statement. *Nat Rev Endocrinol.* 2023;19(12):722-740. PMID: 37670148

Biagetti B, Ferrer Costa R, Alfayate Guerra R, et al. Macroprolactin: from laboratory to clinical practice. *Endocrinol Diabetes Nutr (Engl Ed).* 2022;69(1):63-69. PMID: 35232561

7 ANSWER: E) Stereotactic radiotherapy

This patient has a nonfunctioning gonadotroph pituitary macroadenoma (SF-1 staining tumor, reflecting gonadotroph origin) with residual cavernous sinus disease following surgery. Given that the cavernous sinus portion has grown in a relatively short period, further intervention is needed to address the tumor.

Another surgery (Answer A) is unlikely to be helpful, as the tumor is in the cavernous sinus and is not likely surgically accessible.

Radiation therapy is indicated, and stereotactic radiotherapy (Answer E) is the best choice to control tumor growth, if not shrink it. Because the tumor is not adjacent to the optic chiasm, there is very low risk of chiasmal damage with stereotactic radiotherapy.

Cabergoline (Answer C) has been used in studies of nonfunctioning adenomas, but the overall response is modest. Similarly, studies with bromocriptine (Answer B) have shown a mixed response.

Some studies have used octreotide (Answer D) for management of nonfunctioning adenomas. However, the response is modest, and somatostatin analogues are not currently thought to be sufficiently effective to warrant use in this setting.

EDUCATIONAL OBJECTIVE

Recommend a treatment strategy for nonfunctioning gonadotroph pituitary adenomas.

REFERENCE(S)

Even-Zohar N, Greenman Y. Management of NFAs: medical treatment. *Pituitary.* 2018;21(2):168-175. PMID: 29344905

Minniti G, Flickinger J, Tolu B, Paolini S. Management of nonfunctioning pituitary tumors: radiotherapy. *Pituitary.* 2018;21(2):154-161. PMID: 29372392

Farrell CJ, Garzon-Muvdi T, Fastenberg JH, et al. Management of nonfunctioning recurrent pituitary adenomas. *Neurosurg Clin N Am.* 2019;30(4):473-482. PMID: 31471054

8 ANSWER: D) Switch to pasireotide

This patient has a growing tumor and persistently elevated IGF-1 levels despite octreotide long-acting release at the highest dosage approved by the US FDA. The option with the most rapid response regarding tumor shrinkage and biochemical control is pasireotide (Answer D), the somatostatin receptor ligand. Pasireotide effectively normalizes IGF-1 in approximately 40% to 45% of patients and can shrink tumors. A common adverse event is hyperglycemia, which affects up to two-thirds of patients.

The oral octreotide capsule (Answer E) is indicated in patients with acromegaly who previously responded to and tolerated octreotide or lanreotide. However, this patient is not responding well to parenteral octreotide, so the oral octreotide capsule will not likely be effective.

Adding cabergoline (Answer A) is unlikely to improve biochemical control in a patient with significant biochemical activity and tumor growth.

Adding pegvisomant (Answer B) may result in biochemical control, but given that it is a GH receptor antagonist, it is unlikely to further control tumor growth.

Stereotactic radiotherapy (Answer C) may control both tumor growth and GH hypersecretion, but it could take years to be effective and is unlikely to be helpful in the next 6 months.

EDUCATIONAL OBJECTIVE

Recommend the best management of persistent acromegaly.

REFERENCE(S)

Fleseriu M, Biller BMK, Freda PU, et al. A Pituitary Society update to acromegaly management guidelines. *Pituitary.* 2021;24(1):1-13. PMID: 33079318

Coopmans EC, van Meyel SWF, van der Lely AJ, Neggers SJCMM. The position of combined medical treatment in acromegaly. *Arch Endocrinol Metab.* 2019;63(6):646-652. PMID: 31939490

Coopmans EC, Muhammad A, van der Lely AJ, Janssen JAMJL, Neggers SJCMM. How to position pasireotide LAR treatment in acromegaly. *J Clin Endocrinol Metab.* 2019;104(6):1978-1988. PMID: 30608534

9 ANSWER: D) Repeated clinical assessment and laboratory monitoring in 6 months

This patient has hyperprolactinemia associated with a microlesion of the pituitary gland, consistent with a microprolactinoma. Indications to treat prolactinoma include oligo/amenorrhea, bothersome galactorrhea, infertility, macroadenoma (particularly if associated with local mass effect), and headache. She has mild, nonbothersome galactorrhea, so this is not a clear indication to treat. Surgery could be considered (although this was not a listed answer option), but the decision to proceed with surgery in this setting is debatable, as there is no clear indication for any treatment.

She has regular menstrual cycles, and while ovulation may be affected, she is not currently interested in fertility, so prescribing a dopamine agonist (Answer B) is not indicated now. This may be considered in the future.

Serial dilution of prolactin (Answer C) is performed to rule out the hook effect in the setting of a large—usually giant—lesion and a normal or mildly elevated serum prolactin concentration. The hook effect refers to a falsely low serum prolactin value in the setting of a macroprolactinoma. In patients with a small lesion, assessment for the hook effect is not indicated.

In addition, there is no indication to treat with stereotactic radiotherapy (Answer E), as this may take up to 10 years for effect, there is a reasonable risk of hypopituitarism with this treatment, and there is an approximately 1% risk of malignancy.

Repeating MRI in 6 months (Answer A) is not indicated unless the serum prolactin level increases significantly within that time. Microprolactinomas tend to grow slowly, and only a minority have significant growth over 5 to 10 years. Thus, MRI within 6 months is unlikely to identify findings that would alter therapy.

Given the presented scenario, following this patient with serial monitoring (Answer D) is the best strategy.

EDUCATIONAL OBJECTIVE

Manage microprolactinomas.

REFERENCE(S)

Molitch ME. Diagnosis and treatment of pituitary adenomas: a review. *JAMA*. 2017;317(5):516-524. PMID: 28170483

Chanson P, Maiter D. The epidemiology, diagnosis and treatment of prolactinomas: the old and the new. *Best Pract Res Clin Endocrinol Metab.* 2019;33(2):101290. PMID: 31326373

Honegger J, Nasi-Kordhishti I, Aboutaha N, Giese S. Surgery for prolactinomas: a better choice? *Pituitary.* 2020;23(1):45-51. PMID: 31853793

Petersenn S, Giustina A. Diagnosis and management of prolactinomas: current challenges. *Pituitary.* 2020;23(1):1-2. PMID: 31900881

10 ANSWER: A) Craniopharyngioma

The key feature in this vignette is that the patient has arginine vasopressin deficiency, which indicates a primarily hypothalamic origin of his tumor. One tends to think of craniopharyngiomas as occurring mainly in children, but there is a distinct second peak in older adults (age 50-74 years). Arginine vasopressin deficiency is very uncommon in patients with pituitary adenomas (Answers B, D, and E), but is common in patients with craniopharyngiomas (Answer A). Craniopharyngiomas are typically described on MRI as calcified, solid, and/or cystic lesions, usually with a lobular shape and diameter of 20 to 40 mm. The solid elements are often isointense or hypointense on T1-weighted images, exhibit inhomogeneous high intensity on T2-weighted images, and heterogeneously enhance after gadolinium administration. The cystic elements of adamantinomatous craniopharyngiomas typically display high intensity on T1-weighted images, high or mixed intensity on T2-weighted images, and contrast enhancement of the cyst wall. The squamous-papillary subtype is found in approximately one-third of adults with craniopharyngiomas, and it rarely shows calcification. Overall, the mortality is much higher for patients with craniopharyngiomas than for those with pituitary adenomas. Recent studies suggest that activating pathogenic variants in the gene encoding β-catenin may be involved in the pathogenesis of the adamantinomatous variety of craniopharyngiomas.

The very mild prolactin elevation in this patient is from stalk compression rather than from a prolactinoma (Answer D) and could accompany any of these other tumors/lesions.

Langerhans cell histiocytosis (Answer C) usually presents as an infiltrative disease of the hypothalamus and stalk with stalk thickening on MRI rather than as a mass lesion.

EDUCATIONAL OBJECTIVE

Differentiate among hypothalamic and pituitary mass lesions.

REFERENCE(S)

Mende KC, Kellner T, Petersenn S, et al. Clinical situation, therapy, and follow-up of adult craniopharyngioma. *J Clin Endocrinol Metab.* 2020;105(1):dgz043. PMID: 31589293

Zada G, Lin N, Ojerholm E, Ramkissoon S, Laws ER. Craniopharyngioma and other cystic epithelial lesions of the sellar region: a review of clinical, imaging, and histopathological relationships. *Neurosurg Focus.* 2010;28(4):E4. PMID: 20367361

Erfurth EM, Holmer H, Fjalldal SB. Mortality and morbidity in adult craniopharyngioma. *Pituitary.* 2013;16(1):46-55. PMID: 22961634

Andoniadou CL, Gaston-Massuet C, Reddy R, et al. Identification of novel pathways involved in the pathogenesis of human adamantinomatous craniopharyngioma. *Acta Neuropathol.* 2012;124(2):259-271. PMID: 22349813

11 ANSWER: E) Perform a GH-stimulation test one month after stopping GH

More than two-thirds of children with idiopathic isolated GH deficiency diagnosed by conventional criteria have normal GH secretion as adults. Consequently, retesting such patients as adults with a stimulation test is important before continuing GH treatment. Because one-third of these patients may have persistent GH deficiency, simply discontinuing GH therapy because he has reached peak growth (Answer B) is incorrect. Testing should be done one month after stopping GH. In this setting, IGF-1 measurement alone (Answer C) is not sufficient to document persistent GH deficiency, and a GH-stimulation test is needed (Answer E). Measuring a morning GH level following discontinuation of GH therapy (Answer D) is not useful diagnostically to assess for ongoing GH deficiency.

GH treatment can be resumed at a lower dosage than that used in childhood because of its known benefits on body composition (Answer A), but only if GH deficiency is documented to still be present.

EDUCATIONAL OBJECTIVE

Perform GH-stimulation testing in a young adult with a childhood diagnosis of GH deficiency to determine whether therapy is still needed.

REFERENCE(S)

Tauber M, Moulin P, Pienkowski C, Jouret B, Rochiccioli P. Growth hormone (GH) retesting and auxological data in 131 GH-deficient patients after completion of treatment. *J Clin Endocrinol Metab.* 1997;82(2):352-356. PMID: 9024217

Molitch ME, Clemmons DR, Malozowski S, Merriam GR, Vance ML; Endocrine Society. Evaluation and treatment of adult growth hormone deficiency: an Endocrine Society clinical practice guideline. *J Clin Endocrinol Metab.* 2011;96(6):1587-1609. PMID: 21602453

12 ANSWER: D) Osilodrostat

This patient has Cushing disease, with residual disease despite 2 attempts at transsphenoidal resection. Medical therapy is indicated. Osilodrostat (Answer D) is a potent oral 11β-hydroxylase inhibitor that was recently approved for adults with Cushing disease who either cannot undergo pituitary gland surgery or have undergone surgery but still have the disease. Osilodrostat effectively reduces cortisol levels. It is well tolerated overall, but in some women, it has been associated with hirsutism (noted in this patient), acne, and elevated serum testosterone levels.

Mifepristone (Answer B) is a glucocorticoid-receptor blocker that is effective in the treatment of patients with all forms of Cushing syndrome. Because it blocks the glucocorticoid receptor, cortisol and ACTH levels may actually rise during treatment (the cortisol level fell in this vignette). Mifepristone effectively improves the clinical manifestations of Cushing syndrome, as well as improves glucose control.

Ketoconazole (Answer A) is a steroidogenesis blocker, and it is useful for lowering cortisol. Patients with Cushing syndrome are at risk for liver dysfunction that may be associated with a rise in ACTH levels. However, ketoconazole is not associated with an increase in androgen levels, as noted in this vignette.

Pasireotide (Answer E) is a somatostatin analogue that can reduce ACTH secretion and lead to cortisol control in approximately 20% to 25% of patients, and it is frequently associated with hyperglycemia (not noted in this patient).

Mitotane (Answer C) is an adrenolytic drug used for both Cushing syndrome and adrenocortical carcinoma. Mitotane can normalize hypercortisolism in up to 60% of patients, but adverse effects such as nausea and anorexia limit its use, and it was therefore not recommended for this patient.

EDUCATIONAL OBJECTIVE

Describe the effects of medical therapy in the treatment of Cushing disease.

REFERENCE(S)

Fleseriu M, Pivonello R, Young J, et al. Osilodrostat, a potent oral 11β-hydroxylase inhibitor: 22-week, prospective, Phase II study in Cushing's disease. *Pituitary.* 2016;19(2):138-148. PMID: 26542280

Hinojosa-Amaya JM, Cuevas-Ramos D, Fleseriu M. Medical management of Cushing's syndrome: current and emerging treatments. *Drugs.* 2019;79(9):935-956. PMID: 31098899

13 ANSWER: E) Maintenance of normal IGF-1 levels

An oral octreotide capsule has been approved to treat acromegaly in patients who previously responded to and tolerated treatment with injectable octreotide or lanreotide. In a recent phase 3 randomized, double-blind, placebo-controlled trial, IGF-1 levels were maintained in 78% of patients on the study drug vs in 19% of patients taking placebo. IGF-1 levels are thus expected to be maintained in most patients (Answer E). IGF-1 levels are not expected to increase (Answer D) in patients taking the oral octreotide capsule.

Gastrointestinal adverse effects (Answer A) and occurrence of hyperglycemia (Answer C) are similar between the oral octreotide capsule and injectable analogues.

As the oral octreotide capsule is a somatostatin analogue, GH levels decrease, not increase (Answer B), on the medication.

EDUCATIONAL OBJECTIVE

Describe the use of the oral octreotide capsule in the treatment of acromegaly.

REFERENCE(S)

Melmed S, Popovic V, Bidlingmaier M, et al. Safety and efficacy of oral octreotide in acromegaly: results of a multicenter phase III trial. *J Clin Endocrinol Metab.* 2015;100(4):1699-1708. PMID: 25664604

Samson SL, Nachtigall LB, Fleseriu M, et al. Maintenance of acromegaly control in patients switching from injectable somatostatin receptor ligands to oral octreotide. *J Clin Endocrinol Metab.* 2020;105(10):e3785-e3797. PMID: 32882036

14 ANSWER: B) Perform a glucagon-stimulation test to assess GH levels

This patient is at risk for GH deficiency given his history of pituitary adenoma, sellar radiation therapy, and panhypopituitarism. He has signs and symptoms of GH deficiency, including increased abdominal girth, fatigue, and reduced short-term memory and attention span. In the setting of at least 3 deficient axes, the presence of a serum IGF-1 value less than 85 ng/dL (<15.1 nmol/L) is consistent with GH deficiency. However, IGF-1 can be normal or low-normal in persons with GH deficiency. The next step would be to perform a provocative GH test, and of the listed answer choices, a glucagon-stimulation test (Answer B) would be best. Although an insulin tolerance test (Answer C) is considered the gold standard test for assessment of GH deficiency, this patient's history of seizures precludes its use given the risk of profound hypoglycemia.

Measuring a random GH level (Answer A) is not useful in the diagnosis of GH deficiency.

Patients with GH deficiency may have mild depression, and although referral for psychiatry (Answer E) is not incorrect, addressing the underlying cause is a better first step.

Similarly, while diet and exercise modification (Answer D) is a good idea, it would not address the possible deficiency.

EDUCATIONAL OBJECTIVE

Determine the most appropriate approach to diagnose GH deficiency.

REFERENCE(S)

Yuen KCJ, Biller BMK, Radovick S, et al. American Association of Clinical Endocrinologists and American College of Endocrinology guidelines for management of growth hormone deficiency in adults and patients transitioning from pediatric to adult care. *Endocr Pract.* 2019;25(11):1191-1232. PMID: 31760824

Yuen KC, Tritos NA, Samson SL, Hoffman AR, Katznelson L. American Association of Clinical Endocrinologists and American College of Endocrinology disease state clinical review: update on growth hormone stimulation testing and proposed revised cut-point for the glucagon stimulation test in the diagnosis of adult growth hormone deficiency. *Endocr Pract.* 2016;22(10):1235-1244. PMID: 27409821

Ramos-Leví AM, Marazuela M. Treatment of adult growth hormone deficiency with human recombinant growth hormone: an update on current evidence and critical review of advantages and pitfalls. *Endocrine.* 2018;60(2):203-218. PMID: 29417370

15 ANSWER: C) Octreotide long-acting release

This patient has hyperthyroidism, a thyroid gland with increased iodine uptake, a pituitary lesion, and the unexpected finding of a TSH value that is not suppressed—an indication that a TSH-secreting tumor is the cause of her hyperthyroidism. Surgery would be the best option, but she prefers not to undergo this now.

Somatostatin inhibits both GH and TSH, and somatostatin analogues can inhibit TSH secretion from the tumor, as well as decrease tumor size. Given her history of atrial fibrillation, control of hyperthyroidism is the first step. Thus, octreotide long-acting release (Answer C), a somatostatin analogue, is the correct treatment to administer now. Octreotide is generally successful at normalizing thyroid hormone levels and can reduce tumor size (which is important since it is invading the cavernous sinus). Surgery to debulk the pituitary tumor may be considered on an elective basis when she is clinically stable.

Cabergoline (Answer A) has not been shown to be effective for TSH-secreting tumors.

Methimazole (Answer B) could decrease thyroid hormone levels and help manage hyperthyroidism, but it would have either no effect on the size of the TSH-secreting tumor or it could potentially facilitate tumor growth.

Radiation therapy (Answer D) may take up to 10 years for effect and is associated with hypopituitarism in approximately 30% to 40% of cases.

Although radioactive iodine (Answer E) could treat her hyperthyroidism, it would take months to work and would not treat her TSH-secreting pituitary tumor.

EDUCATIONAL OBJECTIVE

Treat TSH-secreting tumors on the basis of the physiology and regulation of TSH secretion.

REFERENCE(S)

Teramoto A, Sanno N, Tahara S, Osamura YR. Pathological study of thyrotropin-secreting pituitary adenoma: plurihormonality and medical treatment. *Acta Neuropathol.* 2004;108(2):147-153. PMID: 15185102

Beck-Peccoz P, Persani L, Mannavola D, Campi I. TSH-secreting adenomas. *Best Pract Res Clin Endocrinol Metab.* 2009;23(5);597-606. PMID: 19945025

Beck-Peccoz P, Giavoli C, Lania A. A 2019 update on TSH-secreting pituitary adenomas. *J Endocrinol Invest.* 2019;42(12):1401-1406. PMID: 31175617

16 ANSWER: A) Another transsphenoidal surgery

In patients truly cured of Cushing disease, ACTH and cortisol levels are very low because they have been suppressed by the previously high cortisol levels. Although this patient's current cortisol level is considered normal, it is expected that adrenal insufficiency will be detected following curative surgery. This patient's cortisol concentration never fell to a level consistent with adrenal insufficiency. Therefore, she has residual disease. Repeated surgery (Answer A) should be considered.

She is not currently truly hypocortisolemic or hypercortisolemic, so hydrocortisone replacement therapy (Answer C) is not indicated now.

Medical therapy could be considered for management of hypercortisolism, but mitotane (Answer D) is not generally used as first- or second-line medical therapy in this setting. Furthermore, an attempt should be made to cure her surgically before committing to medical therapy.

Stereotactic radiosurgery (Answer E) would be indicated only if repeated surgery, and perhaps medical therapy, has failed. Cortisol levels are usually less than 5 μg/dL (<137.9 nmol/L) when patients are surgically cured and hydrocortisone is generally needed for several months, initially for both maintenance therapy and stress management, and then later just for stress.

Cosyntropin-stimulation testing (Answer B) is not useful in the immediate postoperative period because the adrenal glands themselves are not suppressed and should respond vigorously to exogenous ACTH, thereby giving a falsely reassuring result.

EDUCATIONAL OBJECTIVE

Assess patients with Cushing disease postoperatively.

REFERENCE(S)

Esposito F, Dusick JR, Cohan P, et al. Clinical review: early morning cortisol levels as a predictor of remission after transsphenoidal surgery for Cushing's disease. *J Clin Endocrinol Metab.* 2006;91(1):7- 13. PMID: 16234305

Hameed N, Yedinak CG, Brzana J, et al. Remission rate after transsphenoidal surgery in patients with pathologically confirmed Cushing's disease, the role of cortisol, ACTH assessment and immediate reoperation: a large single center experience. *Pituitary.* 2013;16(4):452-458. PMID: 23242860

Salmon PM, Loftus PD, Dodd RL, et al. Utility of adrenocorticotropic hormone in assessing the response to transsphenoidal surgery for Cushing's disease. *Endocr Pract.* 2014;20(11):1159-1164. PMID: 24936567

17 ANSWER: B) Discuss surgery

Of concern in this patient is the discrepancy between her prolactin concentration of only 152 ng/mL (6.61 nmol/L) and the size of the adenoma—2.4 cm. Although this discrepancy could be due to inefficient production of prolactin by a prolactinoma, it is more likely due to stalk dysfunction caused by a nonfunctioning adenoma or some other mass lesion such as a meningioma or Rathke cleft cyst. A dopamine agonist could indeed reduce, if not normalize, prolactin levels and correct amenorrhea and galactorrhea but have minimal to no effect on the growth of a mass lesion that is not a prolactinoma. Given the size of the lesion and its proximity to the optic chiasm, transsphenoidal surgery should be strongly considered and discussed (Answer B).

Given that this lesion is most likely not a prolactinoma, increasing the bromocriptine dosage (Answer C) or switching from bromocriptine to cabergoline (Answer E) is not indicated, as neither option would be likely to further shrink the tumor.

Performing a pituitary-directed MRI in 6 months (Answer D) to assess for an increase in tumor size could be considered, but because of the tumor's proximity to the chiasm, surgery is the best next step.

The somatostatin analogues octreotide (Answer A) and lanreotide are not useful in the management of prolactinomas.

EDUCATIONAL OBJECTIVE

Distinguish prolactinomas from clinically nonfunctioning adenomas and recommend appropriate management.

REFERENCE(S)

Melmed S, Casanueva FF, Hoffman AR, et al; Endocrine Society. Diagnosis and treatment of hyperprolactinemia: an Endocrine Society clinical practice guideline. *J Clin Endocrinol Metab.* 2011;96(2):273-288. PMID: 21296991

Karavitaki N, Thanabalasingham G, Shore HC, et al. Do the limits of serum prolactin in disconnection hyperprolactinaemia need re-definition? A study of 226 patients with histologically verified non-functioning pituitary macroadenoma. *Clin Endocrinol (Oxf).* 2006;65(4):524-529. PMID: 16984247

18 ANSWER: A) Stop testosterone and obtain a semen analysis

The first thing to establish in this patient is whether he is truly infertile. Although one might expect that he would be, given his panhypopituitarism and being on testosterone replacement, he may have adequate sperm counts and morphology for fertility. Treatment with testosterone is often initiated based on low-normal testosterone or mildly deficient testosterone. Often these values are still associated with adequate spermatogenesis. Therefore, evaluating sperm production (Answer A) is indicated before fertility treatment is initiated.

If he has azoospermia or oligospermia, he might respond to hCG injections and may also need FSH injections. Trying these therapies (Answers D and E) before assessing his fertility status would be inappropriate.

Clomiphene (Answer C), an estrogen receptor antagonist, would not be expected to be useful in stimulating gonadotropin production in a patient with hypopituitarism.

The chances for fertility in a patient such as this are well over 50% and suggesting adoption at this point (Answer B) would be premature.

EDUCATIONAL OBJECTIVE

Evaluate for infertility in men with hypopituitarism.

REFERENCE(S)

Drincic A, Arseven OK, Sosa E, Mercado M, Kopp P, Molitch ME. Men with acquired hypogonadotropic hypogonadism treated with testosterone may be fertile. *Pituitary.* 2003;6(1):5-10. PMID: 14674718

Farhat R, Al-zidjali F, Alzahrani AS. Outcome of gonadotropin therapy for male infertility due to hypogonadotrophic hypogonadism. *Pituitary.* 2010;13(2):105-110. PMID: 19838805

19 ANSWER: C) Pathogenic variant in the *POU1F1* gene

This patient has childhood-onset GH deficiency, recent-onset central hypothyroidism, and hypoprolactinemia. Her history and biochemical assessment are notable for the presence of menses, consistent with adequate gonadotropin function, as well as normal adrenal reserve. These findings suggest that she has a pathogenic variant in the gene encoding the transcription factor POU1F1 (*POU1F1* [formerly *PIT1*]) (Answer C). POU1F1 is important for the development of the somatotroph, lactotroph, and thyrotroph lineages, and *POU1F1* pathogenic variants lead to deficiencies of their respective hormones. The secretion of ACTH, FSH, and LH is preserved.

In patients with pathogenic variants in *PROP1* (Answer D), which is the most common cause of congenital combined pituitary hormone deficiency, gonadotropin deficiency is usually present as well. This is not the case in this patient. POU1F1 is the transcription factor that acts temporally just after PROP1.

Patients with pathogenic variants in *TBX19 (TPIT)* (Answer E) present with isolated ACTH deficiency (not present in this case), as the *TBX19* gene product is necessary for differentiation of corticotroph cells.

Histiocytosis (Answer B) is not this patient's diagnosis, as she does not have arginine vasopressin deficiency and the imaging does not reveal an enhancing posterior sellar mass.

Acute trauma causing pituitary infarction can result in hypopituitarism, and imaging may reveal subsequent empty sella, but this patient does not have a history of significant trauma and the hypopituitarism predated the concussion (Answer A).

EDUCATIONAL OBJECTIVE

Determine the cause of childhood-onset combined hypopituitarism.

REFERENCE(S)

Prince KL, Walvoord EC, Rhodes SJ. The role of homeodomain transcription factors in heritable pituitary disease. *Nat Rev Endocrinol.* 2011;7(12):727-737. PMID: 21788968

Bertko E, Klammt J, Dusatkova P, et al. Combined pituitary hormone deficiency due to gross deletions in the POU1F1 (PIT-1) and PROP1 genes. *J Hum Genet.* 2017;62(8):755-762. PMID: 28356564

Majdoub H, Amselem S, Legendre M, Rath S, Bercovich D, Tenenbaum-Rakover Y. Extreme short stature and severe neurological impairment in a 17-year-old male with untreated combined pituitary hormone deficiency due to POU1F1 mutation. *Front Endocrinol (Lausanne).* 2019;10:381. PMID: 31316460

Mendonca BB, Osorio MG, Latronico AC, Estefan V, Lo LS, Arnhold IJ. Longitudinal hormonal and pituitary imaging changes in two females with combined pituitary hormone deficiency due to deletion of A301,G302 in the PROP1 gene. *J Clin Endocrinol Metab.* 1999;84(3):942-945. PMID: 1008457

20 ANSWER: E) Temozolomide

This patient has a rapidly enlarging macroprolactinoma that has been unresponsive to cabergoline, surgery, and stereotactic radiosurgery. The tumor is certainly acting in a malignant fashion. However, distant metastases would have to be demonstrated for this to qualify as a true malignancy. About 75% of these very aggressive tumors, and some true pituitary carcinomas, respond to temozolomide (Answer E), an alkylating agent used primarily for the treatment of glioblastomas. However, even patients who respond to this agent for a while may have, over time, a bad outcome.

Additional radiotherapy (Answer B) within 2 years after previous radiation may lead to excessive radiation exposure to the local brain structures, so this would not be advised now.

Surgery (Answer A) is unlikely to help given the tumor location.

No data have been published regarding the use of pasireotide (Answer D) to treat prolactinomas, nor are there sufficient data on the use of octreotide long-acting release (Answer C) in this setting.

EDUCATIONAL OBJECTIVE

Recommend a treatment strategy for aggressive pituitary tumors and pituitary carcinomas.

REFERENCE(S)

Di Ieva A, Rotondo F, Syro LV, Cusimano MD, Kovacs K. Aggressive pituitary adenomas--diagnosis and emerging treatments. *Nat Rev Endocrinol.* 2014;10(7):423-435. PMID: 24821329

McCormack AI, Wass JA, Grossman AB. Aggressive pituitary tumours: the role of temozolomide and the assessment of MGMT status. *Eur J Clin Invest.* 2011;41(10):1133-1148. PMID: 21496012

Whitelaw BC, Dworakowska D, Thomas NW, et al. Temozolomide in the management of dopamine agonist-resistant prolactinomas. *Clin Endocrinol (Oxf).* 2012;76(6):877-886. PMID: 22372583

21 ANSWER: D) Give hypertonic saline to raise the serum sodium by 6 mEq/L (6 mmol/L) over 6 hours

Even a standard dose of desmopressin can cause hyponatremia if a person continues to drink; usually progressive nausea limits the intake. Unfortunately, in this case, the patient is unconscious and cannot control her fluid intake. The treatment at this point is tricky. One cannot judge any mental symptoms from the hyponatremia because she is unconscious, but she is at high risk for developing brain edema and is at risk for seizures and brain herniation because of the presumed rapid development of the hyponatremia.

Therefore, hypertonic saline at a rate of 1 mL/kg per h should be given over a few hours to raise her serum sodium about 4 to 6 mEq/L (4-6 mmol/L) to remove her from acute danger (Answer D). Since the hyponatremia developed during a short time frame, the correction does not need to be excessively slow, so Answer E is not the best choice. Although desmopressin should be held initially, the urine output must be observed very carefully; when it wears off, she will start to excrete high volumes of dilute urine and might experience an overly rapid correction of hyponatremia. Correcting hyponatremia at rates that result in an increase of more than 12 mEq/L (12 mmol/L) over 24 hours could put her at risk for central pontine myelinolysis. However, the degree of hyponatremia is severe and has developed rapidly, so one cannot simply change the D5W to saline and wait for the desmopressin to wear off (Answers A, B, and C). Therefore, her urine output and serum sodium must be monitored every 2 to 4 hours to avoid a correction that is too rapid. Waiting 12 hours is insufficiently close monitoring. Reinstitution of desmopressin when urine output increases may then be indicated, but not when she is first seen.

EDUCATIONAL OBJECTIVE

Treat the acute development of severe hyponatremia.

REFERENCE(S)

Verbalis JG, Goldsmith SR, Greenberg A, et al. Diagnosis, evaluation, and treatment of hyponatremia: expert panel recommendations. *Am J Med.* 2013;126(10 Suppl 1):S1-S42. PMID: 24074529

Sterns RH. Disorders of plasma sodium--causes, consequences, and correction. *N Engl J Med.* 2015;372(1):55-65. PMID: 25551526

22 ANSWER: C) Lymphocytic hypophysitis

The most likely lesion in this patient is lymphocytic hypophysitis (Answer C). The key historical point is that these lesions usually develop in the intrapartum or postpartum period and present as mass lesions towards the latter part of pregnancy. A symmetrically enlarged pituitary on MRI is characteristic of hypophysitis, often with extension up the stalk as in this case. Gadolinium was not administered because she is pregnant. ACTH insufficiency occurs in two-thirds of patients with these lesions and should be investigated and treated if found, as adrenal insufficiency is a major cause of death in this setting. In this patient, the progressive, severe fatigue and weight loss point to the possibility of ACTH deficiency. Expectant management will usually suffice for lymphocytic hypophysitis, as the size of most lesions decreases after delivery.

Nonsecreting and prolactin-secreting pituitary adenomas are far more common sellar lesions in women in this age group, but nonsecreting pituitary adenomas (Answer A) generally do not enlarge and cause symptoms during pregnancy. Prolactinomas (Answer E) can, of course, enlarge during pregnancy. However, this patient was previously well, had regular menses before pregnancy, and had no difficulty getting pregnant, implying that she had not been having difficulty with fertility as might be expected with a prolactinoma. The prolactin concentration in this case is also helpful in that a patient with a macroprolactinoma should have prolactin levels exceeding 500 ng/mL (>21.7 nmol/L), but a patient with lymphocytic hypophysitis usually has prolactin levels less than 200 ng/mL (<8.7 nmol/L).

Although craniopharyngiomas (Answer B) do occur in this age group, they are much less common, and they typically do not change in size during pregnancy.

Pituitary hyperplasia of pregnancy (Answer D) is the usual enlargement of the pituitary as an adaptation during pregnancy with maximum diameter not exceeding 10 mm. Her presentation of gradually worsening headaches is more consistent with enlargement from infiltration and not hyperplasia.

EDUCATIONAL OBJECTIVE

Construct the differential diagnosis of mass lesions in pregnancy.

REFERENCE(S)

Carmichael JD. Update on the diagnosis and management of hypophysitis. *Curr Opin Endocrinol Diabetes Obes.* 2012;19(4):314-321. PMID: 22543347

Joshi MN, Whitelaw BC, Carroll PV. Mechanisms in endocrinology: hypophysitis: diagnosis and treatment. *Eur J Endocrinol.* 2018;179(3):R151-R163. PMID: 29880706

Allix I, Rohmer V. Hypophysitis in 2014. *Ann Endocrinol (Paris)*. 2015;76(5):585-594. PMID: 26514950

Elster AD, Sanders TG, Vines FS, Chen MY. Size and shape of the pituitary gland during pregnancy and post partum: measurement with MR imaging. *Radiology*. 1991;181(2):531-535. PMID: 1924800

Thyroid, Section 1 Board Review

Jacqueline Jonklaas, MD, PhD, MPH

1 ANSWER: E) TSH measurement

Statin-induced myopathy is a well-recognized entity. Up to 29% of patients taking statins experience muscle symptoms, some of which are due to a self-limited toxic myopathy that improves with drug withdrawal. In addition, some of these patients have an immune-related necrotizing myopathy due to anti-HMGCR antibodies. However, there can be other causes of myopathy during the course of statin treatment, such as neurogenic etiologies, vacuolar myopathy, and, as illustrated here, severe hypothyroidism. It has also been postulated that statin therapy and hypothyroidism synergistically increase the risk of myopathy. When measured, this patient's serum TSH concentration (Answer E) was 156 mIU/L.

Measurement of the erythrocyte sedimentation rate (Answer C) is a nonspecific assessment of inflammation and is not helpful in determining a specific etiology. Similarly, aldolase measurement (Answer A) can suggest muscle damage, but it does not point to a specific etiology. Studies such as electromyography (Answer B) and MRI of the lower extremities (Answer D) can suggest myopathy, muscle edema, and muscle atrophy, but they do not pinpoint a specific cause.

Hypothyroidism induces a metabolic myopathy with global inhibition of oxidative pathways, alteration of the actin-myosin units so that contractility is poor, and ensuing muscle impairment. Histopathologic examination shows local alterations in muscle fibers from fast twitching type II to slow twitching type I fibers, deposition of glycosaminoglycans, low myosin ATPase activity, and low ATP turnover. Severe hypothyroidism is associated with proximal muscle weakness, elevated creatine kinase levels, and a biopsy showing muscle necrosis. In patients with hypothyroidism-induced myopathy, thyroid hormone replacement and normalization of TSH are associated with normalization of creatine kinase and reduction of creatinine concentrations, if elevated.

Recognizing the contribution of hypothyroidism to this patient's muscle dysfunction is important because treatment of her hypothyroidism would allow statin therapy to continue and thus provide needed treatment for dyslipidemia.

EDUCATIONAL OBJECTIVE

Recognize that hypothyroidism-induced myopathy may present in a similar manner to statin-induced myopathy.

REFERENCE(S)

Antoniol MN, Moreno PJ, Milisenda JC, Selva O'Callaghan A, Grau JM, Padrosa J. Statin use and myopathy. Not always guilty. *Rheumatology (Oxford)*. 2020;59(12):3853-3857. PMID: 32500148

Mammen AL. Which nonautoimmune myopathies are most frequently misdiagnosed as myositis? *Curr Opin Rheumatol*. 2017;29(6):618-622. PMID: 28832350

Sindoni A, Rodolico C, Pappalardo MA, Portaro S, Benvenga S. Hypothyroid myopathy: A peculiar clinical presentation of thyroid failure. Review of the literature. *Rev Endocr Metab Disord*. 2016;17(4):499-519. PMID: 27154040

Scott KR, Simmons Z, Boyer PJ. Hypothyroid myopathy with a strikingly elevated serum creatine kinase level. *Muscle Nerve*. 2002;26(1):141-144. PMID: 12115960

2 ANSWER: D) Decrease to prepregnancy dosage of 88 mcg daily

Individuals with hypothyroidism typically require at least a 30% increase in their levothyroxine dosage during pregnancy. This is especially the case in individuals with postsurgical hypothyroidism in whom there is essentially no endogenous thyroid function. This patient required closer to a 40% increase in her levothyroxine dosage. In general, patients' regimens should be returned to their prepregnancy levothyroxine dosage after delivery (Answer D). Thyroid function can then be checked 6 weeks later to confirm that this dosage remains adequate. Alternating 112 and 125 mcg daily (Answer A), continuing 125 mcg daily (Answer B), or decreasing to the first-trimester dosage of 112 mcg daily (Answer C) would treat the patient with more than her prepregnancy dosage and most likely result in overtreatment.

The fact that the patient is planning to breastfeed does not affect her levothyroxine requirement. Euthyroidism is important to ensure successful lactation. Sufficient levothyroxine does not enter breast milk to cause any concerns for fetal exposure.

Although the patient may not have returned to her prepregnancy weight at 6 weeks post partum, assessment of her weight (Answer E) would probably not be helpful in predicting the best postpartum dosage, as it is ideal body weight or lean body mass that is a better predictor of levothyroxine requirement than actual weight.

Sometimes individuals require a higher levothyroxine requirement post partum. This has been described in patients with Hashimoto hypothyroidism who still have some residual thyroid at the beginning of their pregnancy. However, progression of autoimmune destruction during the course of pregnancy may leave the individual with less endogenous thyroid function, and they may need a higher postpartum levothyroxine dosage than was required before pregnancy.

EDUCATIONAL OBJECTIVE

Explain that the increased levothyroxine requirement seen during pregnancy in a woman with hypothyroidism typically resolves following delivery, such that the prepregnancy dosage of levothyroxine is recommended.

REFERENCE(S)

Pearce EN. Management of hypothyroidism and hypothyroxinemia during pregnancy. *Endocr Pract.* 2022;28(7):711-718. PMID: 35569735

Alexander EK, Pearce EN, Brent GA, et al. 2017 guidelines of the American Thyroid Association for the diagnosis and management of thyroid disease during pregnancy and the postpartum. *Thyroid.* 2017;27(3):315-389. PMID: 28056690

Galofré JC, Haber RS, Mitchell AA, Pessah R, Davies TF. Increased postpartum thyroxine replacement in Hashimoto's thyroiditis. *Thyroid.* 2010;20(8):901-908. PMID: 20615129

3 ANSWER: C) ^{123}I thyroid scan and uptake

Although thyroid hormone is not the hormone most commonly abused by athletes, its use by athletes does need to be considered. Thyroid hormone is most often used in image-based sports in which fat loss is a priority. It is combined with testosterone or, more commonly, other anabolic steroids, to avoid loss of muscle mass. However, it may also be used in other sports such as weightlifting, rowing, etc, in which the athlete is seeking to qualify for a lower weight category. Because thyroid hormone also increases SHBG, some athletes erroneously believe that testosterone action will be enhanced. Elevated SHBG is actually associated with reduced testosterone action in target tissues due to its increased residence time in the circulation. There is no evidence that thyroid hormones improve performance, boost androgen action, or have desirable effects by overcoming low T_3 concentrations. Many of the drug regimens used by athletes are taken in a cyclic manner either to avoid detection or because they think that this improves sensitivity of, or synergy between, agents.

In this particular individual, it appears that there was previous thyroid hormone use, possibly with a T_3-predominant regimen, or that there is current T_3 use and the timing of the laboratory evaluation has not sampled the peak of the T_3 level. At the time of laboratory evaluation, his TSH remains low. The best means of demonstrating exogenous thyroid hormone use would be a ^{123}I thyroid scan and uptake (Answer C), which should show low uptake because the TSH is currently low.

Measuring free T_3 (Answer A) would not be helpful, as it, like total T_3, would be declining from the time of the last dose of liothyronine or other T_3-containing product. The peak free T_3 or total T_3 level may not be captured.

Measuring free T_4 using a different methodology (Answer D) would only be helpful if an assay problem were suspected. The free T_4 value in this vignette may be on the low side due to a T_3-predominant thyroid hormone regimen, rather than due to an assay issue.

Measuring hCG (Answer B) would be part of the workup for an hCG-secreting germ-cell tumor and could be considered if the free T_4 were high and exogenous thyroid hormone ingestion were not a more likely explanation.

Thyroid ultrasonography (Answer E) may be somewhat helpful in showing reduced vascularity of the thyroid gland, but it is not the most specific and definitive test.

If measured, serum thyroglobulin would be low if the patient were taking synthetic thyroid hormones and would be helpful in pointing to a diagnosis of iatrogenic thyrotoxicosis.

EDUCATIONAL OBJECTIVE

Determine the appropriate diagnostic test to support the diagnosis of factitious hyperthyroidism.

REFERENCE(S)

Gild ML, Stuart M, Clifton-Bligh RJ, Kinahan A, Handelsman DJ. Thyroid hormone abuse in elite sports: the regulatory challenge. *J Clin Endocrinol Metab.* 2022;107(9):e3562-e3573. PMID: 35438767

Sagoe D, McVeigh J, Bjørnebekk A, Essilfie MS, Andreassen CS, Pallesen S. Polypharmacy among anabolic-androgenic steroid users: a descriptive metasynthesis. *Subst Abuse Treat Prev Policy.* 2015;10:12. PMID: 25888931

Persani L, dell'Acqua M, Ioakim S, Campi I. Factitious thyrotoxicosis and thyroid hormone misuse or abuse. *Ann Endocrinol (Paris).* 2023;84(3):367-369. PMID: 36963754

Irwig MS, Fleseriu M, Jonklaas J, et al. Off-label use and misuse of testosterone, growth hormone, thyroid hormone, and adrenal supplements: risks and costs of a growing problem. *Endocr Pract.* 2020;26(3):340-353. PMID: 32163313

4 ANSWER: D) Oral conjugated estrogens

Transgender women may elect to undergo hormone therapy and possibly surgery to reduce gender dysphoria and achieve physical and psychological features consistent with their desired gender. This can be initiated with estrogen supplementation alone, which when given at physiologic concentrations will feedback on the hypothalamic-pituitary-gonadal axis and reduce testosterone into the low-normal range for a man. Unless pharmacologic dosages of estrogen are administered, further inhibition of testosterone production would require use of a second agent to suppress testosterone secretion or antagonize the androgen receptor. Gender-affirming surgery can subsequently be considered.

Estrogen has well-documented effects on thyroid function in individuals taking levothyroxine. Oral conjugated estrogens (Answer D) increase the concentration of thyroxine-binding globulin, which increases total T_4, reduces free T_4, and increases TSH. These changes are observed in this patient's laboratory results 3 months after starting the hormonal regimen. Thus, she is most likely taking oral conjugated estrogens. She will need an increase in her levothyroxine dosage.

Transdermal estrogen, delivered via patch or gel (Answers B and C), does not cause the same stimulation of thyroxine-binding globulin production as it bypasses the liver and avoids first-pass metabolism. Thyroid function should remain unchanged with either estrogen gel or patch.

Effects of progesterone (Answer E) on thyroid function have not been well documented.

Cyproterone acetate (Answer A), a progestin with antiandrogenic effects, has also not been described to affect thyroid function, although this has not been well studied.

EDUCATIONAL OBJECTIVE

Predict the changes in thyroid hormone and TSH concentrations that can occur with estrogen treatment.

REFERENCE(S)

Tangpricha V, den Heijer M. Oestrogen and anti-androgen therapy for transgender women. *Lancet Diabetes Endocrinol.* 2017;5(4):291-300. PMID: 27916515

Mazer NA. Interaction of estrogen therapy and thyroid hormone replacement in postmenopausal women. *Thyroid.* 2004;14(Suppl 1):S27-S34. PMID: 15142374

Torre F, Calogero AE, Condorelli RA, Cannarella R, Aversa A, La Vignera S. Effects of oral contraceptives on thyroid function and vice versa. *J Endocrinol Invest.* 2020;43(9):1181-1188. PMID: 32219692

Tahboub R, Arafah BM. Sex steroids and the thyroid. *Best Pract Res Clin Endocrinol Metab.* 2009;23(6):769-780. PMID: 19942152

5 ANSWER: B) ^{123}I thyroid scan and uptake

In this individual who previously underwent thyroidectomy and required a full dosage of levothyroxine, there are several possible causes for development of hyperthyroidism: an alternative source of ingested thyroid hormone, such as in a supplement, or the presence of ectopic thyroid tissue that has gradually become overfunctioning since the patient's thyroidectomy. His physical examination is notable for a mass in the midline at the level of the hyoid bone. An additional piece of information is that the mass was noted to move with tongue protrusion. This examination finding is suggestive of a thyroglossal duct cyst. A thyroglossal duct cyst is a remnant that can remain after embryonic development of the thyroid gland is complete. It usually involutes during gestation, leaving a mucosal depression in the foramen cecum and possibly a pyramidal lobe of the thyroid gland. The thyroid follicular cells present in a thyroglossal duct cyst can rarely, if acted upon by stimulatory antibodies, be a source of hyperthyroidism.

Questioning the patient about supplement use (Answer A) would be appropriate if exogenous use of thyroid hormone were being considered. However, this diagnosis is less likely given his physical examination findings. If this line of inquiry were being pursued, serum thyroglobulin measurement (Answer D) would be helpful to distinguish endogenous hyperthyroidism (thyroglobulin likely elevated) from exogenous thyroid hormone (thyroglobulin low).

hCG-dependent hyperthyroidism could theoretically be produced by high levels of hCG from a germ-cell tumor acting on the thyroid gland or ectopic thyroid tissue, but the latter has not been described. Thus, measuring hCG (Answer C) is incorrect.

Iodine scanning with ^{123}I would be the best approach to identify the location of the functioning thyroid tissue in this patient. Given the suggestive physical examination finding, thyroid scan and uptake encompassing the neck region (Answer B) should be sufficient to identify the functioning tissue. Whole-body ^{123}I scan (Answer E) could be used if ectopic thyroid tissue were present in a more remote location such as the mediastinum.

Although either methimazole or radioactive iodine therapy could be used to treat this patient's hyperthyroidism, the most definitive treatment would be surgical removal of the thyroglossal duct cyst via a Sistrunk procedure. This would also prevent the risk of infection, which is a problem observed with thyroglossal duct cysts that are not surgically removed.

EDUCATIONAL OBJECTIVE

Identify ectopic thyroid tissue as a source of thyroid hormone production in an individual who has had a thyroidectomy.

REFERENCE(S)

Vaz-Pereira R, Santos C, Monteiro A, Pinto de Sousa J. Recurrence of Graves' disease in the thyroglossal duct after total thyroidectomy. *BMJ Case Rep.* 2022;15(2):e248166. PMID: 35135806

Basili G, Andreini R, Romano N, Lorenzetti L, Monzani F, Naccarato G, Goletti O. Recurrence of Graves' disease in thyroglossal duct remnants: relapse after total thyroidectomy. *Thyroid.* 2009;19(12):1427-1430. PMID: 19916864

Baghaffar MH, Samargandy S. A case of recurrent thyrotoxicosis in a thyroglossal duct cyst 18 years following thyroid surgery. *Cureus.* 2023;15(6):e39829. PMID: 37397661

Buckingham H, Sauerwein TJ, Golding AC. Graves' disease in the cervical thyroid and thyroglossal duct remnant: case report and review of literature. *Endocr Pract.* 2006;12(4):401-405. PMID: 16901795

6 ANSWER: C) Restoration of ovulatory menstrual cycles

Patient education is important at the time of hypothyroidism diagnosis. Overt hypothyroidism is frequently associated with irregular menses, which should normalize with treatment (Answer C). This patient should be counseled to avoid pregnancy until hypothyroidism is well controlled, since overt hypothyroidism is associated with adverse obstetric and fetal outcomes, including miscarriage, stillbirth, gestational hypertension, preterm delivery, low birth weight, and decreased child intelligence.

Contrary to popular opinion, weight loss following initiation of treatment for overt hypothyroidism is modest and is primarily due to diuresis rather than loss of fat mass (Answer D).

Restoration of euthyroidism should lead to a rapid decrease in total and LDL-cholesterol levels. Serum HDL cholesterol (Answer A) is also typically decreased by treatment of hypothyroidism. Because hyperlipidemia often resolves with treatment of hypothyroidism and there is a theoretical concern for increased rhabdomyolysis risk when statins are used in the setting of overt hypothyroidism, levothyroxine should be initiated before considering statin therapy in any overtly hypothyroid patient.

Overt hypothyroidism is associated with hyperhomocysteinemia, which improves, not worsens (Answer B), with treatment.

Driving simulation studies show that severe hypothyroidism slows speed in executive functioning tests and slows reaction times in braking tests (thus, Answer E is incorrect). This patient should be advised to avoid driving until her overt hypothyroidism has been treated, which will resolve these deficits.

EDUCATIONAL OBJECTIVE

Educate patients in the setting of newly diagnosed overt hypothyroidism, including counseling regarding the importance of avoiding driving and conception until hypothyroidism resolves.

REFERENCE(S)

Chaker L, Bianco AC, Jonklaas J, Peeters RP. Hypothyroidism. *Lancet.* 2017;390(10101):1550-1562. PMID: 28336049

Karmisholt J, Andersen S, Laurberg P. Weight loss after therapy of hypothyroidism is mainly caused by excretion of excess body water associated with myxoedema. *J Clin Endocrinol Metab.* 2011;96(1):E99-E103. PMID: 20926526

Alexander EK, Pearce EN, Brent GA, et al. 2017 guidelines of the American Thyroid Association for the diagnosis and management of thyroid disease during pregnancy and the postpartum. *Thyroid.* 2017;27(3):315-389. PMID: 28056690

Smith CD, Grondin R, LeMaster W, Martin B, Gold BT, Ain KB. Reversible cognitive, motor, and driving impairments in severe hypothyroidism. *Thyroid.* 2015;25(1):28-36. PMID: 25381990

7 ANSWER: B) TSH, 0.1 mIU/L; free T_4 1.85 ng/dL (23.81 pmol/L); total T_3, 350 ng/dL (5.39 nmol/L)

The goal of antithyroid drug therapy for Graves disease during pregnancy is to keep the serum TSH slightly suppressed and the free T_4 high-normal to mildly elevated. The rationale for these targets is to minimize the amount of antithyroid drug exposure to the fetus by administering the lowest effective dosage. The fetal thyroid is more susceptible than the maternal thyroid to the effects of antithyroid drugs. Both methimazole and propylthiouracil can cross the placenta and affect the fetal thyroid. The values in Answer B are within recommended targets for this patient.

Answer A is incorrect because these values are consistent with overt hyperthyroidism, which is associated with an increased risk of intrauterine growth restriction and fetal demise. Answers C, D, and E each would be associated with a higher dosage of antithyroid drug than the minimally effective dosage. As an aside, it is important to note that the total T_3 level, like the total T_4 level, is affected by the increases in thyroxine-binding globulin that occur during pregnancy, such that total T_3 levels are approximately 50% higher than the nonpregnancy reference range by the end of pregnancy.

EDUCATIONAL OBJECTIVE

Explain the therapeutic goals for Graves disease in pregnancy.

REFERENCE(S)

Alexander EK, Pearce EN, Brent GA, et al. 2017 guidelines of the American Thyroid Association for the diagnosis and management of thyroid disease during pregnancy and the postpartum. *Thyroid.* 2017;27(3):315-389. PMID: 28056690

Pearce EN. Management of thyrotoxicosis: preconception, pregnancy, and the postpartum period. *Endocr Pract.* 2019;25(1):62-68. PMID: 30289300

8 ANSWER: A) Heterophilic antibody interference with the TSH assay

This pattern of laboratory test results is typical of heterophilic antibody interference with the TSH assay (Answer A). The interference occurs in patients who have antibodies that recognize the mouse monoclonal antibody used in the sandwich assay for TSH, creating a link between the capture and signal antibodies in the absence of antigen (in this case, TSH). The human antimouse monoclonal antibodies (HAMA) occur naturally in up to 10% of the general population (not just laboratory workers with mouse exposure, as was first described), and they result in a false elevation of serum TSH. Preincubation of the patient's serum with nonimmune mouse antibodies (intended to eliminate the effect of HAMA) is an added step in the assay. A clue to the presence of HAMA in this case is the unchanged serum TSH despite progressively increasing free T_4 values as the levothyroxine dosage was increased.

If the patient were absorbing levothyroxine poorly (Answer B) or were nonadherent to therapy (Answer C), free T_4 values would not increase with an increasing levothyroxine dosage.

If she had resistance to thyroid hormone (Answer D), the free T_4 level would be elevated, rather than normal, at baseline.

In the setting of a TSH-secreting pituitary adenoma (Answer E), the patient would be expected to be clinically hyperthyroid.

EDUCATIONAL OBJECTIVE

Identify heterophilic antibody interference with the TSH assay.

REFERENCE(S)

SanthanaKrishnan SG, Pathalapati R, Kaplan L, Cobbs RK. Falsely raised TSH levels due to human anti-mouse antibody interfering with thyrotropin assay [published correction appears in *Postgrad Med J.* 2007;83(977):186]. *Postgrad Med J.* 2006;82(973):e27. PMID: 17099084

Ross HA, Menheere PP; Endocrinology Section of SKML (Dutch Foundation for Quality Assessment in Clinical Laboratories), Thomas CM, Mudde AH, Kouwenberg M, Wolffenbuttel BH. Interference from heterophilic antibodies in seven current TSH assays. *Ann Clin Biochem.* 2008;45(Pt 6):616. PMID: 18782812

9 ANSWER: A) Atenolol

This patient has developed what appears to be painless thyroiditis while taking interferon alfa. β-Adrenergic blockade (Answer A) is indicated to control his rapid pulse, but the other measures listed are unnecessary.

Patients with hepatitis C have a higher prevalence of positive TPO antibodies, even before treatment with interferon alfa, than do patients with other forms of viral hepatitis (11.2% vs 3.6%, respectively). The most common thyroid manifestation of interferon alfa therapy is hypothyroidism, which occurs in approximately 5% of all treated patients but in 36% of patients who have positive TPO antibodies before treatment. Women are twice as likely as men to develop this disorder (8.7% vs 3.4% in one study). The percentage of patients with positive TPO antibodies increases after treatment with interferon alfa (from 3.7% to 9.7% in one study).

A smaller number of patients develop thyrotoxicosis during interferon alfa therapy; this is more often painless thyroiditis than Graves disease, although both have been described. Thyroid symptoms improve in most patients (60%) with interferon alfa–associated thyroid dysfunction after drug discontinuation.

Methimazole therapy (Answer C) would not be effective for thyroiditis, as thyroid hormone is being released from the damaged thyroid gland rather than reaching the blood stream from ongoing synthesis.

Propylthiouracil (Answer E) would also be ineffective in the setting of thyroiditis for the same reason. In addition, even in patients with hyperthyroidism due to Graves disease or toxic nodular disease, propylthiouracil is not generally a first-line drug.

Prednisone therapy (Answer D) is sometimes used to treat painful subacute thyroiditis, but it is not indicated for painless drug-induced thyroiditis.

Intravenous immunoglobulin (Answer B) is not indicated for the treatment of thyroiditis.

EDUCATIONAL OBJECTIVE

Diagnose and manage drug-induced thyroiditis during the hyperthyroid phase.

REFERENCE(S)

Nair Kesavachandran C, Haamann F, Nienhaus A. Frequency of thyroid dysfunctions during interferon alpha treatment of single and combination therapy in hepatitis C virus-infected patients: a systematic review based analysis. *PLoS One.* 2013;8(2):e55364. PMID: 23383326

Carella C, Mazziotti G, Amato G, Braverman LE, Roti E. Clinical review 169: interferon-alpha related thyroid disease: pathophysiological, epidemiological, and clinical aspects. *J Clin Endocrinol Metab.* 2004;89(8):3656-3661. PMID: 15292282

Wang L, Li B, Zhao H, Wu P, Wu Q, Chen K, Mu Y. A systematic review and meta-analysis of endocrine-related adverse events associated with interferon. *Front Endocrinol (Lausanne).* 2022;13:949003. PMID: 35992107

10 ANSWER: A) Levothyroxine, 70 mcg intravenously once daily

When given orally, approximately 62% to 82% of the levothyroxine dose is absorbed in the jejunum or ileum. Absorption is better in the fasting state (78%-79%) than in the nonfasting state (59%-68%). Given that 100% of an intravenous dose of levothyroxine reaches the blood stream, when levothyroxine is converted from oral to intravenous dosing, the dose can be reduced. Intravenous levothyroxine dosing is generally started at 70% to 75% of the patient's usual oral therapy dosing (Answer A). The other choices either recommend a levothyroxine dosage that is too high (Answers B and C) or inappropriately substitute liothyronine (Answer E).

Although case studies have been published describing successful use of intramuscular levothyroxine (Answer D), the US FDA has not approved this route of administration, and the dosage listed is incorrect. Similarly, subcutaneous administration of levothyroxine has been attempted. Liquid levothyroxine preparations may result in improved absorption compared with tablet preparations when tube feeds are being administered. In a hospitalized patient such as this one who is in intensive care and may have bowel edema, intravenous levothyroxine is the appropriate route to ensure that a euthyroid state can be maintained.

EDUCATIONAL OBJECTIVE

Guide the transition from oral to intravenous levothyroxine in a patient with hypothyroidism.

REFERENCE(S)

Hays MT. Parenteral thyroxine administration. *Thyroid.* 2007;17(2):127-129. PMID: 17316114

Wenzel KW, Kirschsieper HE. Aspects of the absorption of oral L-thyroxine in normal man. *Metabolism.* 1977;26(1):1-8. PMID: 834138

Liu H, Li W, Zhang W, Sun S, Chen C. Levothyroxine: conventional and novel drug delivery formulations. *Endocr Rev.* 2023;44(3):393-416. PMID: 36412275

11 ANSWER: A) Repeat laboratory tests in 3 months

This patient has subclinical hyperthyroidism, most likely due to TSH receptor–stimulating antibodies. Her family history of autoimmune thyroid disease, her diffuse goiter, and her mildly positive thyroid-stimulating immunoglobulin are all consistent with this etiology. Patients with mild degrees of subclinical hyperthyroidism, particularly when it is due to thyroiditis or mild Graves disease, very often experience spontaneous resolution. Thus, the best course of action for this patient would be to repeat laboratory tests in 3 months (Answer A). In this patient's case, the symptom that prompted screening for thyroid disease (difficulty losing weight) did not lead to the anticipated diagnosis. This illustrates that symptoms overlapping with those of thyroid disease, such as weight gain and fatigue, are often nonspecific.

Predictors of reversibility of hyperthyroidism include having detectable (albeit subnormal) TSH values and having etiologies other than nodular hyperthyroidism (toxic adenoma or toxic multinodular goiter), such as thyroiditis or mild Graves disease, as is illustrated by the current case. Among patients with subclinical hyperthyroidism, the rate of progression to overt hyperthyroidism is 0.5% to 7% annually. Up to half of patients spontaneously revert to normal TSH levels over time.

It is premature to start methimazole (Answer D) in this young patient who has a high likelihood of remission, but this could be considered in an elderly patient with similar findings because of the increased risk of arrhythmia or the concern about adverse effects on bone density, although the dosage of 20 mg daily would be excessive for this situation.

This patient does not require atenolol (Answer C) because she is asymptomatic and has a resting pulse rate less than 90 beats/min.

Although treatment with radioactive iodine (Answer E) could be considered, it would most likely result in permanent hypothyroidism, and she may not require therapy at all.

Most individuals in the United States do not necessarily require vitamin or iodine supplementation (Answer B) to achieve iodine sufficiency, although many may choose to take a multivitamin. However, this would not be a specific part of the management of her subclinical hyperthyroidism.

EDUCATIONAL OBJECTIVE

Describe the natural history of nonnodular causes of subclinical hyperthyroidism.

REFERENCE(S)

Mai VQ, Burch HB. A stepwise approach to the evaluation and treatment of subclinical hyperthyroidism. *Endocr Pract.* 2012;18(5):772-780. PMID: 22784850

Ross DS, Burch HB, Cooper DS, et al. 2016 American Thyroid Association guidelines for diagnosis and management of hyperthyroidism and other causes of thyrotoxicosis. *Thyroid.* 2016;26(10):1343-1421. PMID: 27521067

Das G, Ojewuyi TA, Baglioni P, Geen J, Premawardhana LD, Okosieme OE. Serum thyrotrophin at baseline predicts the natural course of subclinical hyperthyroidism. *Clin Endocrinol (Oxf).* 2012;77(1):146-151. PMID: 22283624

12 ANSWER: D) Thyroid-stimulating immunoglobulin level

Overall, without considering individual risk factors, the chance of hyperthyroidism remission after 12 to 18 months of antithyroid drug therapy is 30% to 50%. Men, persons older than 40 years, individuals with large goiters, cigarette smokers, and those with higher baseline thyroid hormone levels are less likely to achieve remission. This patient is younger than 40 years, does not have a large goiter, and is a nonsmoker (thus, Answers A, B, and C are incorrect).

After 12 to 18 months of antithyroid drug treatment, thyroid-stimulating immunoglobulin levels (Answer D) can be used to refine estimates for the likelihood of remission. Patients with negative thyroid receptor antibodies after 18 months of antithyroid drug treatment are more likely to remit than those in whom thyroid receptor antibodies remain detectable. In this patient who is euthyroid on methimazole but whose thyroid-stimulating immunoglobulin level remains high, the likelihood of long-term remission is approximately 15%.

TPO antibody titer (Answer E) is not associated with the probability of remission.

The recommendation from the 2016 American Thyroid Association guidelines for treating hyperthyroidism is as follows: "If MMI [methimazole] is chosen as the primary therapy for GD [Graves disease], the medication should be continued for approximately 12-18 months, then discontinued if the TSH and TRAb levels are normal at that time."

EDUCATIONAL OBJECTIVE

List predictors of remission in Graves hyperthyroidism.

REFERENCE(S)

Franklyn JA, Boelaert K. Thyrotoxicosis. *Lancet.* 2012;379(9821):1155-1166. PMID: 22394559

Barbesino G, Tomer Y. Clinical review: clinical utility of TSH receptor antibodies. *J Clin Endocrinol Metab.* 2013;98(6):2247-2255. PMID: 23539719

Carella C, Mazziotti G, Sorvillo F, et al. Serum thyrotropin receptor antibodies concentrations in patients with Graves' disease before, at the end of methimazole treatment, and after drug withdrawal: evidence that the activity of thyrotropin receptor antibody and/or thyroid response modify during the observation period. *Thyroid.* 2006;16(3):295-302. PMID: 16571093

Ross DS, Burch HB, Cooper DS, et al. 2016 American Thyroid Association guidelines for diagnosis and management of hyperthyroidism and other causes of thyrotoxicosis. *Thyroid.* 2016;26(10):1343-1421. PMID: 27521067

13 ANSWER: C) Primary hypothyroidism

Sunitinib is a tyrosine kinase inhibitor used to treat certain malignancies such as renal cell carcinoma and gastrointestinal stromal tumors. Studies show that sunitinib can induce primary hypothyroidism (Answer C) in up to 85% of patients. Furthermore, sunitinib seems to increase the levothyroxine dosage requirement in hypothyroid patients. Sunitinib therapy would not be expected to result in secondary hypothyroidism (Answer E), primary hyperthyroidism (Answer B), or secondary hyperthyroidism (Answer D). As described, the patient does not appear to have an illness that would lead to him currently having euthyroid sick syndrome (Answer A). Many other tyrosine kinase inhibitors, including sorafenib, cabozantinib, nilotinib, and pazopanib, are also associated with the development of hypothyroidism.

Various mechanisms have been suggested to explain the development of hypothyroidism. In animal studies, hepatic type 3 deiodinase activity is increased and thyroid histologic examination shows marked capillary regression. In patients being treated with sunitinib, there is also evidence of altered T_4/T_3 metabolism and some of those who develop hypothyroidism also develop TPO-antibody positivity. Interestingly, the development of hypothyroidism appears to be associated with improved overall survival in patients with nonthyroidal cancers.

EDUCATIONAL OBJECTIVE

Predict the most common effect that sunitinib has on thyroid function.

REFERENCE(S)

Illouz F, Braun D, Briet C, Schweizer U, Rodien P. Endocrine side-effects of anti-cancer drugs: thyroid effects of tyrosine kinase inhibitors. *Eur J Endocrinol.* 2014;171(3):R91-R99. PMID: 24833135

Lechner MG, Vyas CM, Hamnvik OR, et al. Hypothyroidism during tyrosine kinase inhibitor therapy is associated with longer survival in patients with advanced nonthyroidal cancers. *Thyroid.* 2018;28(4):445-453. PMID: 29652597

Kappers MHW, van Esch JHM, Smedts FMM, et al. Sunitinib-induced hypothyroidism is due to induction of type 3 deiodinase activity and thyroidal capillary regression. *J Clin Endocrinol Metab.* 2011;96(10):3087-3094. PMID: 21816788

Pani F, Atzori F, Baghino G, et al. Thyroid dysfunction in patients with metastatic carcinoma treated with sunitinib: is thyroid autoimmunity involved? *Thyroid.* 2015;25(11):1255-1261. PMID: 26414109

14 ANSWER: D) Plasmapheresis

This patient has developed thyroid storm after discontinuing methimazole. The diagnosis of thyroid storm can be made empirically with additional guidance from the use of diagnostic scoring systems. Both the Burch-Wartofsky point score (75 points) and the Japan Thyroid Association system ("Thyroid storm-1, Combination-2") would categorize this patient as having thyroid storm. Emergent thyroidectomy has been used in patients with a similar deteriorating presentation when other conventional medical therapies fail.

Because antithyroid drugs cannot be started in this patient, other means must be used to prepare him for thyroidectomy. Plasmapheresis (Answer D), plasma exchange, and charcoal hemoperfusion have been used successfully in this setting in the immediate preoperative period since they remove plasma-containing proteins such as immunoglobulins and thyroxine-binding globulin, along with its bound thyroid hormones.

Hemodialysis (Answer C) does not remove the majority of thyroid hormone because it is bound to binding proteins.

Changing from intravenous propranolol to intravenous esmolol would make sense because of the ability to rapidly titrate the latter. However, changing to atenolol (Answer E), which is even less titratable than propranolol and does not provide propranolol's beneficial effect on blocking conversion of T_4 to T_3, would be incorrect.

Intravenous immunoglobulin therapy (Answer B) has not been used effectively in the treatment of thyroid storm.

Cholestyramine (Answer A) can be used to treat hyperthyroidism and it acts by blocking the recirculation of thyroid hormones. However, its action is not likely to be of sufficient magnitude or of rapid enough onset to be helpful in this urgent situation.

EDUCATIONAL OBJECTIVE

Manage life-threatening thyrotoxicosis and recommend plasmapheresis in patients unable to take antithyroid drugs.

REFERENCE(S)

Warnock AL, Cooper DS, Burch HB. Life-threatening thyrotoxicosis: thyroid storm and adverse effects of antithyroid drugs. In: Mattfin G, ed. *Endocrine Medical Emergencies.* Endocrine Press: 2014.

Ross DS, Burch HB, Cooper DS, et al. 2016 American Thyroid Association guidelines for diagnosis and management of hyperthyroidism and other causes of thyrotoxicosis. *Thyroid.* 2016;26(10):1343-1421. PMID: 27521067

Akamizu T, Satch T, Isozaki O, et al; Japan Thyroid Association. Diagnostic criteria, clinical features, and incidence of thyroid storm based on nation-wide surveys. *Thyroid.* 2012;22(7):661-679. PMID: 22690898

Vyas AA, Vyas P, Fillipon NL, Vijayakrishnan R, Trivedi N. Successful treatment of thyroid storm with plasmapheresis in a patient with methimazole-induced agranulocytosis. *Endocr Pract.* 2010;16(4):673-676. PMID: 20439250

Carhill A, Gutierrez A, Lakhia R, Nalini R. Surviving the storm: two cases of thyroid storm successfully treated with plasmapheresis. *BMJ Case Rep.* 2012. PMID: 23087271

15 ANSWER: C) Serum thyroglobulin measurement

The differential diagnosis for patients with thyrotoxicosis and low radioactive iodine uptake includes painless and postpartum thyroiditis, subacute thyroiditis, struma ovarii (with low radioactive iodine uptake in the neck, but uptake in the pelvis on whole-body scan), factitious or iatrogenic thyroiditis, amiodarone use, and recent high-dose iodine exposure. In this male patient, struma ovarii and postpartum thyroiditis are not possibilities. He is not taking amiodarone. Subacute thyroiditis is less likely given the lack of a viral prodrome, fever, or thyroid tenderness, so assessing his erythrocyte sedimentation rate (Answer A) is incorrect. The urinary iodine concentration is not consistent with recent excessive iodine exposure, so repeating the radioactive iodine uptake following a low-iodine diet (Answer B) is unlikely to change results.

In this patient, the most likely diagnoses are factitious thyrotoxicosis or painless thyroiditis. Graves disease has already been ruled out by the low radioactive iodine uptake, so thyroid-stimulating immunoglobulin measurement (Answer D) is incorrect. Thyroid ultrasonography with color Doppler (Answer E) would show absent hypervascularity with both of these entities. However, the serum thyroglobulin concentration (Answer C) would be elevated in painless thyroiditis but low in factitious thyrotoxicosis.

Factitious hyperthyroidism can occur when patients take supplements that contain thyroid hormones or when patients take thyroid hormone to achieve weight loss. Typically, as in this case, doses of thyroid hormones that are associated with weight loss are also associated with other stigmata of thyrotoxicosis.

EDUCATIONAL OBJECTIVE

Construct the differential diagnosis for thyrotoxicosis with low radioiodine uptake.

REFERENCE(S)

De Leo S, Lee SY, Braverman LE. Hyperthyroidism. *Lancet.* 2016;388(10047):906-918. PMID: 27038492

16 ANSWER: D) Reduce the methimazole dosage

This patient has a history of thyrotoxicosis and is being treated with methimazole. Her thyroid scan from 2 years ago clearly shows a pattern of toxic multinodular goiter. Unlike Graves disease, which may enter a lasting remission after completion of a 12- to 18-month course of antithyroid drug therapy, toxic multinodular goiter generally has a natural history of gradual progression. Thus, patients with toxic multinodular goiters usually require either continued medical therapy with low dosages of antithyroid drugs or definitive therapy with radioactive iodine or thyroidectomy. Because the patient is currently biochemically hypothyroid, her methimazole dosage should be reduced (Answer D) or definitive therapy (surgery or radioactive iodine therapy) could be considered. She has stated that she wishes to avoid therapy with radioactive iodine (Answer E), so this avenue should clearly not be pursued.

There is no reason to perform another scan with radioactive iodine uptake (Answer C) because the pattern of uptake and percentage uptake are unlikely to have changed substantially.

Discontinuing methimazole (Answers A and B) would result in resurgent thyrotoxicosis. The 2016 American Thyroid Association guidelines for the management of hyperthyroidism state that long-term therapy with low-dosage antithyroid drugs is an acceptable option for patients who prefer to avoid definitive therapy, and a recent meta-analysis concluded that long-term antithyroid drug use is safe.

EDUCATIONAL OBJECTIVE

Recommend continued therapy with a low-dosage antithyroid drug in a patient with toxic multinodular goiter and distinguish this approach from that used to treat Graves disease, which may enter remission.

REFERENCE(S)

Ross DS, Burch HB, Cooper DS, et al. 2016 American Thyroid Association guidelines for diagnosis and management of hyperthyroidism and other causes of thyrotoxicosis. *Thyroid.* 2016;26(10):1343-1421. PMID: 27521067

Azizi F, Malboosbaf R. Long-term antithyroid drug treatment: a systematic review and meta-analysis. *Thyroid.* 2017;27(10):1223-1231. PMID: 28699478

Thyroid, Section 2 Board Review

Kaniksha Desai, MD

17 ANSWER: C) Radiofrequency ablation of thyroid nodule

This patient is symptomatic and therefore observation (Answer A) would not be recommended.

Radiofrequency ablation (Answer C) is a noninvasive procedure that could ablate this patient's thyroid nodule and shrink it enough to improve his symptoms.

The patient is a poor surgical candidate because he has significant coronary artery disease with a recent myocardial infarction and suboptimally controlled diabetes. Thus, surgery with lobectomy (Answer D) or total thyroidectomy (Answer E) is not recommended.

Radioactive iodine treatment (Answer B) would not work because he is euthyroid, and it is unlikely to shrink the nodule enough to decrease symptoms.

EDUCATIONAL OBJECTIVE

Recommend radiofrequency ablation for treatment of a thyroid nodule in a symptomatic patient who is a poor surgical candidate.

REFERENCE(S)

Orloff LA, Noel JE, Stack BC Jr, et al. Radiofrequency ablation and related ultrasound-guided ablation technologies for treatment of benign and malignant thyroid disease: an international multidisciplinary consensus statement of the American Head and Neck Society Endocrine Surgery Section with the Asia Pacific Society of Thyroid Surgery, Association Medici Endocrinology, British Association of Endocrine and Thyroid Surgeons, European Thyroid Association, Italian Society of Endocrine Surgery Units, Korean Society of Thyroid Radiology, Latin American Thyroid Society, and Thyroid Nodules Therapies Association. *Head Neck*. 2022;44(3):633-660. PMID: 34939714

Muhammad H, Santhanam P, Russell JO. Radiofrequency ablation and thyroid nodules: updated systematic review. *Endocrine*. 2021;72(3):619-632. PMID: 33449296

18 ANSWER: A) Stage 1 high risk

Staging a patient's thyroid cancer appropriately is important in counseling about prognosis. Risk stratifying patients is an important aspect of thyroid cancer management because it determines further treatment with radioactive iodine and TSH goals.

Per the American Joint Committee on Cancer (AJCC) 8th edition, thyroid cancer staging is based on age (*see table, following page*). Age younger than 55 years is categorized as stage 1 or stage 2 (thus, Answer E is incorrect). Stage 1 is disease in the neck (any T and any N). Stage 2 is diagnosed only if the thyroid cancer has spread with distant metastatic disease, M1, which this patient does not have (thus, Answers C and D are incorrect). Per American Thyroid Association thyroid cancer guidelines, patients are risk stratified for cancer recurrence. This is done independent of staging. This patient has a very large lymph node. Having a lymph node that is smaller than 3 cm is intermediate risk, while a lymph node larger than 3 cm is high risk. Since her lymph node is larger than 3 cm, her disease is high risk (thus, Answer B is incorrect). Stage 1 high risk is defined by a patient younger than 55 years with any T and any N but M0, and high risk is defined as a patient who has a lymph node larger than 3 cm (Answer A).

Differentiated thyroid cancer

When age at diagnosis is...	*And T is...*	*And N is...*	*And M is...*	*Then the stage group is...*
< 55 yrs	Any T	Any N	M0	I
	Any T	Any N	M1	II
≥ 55 yrs	T1	N0/NX	M0	I
	T1	N1	M0	II
	T2	N0/NX	M0	I
	T2	N1	M0	II
	T3a/T3b	Any N	M0	II
	T4a	Any N	M0	III
	T4b	Any N	M0	IVA
	Any T	Any N	M1	IVB

Reprinted with permission from Tuttle RM et al. *Thyroid*, 2017; 27(6):751-756. © Mary Ann Liebert, Inc.

EDUCATIONAL OBJECTIVE

Stage and risk stratify thyroid cancer at the time of diagnosis.

REFERENCE(S)

Tuttle RM, Haugen B, Perrier ND. Updated American Joint Committee on Cancer/Tumor-Node-Metastasis Staging System for Differentiated and Anaplastic Thyroid Cancer (Eighth Edition): what changed and why? *Thyroid.* 2017;27(6):751-756. PMID: 28463585

Haugen BR, Alexander EK, Bible KC, et al. 2015 American Thyroid Association management guidelines for adult patients with thyroid nodules and differentiated thyroid cancer: the American Thyroid Association guidelines task force on thyroid nodules and differentiated thyroid cancer. *Thyroid.* 2016;26(1):1-133. PMID: 26462967

19 ANSWER: C) Indeterminate response

After a patient completes initial treatment, in this case total thyroidectomy followed by radioactive iodine, assessing their response to treatment is important. The treatment response determines the patient's TSH goals. An assessment for treatment response can be done once the patient has completed initial treatment. This patient had radioactive treatment 1 year ago, and an adequate amount of time has passed to allow for treatment effect (thus, Answer E is incorrect).

The patient has detectable thyroglobulin (<2.0 ng/mL [<2.0 μg/L]) and a very small hypoechoic nodule, which does not meet criteria for FNA biopsy. This scenario is considered an indeterminate response to treatment (Answer C).

An excellent treatment response (Answer B) is defined as no biochemical or structural evidence of disease. Thyroglobulin would be undetectable, and neck ultrasonography would show no thyroid bed lesions.

A biochemical incomplete response (Answer A) is defined as a persistent abnormal thyroglobulin concentration greater than 2.0 ng/mL (>2.0 μg/L) with no localized disease on imaging.

A structural incomplete response (Answer D) is persistent or newly identified disease either in the neck or as distant metastases. This patient's thyroid ultrasonography shows a small indeterminate nodule that has not been biopsy-proven to be thyroid cancer.

EDUCATIONAL OBJECTIVE

Assess treatment response in a patient with thyroid cancer 1 year after treatment is completed.

REFERENCE(S)

Tuttle RM, Alzahrani AS. Risk stratification in differentiated thyroid cancer: from detection to final follow-up. *J Clin Endocrinol Metab.* 2019;104(9):4087-4100. PMID: 30874735

Haugen BR, Alexander EK, Bible KC, et al. 2015 American Thyroid Association management guidelines for adult patients with thyroid nodules and differentiated thyroid cancer: the American Thyroid Association guidelines task force on thyroid nodules and differentiated thyroid cancer. *Thyroid.* 2016;26(1):1-133. PMID: 26462967

20 ANSWER: A) Lobectomy; >50% chance of requiring thyroid hormone replacement

Current American Thyroid Association guidelines recommend lobectomy for patients with low-risk thyroid cancer. This patient is an ideal candidate for lobectomy because she has a solitary thyroid nodule in the right lobe that has been documented to be papillary thyroid cancer on FNA biopsy. She has no nodules in the contralateral lobe and no abnormal lymphadenopathy. Thus, recommending thyroidectomy (Answer D) is incorrect. Having positive TPO antibodies does increase the risk of hypothyroidism post surgically, but it is not an indication for total thyroidectomy in a patient with low-risk thyroid cancer.

Before surgery, patients should be counseled on requiring thyroid hormone (thus, Answer C is incorrect). If she had a lower TSH concentration and was TPO antibody–negative, then her risk of requiring thyroid hormone would be low (Answer B). Since her TSH value is almost 2.0 mIU/L and she has positive TPO antibodies, she is at high risk of requiring thyroid hormone after surgery (Answer A).

EDUCATIONAL OBJECTIVE

Counsel patients regarding lobectomy for treatment of thyroid cancer and assess the risk of hypothyroidism following surgery.

REFERENCE(S)

Haugen BR, Alexander EK, Bible KC, et al. 2015 American Thyroid Association management guidelines for adult patients with thyroid nodules and differentiated thyroid cancer: the American Thyroid Association guidelines task force on thyroid nodules and differentiated thyroid cancer. *Thyroid.* 2016;26(1):1-133. PMID: 26462967

Cox C, Bosley M, Southerland LB, et al. Lobectomy for treatment of differentiated thyroid cancer: can patients avoid postoperative thyroid hormone supplementation and be compliant with the American Thyroid Association guidelines? *Surgery.* 2018;163(1):75-80. PMID: 29122328

Kim SY, Kim HJ, Kim SM, et al. Thyroid hormone supplementation therapy for differentiated thyroid cancer after lobectomy: 5 years of follow-up. *Front Endocrinol (Lausanne).* 2020;11:520. PMID: 32849303

21 ANSWER: D) Shape

The American Thyroid Association criteria uses pattern recognition to identify high and low risk for malignant characteristics on ultrasonography. TI-RADS (Thyroid Imaging, Reporting, and Data System) uses risk stratification based on general categories: composition, shape, margins, echogenic foci, and echogenicity (*see figures 1 and 2, following page*).

This nodule has a taller-than-wide shape, which is a high-risk ultrasound characteristic according to both American Thyroid Association and TI-RADS criteria (thus, Answer D is correct).

A solid nodule has an intermediate risk for cancer; however, a taller-than-wide nodule has a higher risk of malignancy than a solid nodule (thus, Answer A is incorrect).

Comet tail artifacts are benign calcifications (thus, Answer B is incorrect)

Isoechoic nodules tend to be benign (thus, Answer C is incorrect).

Neither system correlates size directly with malignancy risk, although size is used in combination with other ultrasound characteristics to determine whether FNA biopsy is necessary (thus, Answer E is incorrect).

EDUCATIONAL OBJECTIVE

Identify benign and malignant ultrasound characteristics using TI-RADS and American Thyroid Association criteria.

REFERENCE(S)

Grant EG, Tessler FN, Hoang JK, et al. Thyroid ultrasound reporting lexicon: white paper of the ACR Thyroid Imaging, Reporting and Data System (TIRADS) Committee. *J Am Coll Radiol.* 2015;12(12 Pt A):1272-1279. PMID: 26419308

Haugen BR, Alexander EK, Bible KC, et al. 2015 American Thyroid Association management guidelines for adult patients with thyroid nodules and differentiated thyroid cancer: the American Thyroid Association guidelines task force on thyroid nodules and differentiated thyroid cancer. *Thyroid.* 2016;26(1):1-133. PMID: 26462967

22 ANSWER: A) Familial dysalbuminemic hyperthyroxinemia

Familial dysalbuminemic hyperthyroxinemia (Answer A) is the most common inherited form of hyperthyroxinemia. This condition is found in 0.1% to 1.8% of individuals and is most common in Hispanic populations. Patients with familial dysalbuminemic hyperthyroxinemia are frequently overlooked with the widespread measurement of TSH alone to screen for thyroid dysfunction. Although free T_4 by equilibrium dialysis yields normal values in patients with familial

Figure 1. American Thyroid Association Sonographic Patterns and Risk of Malignancy.

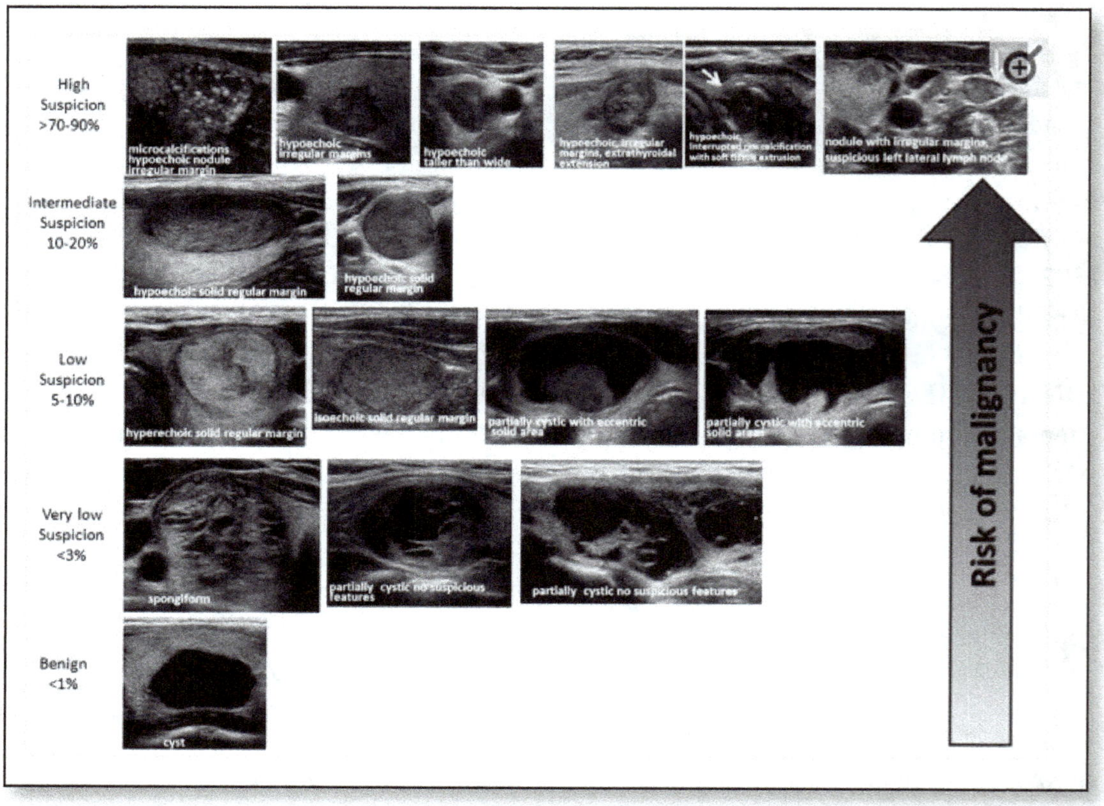

Reprinted with permission from Haugen BR et al. *Thyroid*, 2016; 26(1):1-133. © Mary Ann Liebert, Inc.

Figure 2. ACR TI-RADS

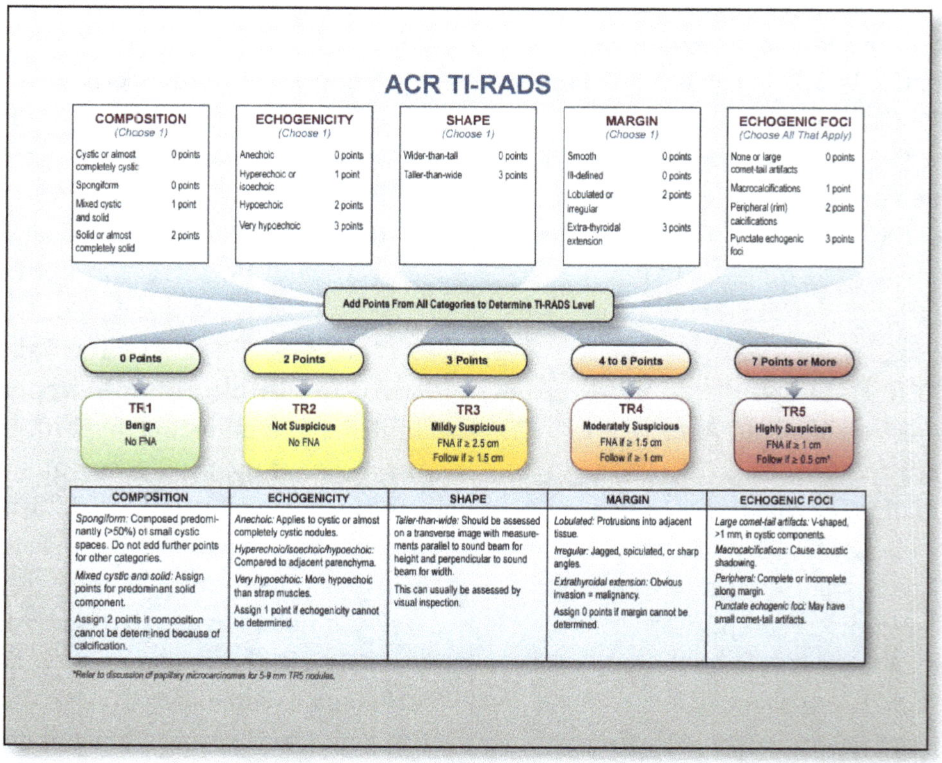

Reprinted from Grant EG et al. *J Am Coll Radiol*, 2015; 12(12 Pt A):1272-9. © The American College of Radiology. Published by Elsevier Inc.

dysalbuminemic hyperthyroxinemia, many free T_4 assays that are more susceptible to binding-protein changes give spurious elevations in free T_4 due to altered protein binding (*see figure*).

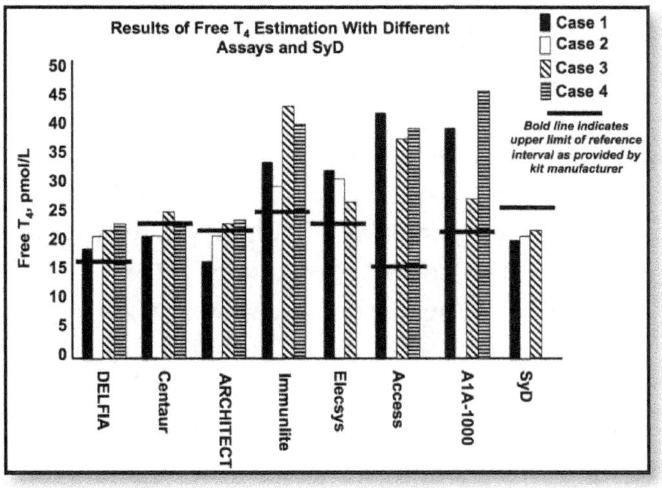

Adapted with permission from Cartwright D et al. *Clin Chem*, 2009; 55(5):1044-1046. © 2009 The American Association for Clinical Chemistry.

Familial dysalbuminemic hyperthyroxinemia is inherited in an autosomal dominant fashion and is the result of gain-of-function pathogenic variants in the *ALB* gene encoding albumin that enhance the affinity of albumin for T_4, but generally not for T_3. As a result, reliance on total T_4 (elevated) or free T_4 index (also elevated, since this is a product of normal T_3 resin and elevated T_4) may be misleading.

A defect in 5′-monodeiodination due to selenium deficiency (Answer C) is much less common than familial dysalbuminemic hyperthyroxinemia.

This patient does not have a TSH-secreting pituitary adenoma (Answer E) given that he is clinically euthyroid and T_3 levels are normal.

This is not thyroid hormone resistance (Answer D) or familial thyroxine-binding globulin excess (Answer B) because the total T_3 value is normal rather than elevated—an elevated total T_3 concentration would be expected in each of these disorders.

EDUCATIONAL OBJECTIVE

Diagnose familial dysalbuminemic hyperthyroxinemia on the basis of clinical findings and thyroid function test results.

REFERENCE(S)

Pappa T, Ferrara AM, Refetoff S. Inherited defects of thyroxine-binding proteins. *Best Pract Res Clin Endocrinol Metab.* 2015;29(5):735-747. PMID: 26522458

Pannain S, Feldman M, Eiholzer U, Weiss RE, Scherberg NH, Refetoff S. Familial dysalbuminemic hyperthyroxinemia in a Swiss family caused by a mutant albumin (R218P) shows an apparent discrepancy between serum concentration and affinity for thyroxine. *J Clin Endocrinol Metab.* 2000;85(8):2786-2792. PMID: 10946882

23 ANSWER: C) Tumor size increase of at least 3 mm

In this vignette, a solitary microcarcinoma was identified. The patient has no evidence of metastatic disease. The risk of tumor persistence or recurrence in unifocal, intrathyroidal micropapillary carcinoma (tumor size ≤1 cm) is extremely low—on the order of 1% to 2%. The risk for tumor-related mortality is essentially zero. The American Thyroid Association guidelines recommend against FNA biopsy for nodules smaller than 1 cm. However, having diagnosed this patient's micropapillary carcinoma, there is a need to determine the best course of action. An active surveillance approach instead of immediate surgery can be considered in carefully selected patients and in appropriate settings. Ideal patients for this approach include euthyroid older individuals (since tumor progression is more likely in patients younger than 40 years) who have papillary microcarcinomas without known metastases or local invasion, and whose tumor is not adjacent to the thyroid capsule or the recurrent laryngeal nerve. Patients must be comfortable with the concept of monitoring a low-risk cancer rather than pursuing immediate intervention, and they must be willing to return for follow-up visits. The availability of high-quality neck ultrasonography is essential.

Cohort studies have demonstrated that among carefully selected patients undergoing active surveillance, clinically significant tumor growth occurs in only 10% to 15%. Protocols for active surveillance typically call for neck ultrasonography and TSH measurement every 6 months, with the follow-up period extended to 12 months if the tumor size remains stable for 2 years. Proceeding to thyroid surgery is warranted for a tumor size increase of at least 3 mm (Answer C), new neck node metastases, a tumor size increase to at least 12 mm, or a tumor volume increase of at least 50% (not 100%, as in Answer D). Serum thyroglobulin values (Answers A and B) are not helpful in active surveillance protocols.

EDUCATIONAL OBJECTIVE

Guide appropriate patient selection and strategies for active surveillance of micropapillary thyroid cancer.

REFERENCE(S)

Tuttle RM, Fagin JA, Minkowitz G, et al. Natural history and tumor volume kinetics of papillary thyroid cancers during active surveillance. *JAMA Otolaryngol Head Neck Surg.* 2017;143(10):1015-1020. PMID: 28859191

Brito JP, Ito Y, Miyauchi A, Tuttle RM. A clinical framework to facilitate risk stratification when considering an active surveillance alternative to immediate biopsy and surgery in papillary micro-carcinoma. *Thyroid.* 2016;26(1):144-149. PMID: 26414743

Kim TY, Shong YK. Active surveillance of papillary thyroid microcarcinoma: a mini-review from Korea. *Endocrinol Metab (Seoul).* 2017;32(4):399-406. PMID: 29271613

24 ANSWER: C) Lenvatinib

This patient has rapidly progressive, metastatic differentiated thyroid cancer that is becoming increasingly symptomatic. He is not a good candidate for additional radioactive iodine treatment because the absence of uptake on his posttreatment scans indicates that his disease is ^{131}I refractory. Although doxorubicin is approved by the US FDA to be used for treatment of metastatic thyroid cancer, cytotoxic chemotherapy (Answer A) is generally of limited utility in differentiated thyroid cancer. Given that his disease is refractory to radioactive iodine and is diffuse, progressive, and symptomatic (which would be expected to produce morbidity or mortality within 6 months), he is a candidate for tyrosine kinase inhibitor therapy. In several trials, this treatment has been shown to improve progression-free survival. Although several other tyrosine kinase inhibitors are currently being studied in differentiated thyroid cancer (*see table*), only 2—lenvatinib (Answer C) and sorafenib (Answer D)—are currently FDA approved for the treatment of differentiated thyroid cancer in patients with extensive local disease or distant metastases. While sorafenib is approved in this setting, lenvatinib is the preferred treatment because patients taking lenvatinib have a longer progression-free survival time than patients taking sorafenib.

Ipilimumab (Answer B) is a monoclonal antibody that blocks the cytotoxic T-cell receptor 4 (CTLA-4) on activated T cells. It is used to treat metastatic melanoma, but it has not been studied in differentiated thyroid cancer.

Vandetanib (Answer E) is approved for the treatment of metastatic medullary thyroid cancer and thus would not be the best agent to use in this patient.

Table. Tyrosine Kinase Inhibitors Currently Approved for Use in Advanced Thyroid Cancer

Tyrosine kinase inhibitor	Type of thyroid cancer	Effectiveness: progression-free survival compared with placebo[a]
Vandetanib	Medullary	30.5 vs 19.3 months
Cabozantinib	Medullary	11.2 vs 4 months
Sorafenib	Differentiated	10.8 vs 5.8 months
Lenvatinib	Differentiated	18.3 vs 3.6 months
Dabrafenib and trametinib	Anaplastic	Open-label trial with 69% overall response rate[b]

[a] Enrolled populations were different; efficacy cannot be compared directly across studies.

[b] Phase II open label trial.

Many other multikinase inhibitors are currently being investigated for use in advanced thyroid cancer.

EDUCATIONAL OBJECTIVE

Recommend treatment options in radioactive iodine–refractory metastatic differentiated thyroid cancer.

REFERENCE(S)

Haugen BR, Alexander EK, Bible KC, et al. 2015 American Thyroid Association management guidelines for adult patients with thyroid nodules and differentiated thyroid cancer: the American Thyroid Association guidelines task force on thyroid nodules and differentiated thyroid cancer. *Thyroid.* 2016;26(1):1-133. PMID: 26462967

Berdelou A, Lamartina L, Klain M, Leboulleux S, Schlumberger M; TUTHTYREF Network. Treatment of refractory thyroid cancer. *Endocr Relat Cancer.* 2018;25(4):R209-R223. PMID: 29371330

25 ANSWER: C) Medullary thyroid cancer

The photograph shows cutaneous lichen amyloidosis, an autosomal dominant condition that has been strongly associated with multiple endocrine neoplasia type 2A, particularly in families harboring a pathogenic variant in codon 634 of the *RET* proto-oncogene, with a prevalence in some families as high as 36%. Cutaneous lichen amyloidosis typically occurs in the location shown (between the spine and the scapula) and is pruritic. It may occur in either or both interscapular areas. This lesion may precede the diagnosis of multiple endocrine neoplasia type 2A by many years. In one study, cutaneous lichen amyloidosis was diagnosed at an average age of 14 years, compared with an average age at diagnosis of medullary thyroid cancer of 31 years. The current theory regarding the pathogenesis of this lesion is that it is due to patient scratching to relieve a neurally mediated pruritus. Of the listed choices, only medullary thyroid cancer (Answer C) is associated with cutaneous lichen amyloidosis.

EDUCATIONAL OBJECTIVE

Identify cutaneous lichen amyloidosis and its association with multiple endocrine neoplasia type 2.

REFERENCE(S)

Verga U, Fugazzola L, Cambiaghi S, et al. Frequent association between MEN 2A and cutaneous lichen amyloidosis. *Clin Endocrinol (Oxf).* 2003;59(2):156-161. PMID: 12864791

Scapineli JO, Ceolin L, Punales MK, Dora JM, Maia AL. MEN 2A-related cutaneous lichen amyloidosis: report of three kindred and systematic literature review of clinical, biochemical and molecular characteristics. *Fam Cancer.* 2016;15(4):625-633. PMID: 26920351

26 ANSWER: C) Perform FNA biopsy after surgery and chemotherapy

The American College of Radiology TI-RADS (Thyroid Imaging, Reporting, and Data System) is used to assess the risk for malignancy of thyroid nodules and to determine whether to proceed to a thyroid nodule biopsy. The TI-RADS system assesses nodules based on their composition, echogenicity, shape, margins, and echogenic foci as visualized on ultrasonography. The incidentally identified thyroid nodule in this vignette is TI-RADS level 5. This highly suspicious category usually leads to a biopsy for thyroid nodules that are 1 cm or larger.

Such incidentally found FDG-PET–positive thyroid nodules are identified in about 2% of FDG-PET scans performed for nonthyroidal malignancies such as breast cancer, lung cancer, melanoma, and colon cancer. While this thyroid nodule appears likely to be thyroid cancer and would be biopsied now (Answer D) in the absence of other diagnoses with a significant adverse impact on the patient's prognosis, this may not be the wisest approach given the gravity of his lung cancer diagnosis and the nodule's small size. This patient has a high mortality risk from his lung cancer and thyroid nodule biopsy could be deferred until his response to lung cancer therapy has been assessed (Answer C). One study of patients from a cancer referral center documented a 5-year survival rate for patients with lung cancer. Not only would proceeding with further treatment for thyroid cancer have a relatively minor effect on this patient's overall survival compared with the impact from his lung cancer, it would also burden him with the stress of having a second malignancy. Thus, this patient's thyroid nodule biopsy can be deferred until initial treatment for his lung cancer has been completed. He could also be a candidate for active surveillance if papillary thyroid cancer is confirmed.

Measuring free T_4 (Answer A) is not necessary because he has a normal TSH concentration.

Serum thyroglobulin measurement (Answer B) would not be indicated before thyroidectomy even if thyroid cancer were confirmed, as it would not provide useful information about thyroid cancer burden with the thyroid gland still in place.

The tissue from the patient's lung biopsy does not need to be stained for thyroglobulin (Answer E) because thyroglobulin-positivity is specific for thyroid cancer.

In a recent study of patients who had an FDG-PET–positive incidental thyroid nodule, thyroid ultrasonography was performed in 42%, biopsy was performed in 32%, and thyroid surgery was performed in 6%.

EDUCATIONAL OBJECTIVE

Consider patient comorbidities and prognosis in decision-making concerning FNA biopsy of small suspicious thyroid nodules.

REFERENCE(S)

Tessler FN, Middleton WD, Grant EG, et al. ACR Thyroid Imaging, Reporting and Data System (TI-RADS): white paper of the ACR TI-RADS Committee. *J Am Coll Radiol.* 2017;14(5):587-595. PMID: 28372962

Piek MW, de Boer JP, Vriens MR, et al. Retrospective analyses of 18FDG-PET/CT thyroid incidentaloma in adults: incidence, treatment, and outcome in a tertiary cancer referral center. *Thyroid.* 2021;31(11):1715-1722. PMID: 34340567

27 ANSWER: D) 70%-90%

The American Thyroid Association guidelines for the treatment of thyroid cancer have defined several risk categories for the likelihood of thyroid cancer associated with patterns observed on thyroid ultrasonography. In addition, the American College of Radiology has created a proposed risk stratification based on ultrasound characteristics (TI-RADS). These systems have good predictive value (thus, Answer E is incorrect). The image shows a nodule with a high risk of malignancy (TI-RADS 5 nodule) (70%-90% [Answer D]).

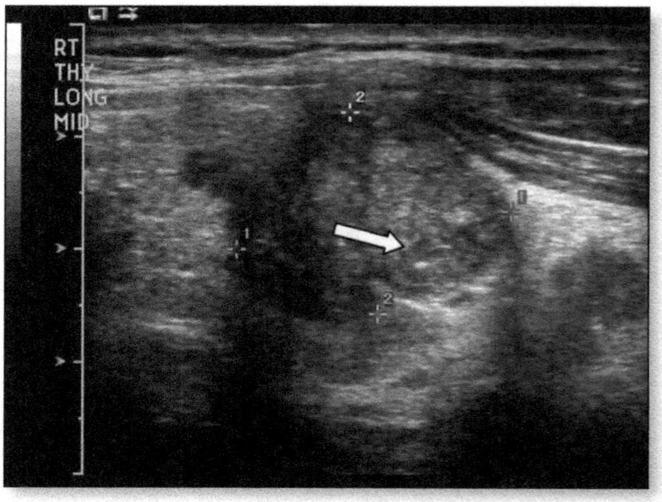

It has classic features associated with papillary thyroid cancer, including hypoechogenicity, irregular margins, and scattered microcalcifications (*arrow*).

Nodules with a very low risk for malignancy (Answer A) include spongiform nodules with clearly defined margins.

Intermediate suspicion patterns associated with a 10% to 20% risk of malignancy (TI-RADS 4) (Answer B) include hypoechoic nodules with smooth margins but without microcalcifications, extrathyroidal extension, or taller-than-wide shape.

There is currently no American Thyroid Association–defined ultrasonography pattern associated with a 20% to 40% malignancy risk (Answer C).

EDUCATIONAL OBJECTIVE

Identify sonographic features consistent with high risk for papillary thyroid carcinoma.

REFERENCE(S)

Haugen BR, Alexander EK, Bible KC, et al. 2015 American Thyroid Association management guidelines for adult patients with thyroid nodules and differentiated thyroid cancer: the American Thyroid Association Guidelines Task Force on Thyroid Nodules and Differentiated Thyroid Cancer. *Thyroid.* 2016;26(1):1-133. PMID: 26462967

Brito JP, Gionfriddo MR, Al Nofal A, et al. The accuracy of thyroid nodule ultrasound to predict thyroid cancer: systematic review and meta-analysis. *J Clin Endocrinol Metab.* 2014;99(4):1253-1263. PMID: 24276450

Grant EG, Tessler FN, Hoang JK, et al. Thyroid ultrasound reporting lexicon: white paper of the ACR thyroid imaging, reporting and data system (TIRADS) committee. *J Am Coll Radiol.* 2015;12(12 Pt A):1272-1279. PMID: 26419308

28 ANSWER: D) Expected changes in euthyroid patients on amiodarone

Amiodarone can have complex effects on the thyroid gland due to both intrinsic drug effects and effects due to its iodine content. Intrinsic drug effects include inhibition of type 1 and 2 5′-deiodinase, decreased T3 binding to its receptor, and thyroid cytotoxicity leading to thyroiditis. Iodine-related effects include development of hypothyroidism in those with underlying Hashimoto disease and induction of hyperthyroidism in those with autonomous nodules or subclinical Graves disease. Drug-induced hyperthyroidism occurs in approximately 5% of treated patients, while hypothyroidism occurs in approximately 7%. Because this patient's TSH value is still in the reference range at this time, the patient does not have overt hypothyroidism and does not need to be started on levothyroxine treatment (thus, Answer A is incorrect).

Amiodarone has dramatic effects on thyroid function tests in clinically euthyroid patients. A large iodine load (74 mg total iodine, 7.4 mg of free iodine per 200-mg tablet) is delivered with each dose. Amiodarone inhibits both peripheral and central (intrapituitary) conversion of T_4 to T_3 through its action on type 1 and type 2 5′-monodeiodinase, respectively. Lastly, amiodarone has T_3 antagonistic effects at the nuclear level. The common pattern observed in euthyroid patients is high free T_4 and total T_4, low-normal T_3, high reverse T_3, and high-normal TSH (thus, Answer D is correct). These changes tend to persist over time, although serum TSH values may gradually normalize in some patients. The pattern of these changes is shown (*see figure*).

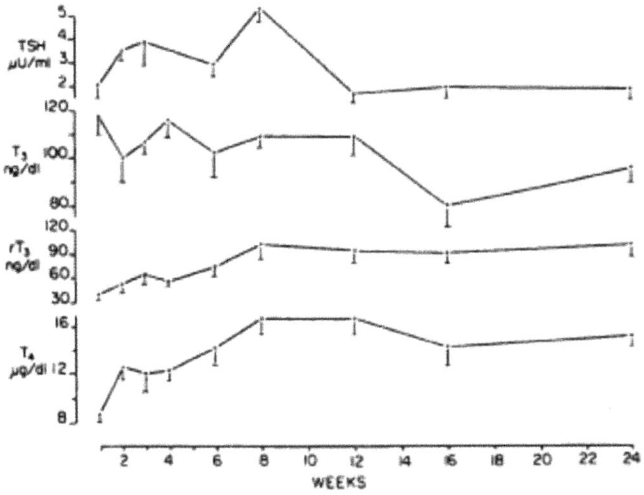

Long-term (6-month) changes in thyroid function in 10 patients on chronic amiodarone treatment. The abscissa indicates the beginning of each week of therapy. By the end of 3 weeks of treatment, each hormone level was significantly different from the pretreatment value, as determined by analysis of variance. Reprinted from Melmed S et al. J Clin Endocrinol Metab, 1981; 53(5):997–1001. © The Endocrine Society.

Amiodarone and its metabolites are not known to cause artifactual interference with thyroid function assays (Answer B).

This patient's normal TSH and lack of symptoms exclude thyrotoxicosis (Answer E).

Also, he is not acutely ill, so euthyroid sick syndrome (Answer C) is incorrect.

EDUCATIONAL OBJECTIVE

Distinguish expected changes in thyroid function parameters in patients taking amiodarone from amiodarone-induced thyroid dysfunction.

REFERENCE(S)

Danzi S, Klein I. Amiodarone-induced thyroid dysfunction. *J Intensive Care Med.* 2015;30(4):179-185. PMID: 24067547

Basaria S, Cooper DS. Amiodarone and the thyroid. *Am J Med.* 2005;118(7):706-714. PMID: 15989900

Melmed S, Nademanee K, Reed AW, Hendrickson JA, Singh BN, Hershman JM. Hyperthyroxinemia with bradycardia and normal thyrotropin secretion after chronic amiodarone administration. *J Clin Endocrinol Metab.* 1981;53(5):997-1001. PMID: 7287882

29 ANSWER: D) Refer for immediate total thyroidectomy with neck dissection

Current guidelines for the management of thyroid disease in pregnancy suggest that, in general, it is safe to wait until after delivery to perform thyroid surgery for thyroid cancer discovered early in pregnancy. The exception, however, is in patients demonstrating a more aggressive course, including growth by 50% of nodule volume (or 20% in 2 dimensions) and appearance of abnormal lymphadenopathy or aggressive baseline features, such as local invasion. This patient had a doubling of her tumor size and the new appearance of metastatic disease to lymph nodes; therefore, thyroidectomy with lymph node dissection (Answer D) is recommended now. Surgery should not be deferred until after delivery (Answer C) because thyroid cancer with extensive lymph nodes can be progressive during pregnancy.

If thyroid surgery is required during pregnancy, the second trimester is thought to be safest because anesthetic agents may have a teratogenic effect during organogenesis in the first trimester, and surgery in the third trimester (Answer A) has the potential to induce premature labor.

Initiating levothyroxine suppressive therapy (Answer E) is not recommended over surgery.

Ethanol ablation of the lymph node (Answer B) is not approved or recommended during pregnancy, and it only addresses the known metastatic node and not the primary tumor, which could continue to progress.

EDUCATIONAL OBJECTIVE

Recommend options for thyroid cancer treatment in pregnant women.

REFERENCE(S)

Alexander EK, Pearce EN, Brent GA, et al. 2017 Guidelines of the American Thyroid Association for the diagnosis and management of thyroid disease during pregnancy and the postpartum. *Thyroid.* 2017;27(3):315-389. PMID: 28056690

Gibelli B, Zamperini P, Proh M, Giugliano G. Management and follow-up of thyroid cancer in pregnant women. *Acta Otorhinolaryngol Ital.* 2011;31(6):358-365. PMID: 22323846

30 ANSWER: C) Perform thyroid lobectomy

Nondiagnostic FNA biopsy results describe samples that contain only cyst fluid or in which there are insufficient cells for diagnosis; this occurs in 2% to 16% of FNA biopsy attempts. Repeated FNA biopsy is typically recommended when this occurs, and repeated aspiration is diagnostic 60% to 80% of the time when nodules are not predominantly cystic. The risk of malignancy in repeatedly nondiagnostic nodules with suspicious sonographic features such as irregular margins, taller-than-wide shape, hypoechogenicity, or microcalcifications is approximately 25%, whereas the risk of malignancy is only about 4% in nodules lacking those concerning features. A diagnostic lobectomy (Answer C) is recommended to rule out malignancy in this patient.

As his nodule is high risk (irregular margins) and has shown growth from 2.3 to 3.1 cm, continued observation with repeat thyroid ultrasonography in 6 to 12 months (Answer D) would not be recommended.

FDG PET-CT uptake (Answer B) in thyroid nodules confers an increased risk for thyroid cancer (about 33%), but this imaging would not provide a definitive diagnosis.

Molecular markers (Answer E) are unlikely to provide additional diagnostic information in the absence of an adequate cellular biopsy.

Whether serum calcitonin (Answer A) should be routinely measured in the workup of thyroid nodules remains controversial, but this will not provide a definitive diagnosis in the case.

EDUCATIONAL OBJECTIVE

Manage thyroid nodules that have repeatedly nondiagnostic cytopathology.

REFERENCE(S)

Haugen BR, Alexander EK, Bible KC, et al. 2015 American Thyroid Association management guidelines for adult patients with thyroid nodules and differentiated thyroid cancer: the American Thyroid Association guidelines task force on thyroid nodules and differentiated thyroid cancer. *Thyroid.* 2016;26(1):1-133. PMID: 26462967

Moon HJ, Kwak JY, Choi YS, Kim EK. How to manage thyroid nodules with two consecutive non-diagnostic results on ultrasonography-guided fine-needle aspiration. *World J Surg.* 2012;36(3):586-592. PMID: 22228400

Park CJ, Kim EK, Moon HJ, Yoon JH, Park VY, Kwak JY. Thyroid nodules with nondiagnostic cytologic results: follow-up management using ultrasound patterns based on the 2015 American Thyroid Association Guidelines. *AJR Am J Roentgenol.* 2018;210(2):412-417. PMID: 29091005

31 ANSWER: A) Follow-up thyroid ultrasonography in approximately 1 year

The results of FNA biopsy cytology may yield benign (Bethesda II) or malignant (Bethesda VI) results. Such results are directly useful for determining a patient's management. However, approximately 25% of thyroid nodule aspirates are classified as indeterminate for malignancy, as occurred in this patient's case. Additional testing can be helpful for cases of indeterminate cytology; genetic testing, RNA-based classifier, and microRNA classifier approaches are all available.

Genetic testing may include testing for strong driver variants (*BRAF* V600E pathogenic variant, *RET* fusions, and *TERT* promoter variants), the more common weak driver variants (*RAS*), as well as other pathogenic variants and fusions with low frequencies and uncertain predictive value for malignancy. The strong driver variants are highly predictive of malignancy, with robust positive predictive values. RNA-based risk classifiers have been particularly useful for ruling out the need for surgery due to their high negative predictive value. MicroRNA testing has shown promise for improving diagnostic accuracy in preliminary testing when it is combined with testing for pathogenic variants.

This patient wishes to avoid surgery if her cancer risk is low, and testing did not reveal any pathogenic variants. Commercial testing panels for pathogenic variants include ThyroSeq v3, ThyroSeq v2, and ThyGeNEXT. The negative predictive values of ThyroSeq v3 and ThyroSeq v2 are reported as 0.96 (95% CI, 0.83-0.88) and 0.95 (95% CI, 0.85-1.00), respectively, in a recent meta-analysis. Results from ThyGeNEXT suggest a negative predictive value of 0.84 (95% CI, 0.77-0.91) with adjustment for disease prevalence in Bethesda II, IV, and V nodules. Preliminary data suggest that combining both ThyGeNEXT testing and microRNA testing in a multiplatform test, as was done for this patient, improves both positive and negative predictive value. Refinements in RNA-based classifiers have also improved the performance of this diagnostic test.

Regardless of which genetic testing was used for this patient, these negative predictive values are sufficiently high for her to avoid total thyroidectomy (Answer E). Furthermore, right lobectomy (Answer D) can also be avoided; the number of false-negative results with ThyroSeq v3 and v2 is extremely low. Follow-up for a TI-RADS 4 nodule is at year 1, 3, and 5 following diagnosis, so follow-up ultrasonography to assess for changes in the size or appearance of the patient's nodule is indicated (Answer A).

Levothyroxine (Answer B) is not recommended to treat patients with low-risk thyroid nodules.

Recommending no further treatment or follow-up (Answer C) would be inappropriate.

EDUCATIONAL OBJECTIVE

Explain the role of genetic testing in informing decisions about management of thyroid nodules.

REFERENCE(S)

Silaghi CA, Lozovanu V, Georgescu CE, et al. Thyroseq v3, Afirma GSC, and microRNA panels versus previous molecular tests in the preoperative diagnosis of indeterminate thyroid nodules: a systematic review and meta-analysis. *Front Endocrinol (Lausanne).* 2021;12:649522. PMID: 34054725

Jug R, Foo W-C, Jones C, Ahmadi S, Jiang XS. High-risk and intermediate-high-risk results from the ThyroSeq v2 and v3 thyroid genomic classifier are associated with neoplasia: independent performance assessment at an academic institution. *Cancer Cytopathol.* 2020;128(8):563-569. PMID: 32339438

Lupo MA, Walts AE, Sistrunk JW, et al. Multiplatform molecular test performance in indeterminate thyroid nodules. *Diagn Cytopathol.* 2020;48(12):1254-1264. PMID: 32767735

Vuong HG, Nguyen TPX, Hassell LA, Jung CK. Diagnostic performances of the Afirma Gene Sequencing Classifier in comparison with the Gene Expression Classifier: a meta-analysis. *Cancer Cytopathol.* 2021;129(3):182-189. PMID: 32726885

32 ANSWER: A) Benign follicular adenoma

RAS variants are the most frequent genetic alteration found in thyroid nodules with indeterminate cytology. They are also the second most common pathogenic variant found in malignant thyroid nodules. The *BRAF* V600E pathogenic variant (not found in this patient's nodule) is a strong predictor of papillary thyroid cancer. However, *RAS* variants do not have a good predictive value for thyroid cancer and, overall, *RAS*-like variants are generally associated with low-risk thyroid cancer. *RAS* variants can be present in benign nodules; noninvasive follicular thyroid neoplasms with papillary-like nuclear features (NIFTP); and cancers such as follicular variant of papillary thyroid cancer, papillary thyroid cancer, and poorly differentiated thyroid cancer. Benign follicular adenomas develop from a clonal process and can acquire additional variants. In thyroid nodules with a *RAS* variant, NIFTP can be considered a precursor lesion for invasive encapsulated follicular variant of papillary thyroid cancer, and follicular adenoma can be thought of as a precursor of follicular thyroid carcinoma. Of the answer options given, benign follicular adenoma (Answer A) is the answer most congruent with having a *RAS* variant present, but not having a *BRAF* V600E pathogenic variant.

RAS tumors typically have the sonographic features shown in this case: regular margins, mixed echogenicity or isoechoic or hyperechoic appearance, and lack of calcifications. *BRAF* tumors are more likely to have irregular margins, hypoechogenicity, calcifications, and abnormal lymph nodes. In a retrospective study of 78 thyroid nodules with indeterminate cytology that underwent resection, 50 had *RAS*-like variants. Of these, 36% were benign, 32% were NIFTP, and 32% were cancer (6% follicular cancer, 10% follicular variant of papillary thyroid cancer, and 16% classic papillary thyroid cancer). Most had low-risk sonographic features. In the same study, 8 nodules had *BRAF*-like variants, most had a high-risk sonographic appearance, and all were papillary thyroid cancer.

Nodules harboring the tall cell variant of papillary thyroid cancer (Answer E) are often microlobulated and hypoechoic, have microcalcifications, and are frequently associated with lymph node metastases. Most tumors have the *BRAF* V600E pathogenic variant.

The sonographic features of the diffuse sclerosing variant of papillary thyroid cancer (Answer C) include an ill-defined hypoechoic nodule and scattered microcalcifications, with the major genetic rearrangement being *RET/PTC.*

The hobnail variant of papillary thyroid cancer (Answer D) is rare, but findings reported on ultrasonography include hypoechogenicity, microcalcifications, and metastatic lymph nodes. The *BRAF* V600E pathogenic variant may be present.

Columnar cell variants (Answer B) are also rare, and their sonographic features include being hypoechoic, having microcalcifications, and having capsular protrusions representing extrathyroidal extension and nodal metastases. The *BRAF* V600E pathogenic variant may be present. The sonographic findings in this vignette are not consistent with this entity.

EDUCATIONAL OBJECTIVE

Predict the type of histology likely to be associated with a thyroid nodule with a *RAS* pathogenic variant and low-risk sonographic appearance.

REFERENCE(S)

Chin PD, Zhu CY, Sajed DP, et al. Correlation of ThyroSeq results with surgical histopathology in cytologically indeterminate thyroid nodules. *Endocr Pathol.* 2020;31(4):377-384. PMID: 32671653

Nikiforov YE. Role of molecular markers in thyroid nodule management: then and now. *Endocr Pract.* 2017;23(8):979-988. PMID: 28534687

Angell TE. RAS-positive thyroid nodules. *Curr Opin Endocrinol Diabetes Obes.* 2017;24(5):372-376. PMID: 28639967

Guan H, Toraldo G, Cerda S, et al. Utilities of *RAS* mutations in preoperative fine needle biopsies for decision making for thyroid nodule management: results from a single-center prospective cohort. *Thyroid.* 2020;30(4):536-547. PMID: 31996097

Shin JH. Ultrasonographic imaging of papillary thyroid carcinoma variants. *Ultrasonography.* 2017;36(2):103-110. PMID: 28222584

33 ANSWER: D) Surgical resection of the cystic mass

This patient has a thyroglossal duct cyst present in the midline superior to the thyroid gland (denoted by arrows on the CT images). The thyroglossal duct is the tract that the developing thyroid follows in its embryologic descent from the base of the tongue to its final anatomic position in the neck. When the tract persists, it is prone to cyst formation along its length. This patient's thyroglossal duct cyst is unlikely to completely resolve spontaneously at this stage. According to the literature, these lesions are prone to bacterial infection at a lifetime rate of approximately 50% if left untreated. Therefore, recommending no treatment now (Answer B) is not the ideal approach. The best means of definitively managing thyroglossal duct cysts is generally surgical resection together with removal of the central portion of the hyoid bone (this surgery is known as the Sistrunk procedure) (Answer D).

The incidence of thyroid cancer within a thyroglossal duct cyst is only 1%. There would be no indication to perform a total thyroidectomy as well as a Sistrunk procedure (Answer E) unless independent evidence suggested a malignancy within the thyroid gland itself.

Thyroglossal duct cysts do not respond to thyroid hormone suppressive therapy (Answer A) or radioiodine therapy (Answer C).

EDUCATIONAL OBJECTIVE

Choose a management approach for a thyroglossal duct cyst based on the risk for cancer and infection.

REFERENCE(S)

Rayess HM, Monk I, Svider PF, Gupta A, Raza SN, Lin HS. Thyroglossal duct cyst carcinoma: a systematic review of clinical features and outcomes. *Otolaryngol Head Neck Surg.* 2017;156(5):794-802. PMID: 28322121

Gioacchini FM, Alicandri-Ciufelli M, Kaleci S, Magliulo G, Presutti L, Re M. Clinical presentation and treatment outcomes of thyroglossal duct cysts: a systematic review. *Int J Oral Maxillofac Surg.* 2015;44(1):119-126. PMID: 25132570

34 ANSWER: B) Excessive dental caries

Salivary gland dysfunction after treatment with radioactive iodine is quite common. This can take the form of sialadenitis, xerostomia, and taste alterations. The incidence of xerostomia is between 15% and 54%, and it tends to improve over time. Prolonged or persistent xerostomia predisposes patients to excessive caries (Answer B).

Alteration of taste, which occurs commonly after radioiodine therapy, is typically transient rather than permanent (Answer E). Patients may describe a metallic or chemical taste that occasionally persists for months after therapy.

Nasolacrimal duct obstruction (Answer D) is an adverse effect of radioactive iodine; however, is less common than salivary gland damage, occurring in about 3% of patients.

Transient depression of sperm count occurs following radioiodine, and there is a cumulative effect on the testes, manifested as an elevation in serum FSH and slight decrease in sperm count, but not azoospermia (Answer A). Men desiring future fertility and receiving radioiodine doses greater than 400 mCi should be counseled about sperm cryopreservation.

Leukemia (Answer C) is a potential consequence of receiving very high doses of radioiodine, with a frequency of 0.3%, typically occurring in older patients receiving a cumulative dose greater than 800 mCi. Patients who receive the highest doses over the shortest intervals are most likely to develop this rare complication, with a latency period of less than 10 years. Ideally, patients requiring repeated treatments with radioiodine should receive treatment at intervals of at least 1 year, but patients with aggressive radioiodine-avid disease should not be denied therapy at shorter intervals when appropriate.

EDUCATIONAL OBJECTIVE

Anticipate the most likely adverse effects of high-dose radioactive iodine treatment.

REFERENCE(S)

Clement SC, Peeters RP, Ronckers CM, et al. Intermediate and long-term adverse effects of radioiodine therapy for differentiated thyroid carcinoma--a systematic review. *Cancer Treat Rev.* 2015;41(10):925-934. PMID: 26421813

Singer MC, Marchal F, Angelos P, et al. Salivary and lacrimal dysfunction after radioactive iodine for differentiated thyroid cancer: American Head and Neck Society Endocrine Surgery Section and Salivary Gland Section joint multidisciplinary clinical consensus statement of otolaryngology, ophthalmology, nuclear medicine and endocrinology. *Head Neck.* 2020;42(11):3446-3459. PMID: 32812307

www.ingramcontent.com/pod-product-compliance
Lightning Source LLC
LaVergne TN
LVHW080157080226
831114LV00036B/160
9781936704439